*Essentials of*
# Dental Anatomy and Oral Histology

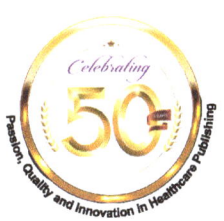

# Essentials of
# Dental Anatomy and Oral Histology

## Third Edition

**Kabita Chatterjee** BDS (Cal) MDS (Mang)
*Former* Professor and Head
Department of Oral and Maxillofacial Pathology
Buddha Institute of Dental Sciences and Hospital
Patna, Bihar, India

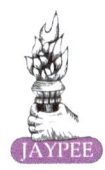

**JAYPEE BROTHERS MEDICAL PUBLISHERS**
*The Health Sciences Publisher*
New Delhi | London

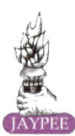 **Jaypee Brothers Medical Publishers (P) Ltd**

**Headquarters**
Jaypee Brothers Medical Publishers (P) Ltd
EMCA House, 23/23-B
Ansari Road, Daryaganj
New Delhi - 110 002, INDIA
Landline: +91-11-23272143, +91-11-23272703, +91-11-23282021, +91-11-23245672
Head Office: 011-43574357
Email: jaypee@jaypeebrothers.com

**Corporate Office**
Jaypee Brothers Medical Publishers (P) Ltd
4838/24, Ansari Road, Daryaganj
New Delhi 110 002, India
Phone: +91-11-43574357
Fax: +91-11-43574314
Email: jaypee@jaypeebrothers.com

**Overseas Office**
J.P. Medical Ltd
83 Victoria Street, London
SW1H 0HW (UK)
Phone: +44 20 3170 8910
Fax: +44 (0)20 3008 6180
Email: info@jpmedpub.com

Website: www.jaypeebrothers.com
Website: www.jaypeedigital.com

© 2021, Jaypee Brothers Medical Publishers

The views and opinions expressed in this book are solely those of the original contributor (s)/author (s) and do not necessarily represent those of editor (s) of the book.

All rights reserved. No part of this publication may be reproduced, stored or transmitted in any form or by any means, electronic, mechanical, photocopying, recording or otherwise, without the prior permission in writing of the publishers/editors.

All brand names and product names used in this book are trade names, service marks, trademarks or registered trademarks of their respective owners. The publisher is not associated with any product or vendor mentioned in this book.

Medical knowledge and practice change constantly. This book is designed to provide accurate, authoritative information about the subject matter in question. However, readers are advised to check the most current information available on procedures included and check information from the manufacturer of each product to be administered, to verify the recommended dose, formula, method and duration of administration, adverse effects and contraindications. It is the responsibility of the practitioner to take all appropriate safety precautions. Neither the publisher nor the author (s)/editor (s) assume any liability for any injury and/or damage to persons or property arising from or related to use of material in this book.

This book is sold on the understanding that the publisher is not engaged in providing professional medical services. If such advice or services are required, the services of a competent medical professional should be sought.

Every effort has been made where necessary to contact holders of copyright to obtain permission to reproduce copyright material. If any have been inadvertently overlooked, the publisher will be pleased to make the necessary arrangements at the first opportunity. The **CD/DVD-ROM** (if any) provided in the sealed envelope with this book is complimentary and free of cost. **Not meant for sale.**

Inquiries for bulk sales may be solicited at: jaypee@jaypeebrothers.com

*Essentials of Dental Anatomy and Oral Histology*

*First Edition*: 2006

*Second Edition*: 2014

Third Edition: **2021**

ISBN: 978-93-90595-96-9

**Dedicated to**

*My parents
Dr Kamal Bose
and
Ashoka Bose*

# Preface to the Third Edition

The third edition of the book follows the form and principles of earlier editions. All the chapters have been reviewed. Some minor changes and corrections were deemed necessary. Review questions are added at the end of histology chapters for the convenience of the students.

I assume all the responsibilities for errors and omissions in this book.

Finally, I am as ever grateful to the readers who have provided comments and criticisms.

**Kabita Chatterjee**

# Preface to the First Edition

The oral cavity or stomatodeum is considered as the mirror of the body. Many systemic diseases have their oral manifestations. So a good clinician should have a firm knowledge of oral histology which is the fundamental science for understanding the intricate morphologies of oral and paraoral tissues.

There are several excellent textbooks available on oral histology. *Essentials of Oral Histology* has been written with a view to present the subject to the undergraduate dental students in a more simplified manner for their easy assimilation. It is a humble attempt to fill the niche for the students of dentistry with the current information about the development, structure, and function of teeth and associated tissues.

I assume all the responsibilities for errors and omissions in this book. I sincerely welcome the constructive suggestions from the students and the teachers for further improvement of this maiden effort.

**Kabita Chatterjee**

# Acknowledgments

I take this opportunity to express my deep sense of gratitude to my respected teachers Prof Dr HM Dholakia, Prof BB Dutta, Prof RR Paul, and Prof D Gadewar for teaching me with their personal attention and valuable guidance.

I would like to acknowledge with sincere thanks for the assistance of my husband Dr DK Chattopadhyay and my son Dr Dipmalya Chatterjee for drawing the illustrations, proofreading, and meticulous attention to details.

I gratefully acknowledge the contribution made by my aunt Miss Sati Mitra for typing the manuscript.

I very much appreciate the constant support given to me by Dr Sourav Bhattacharya, Dr Anjana Majumdar, and my daughter Miss Dipanwita Chatterjee.

I am deeply indebted to all the authors who have contributed to my knowledge of oral anatomy and histology.

It is my proud privilege to thank the administrator, colleagues, and students of Buddha Institute of Dental Sciences and Hospital for their support and encouragement.

I am immensely grateful to Shri Jitendar P Vij (Group Chairman), Mr Ankit Vij (Managing Director), Mr MS Mani (Group President), Dr Madhu Choudhary (Publishing Head–Education), Ms Pooja Bhandari (Production Head), Ms Samina Khan (Executive Assistant to Publishing Head–Education), Dr Akanksha Singh (Development Editor), Ms Seema Dogra (Cover Visualizer), Mr Narsingh (Proofreader), Mr Deepak Saxena (Operator), Mr Nitin Bhardwaj (Graphic Designer) and the whole team of M/s Jaypee Brothers Medical Publishers (P) Limited, for the assistance, guidance and their support in the preparation of the manuscript. Without their cooperation, I could not have completed this project.

Lastly, I extend my special thanks and appreciation to Mr Bhuban Sarkar and Mr Bamdeb Mondal, technicians of my laboratory for their meticulous laboratory technique in jaw bone and tooth decalcification as well as soft tissue processing.

# Contents

1. **Introduction**     1
   Incisors    2
   Canines    2
   Premolars    2
   Molars    2
   Functions of Teeth    3
   Dental Formula    3
   Fédération Dentaire Internationale (FDI) Approved System    4
   Morphology of Teeth    4
   Surfaces of Tooth    4
   Glossary    4

2. **The Deciduous (Primary) Teeth**     10
   Importance of Deciduous Teeth    10
   The Deciduous Incisors    11
   The Deciduous Canine    14
   The Deciduous Molars    16

3. **The Permanent Teeth**     24
   The Permanent Incisors    24
   The Permanent Canines    29
   The Premolars    32
   The Permanent Molars    39

4. **Method of Tooth Carving**     52
   Equipment    52
   Carving of Permanent Maxillary Central Incisor    52
   Carving of Permanent Maxillary Canine    52
   Carving of Maxillary Premolar    54
   Carving of Maxillary First Molar    55

5. **Vasculature and Innervations of the Teeth and Associated Structures**     56
   Arterial Supply of the Teeth and Associated Structures    56
   Venous Drainage of Orodental Tissues    58
   Innervation of Orodental Tissues    58

6. **The Temporomandibular Joint and Muscles of Mastication**     61
   Anatomy in Brief    61
   Articular Fibrous Covering    64
   Articular Disk    65
   Articular Capsule    65
   Clinical Considerations    65
   Muscles of Mastication    66

7. **The Maxillary Sinus**     69
   Enumeration    69
   Functions    69
   Maxillary Sinus    69
   Applied Anatomy    72

8. **Occlusion**     73
   Definition    73
   Few Terminologies    73
   Development of Occlusion    75

9. **Histological Techniques for Study of Oral Tissues**     82
   Microscopy    82
   Few Analytical Methods    85
   Routine Laboratory Techniques for Histologic Study    85

10. **Development of Face and Oral Cavity**     90
    Zygote    90
    Morula    90
    Blastocyst    90
    Placenta    91
    Bilaminar Germ Disk    91
    Amniotic Cavity    91
    Yolk Sac    91
    Prochordal Plate    91
    Primitive Streak    91
    Mesoderm    92
    Notochord    92
    Derivatives of Three Germ Layers    92
    Subdivisions of Mesoderm    93
    Folding of Embryo    94
    Early Orofacial Development    95
    Branchial Arches    96
    The Branchial Grooves and Pharyngeal Pouches    97
    Formation of the Tongue    99
    Development of Palate    101
    Development of the Jaws    101

Development of Maxilla  105
Development of the
  Temporomandibular Joint  105
Development of the Skull  105
Development of Salivary Gland  107
Clinical Considerations  108

## 11. Development of Tooth  110
Primary Epithelial Band  110
Different Stages of Tooth
  Development  112
Histodifferentiation of Tooth Germ Prior
  to Enamel and Dentin Formation  119

## 12. Eruption and Shedding of Tooth  133
Eruption  133
Histology of Tooth Movement  135
Mechanism of Eruption of Tooth  137
Shedding of the Deciduous Teeth  139
Clinical Considerations  141

## 13. Enamel  143
Physical Characteristics  143
Chemical Composition  143
Structure of Enamel  144
Age Changes of Enamel  155
Clinical Considerations  155

## 14. Dentin  157
Physical Characteristics  157
Chemical Composition  157
Structure of Dentin  157
Peritubular (Intratubular) Dentin  159
Intertubular Dentin  159
Predentin  160
Odontoblast Process  160
Different Forms of Dentin  160
Theories of Pain Transmission
  through Dentin  163
Age and Functional Changes  164
Clinical Considerations  166

## 15. Pulp  168
Functions  168
Anatomy  168
Development  169
Structural Features  170
Clinical Considerations  175

## 16. Cementum  177
Physical Characteristics  177
Chemical Composition  177
Function  177
Structure  178
Scanning Electron Microscopy  181
Classification of Cementum
  based on the Nature and
  Origin of the Organic Matrix  182
Cementodentinal Junction  183
Cementoenamel Junction  183
Clinical Considerations  184

## 17. Periodontium  186
Periodontal Ligament  186
Fibers of the Periodontal Ligament  187
Ground Substance of the
  Periodontal Ligament  191
Cells of the Periodontal Ligament  191
Blood Vessels and Nerves of the
  Periodontal Ligament  194
Clinical Considerations  194

## 18. Alveolar Bone  197
Function  197
Structure of Bone  197
Types of Bone Tissues  199
Physiologic Changes in Alveolar
  Process  204
Internal Reconstruction of Bone  204
Clinical Considerations  206

## 19. Oral Mucous Membrane  207
Functions of the Oral Mucosa  207
Organization of the Oral Mucosa  208
Classification of Oral Mucosa
  (According to Function)  208
Clinical Appearance  208
Component Tissues of Oral Mucosa  209
Structure of Mucosa in Different
  Regions of the Oral Cavity  216
Age Changes  225
Clinical Considerations  226

## 20. Salivary Glands  227
Definition of Gland  227
Classification of Glands  227
Classification of Salivary Glands  227
Structural Pattern of the Salivary
  Gland  228
Ductal System  233
Saliva  235
Clinical Considerations  238

*Index*  239

# CHAPTER 1

# Introduction

Oral and paraoral tissues comprise oral mucous membrane, three pairs of major and innumerable minor salivary glands, jaw bones bearing deciduous and permanent sets of dentitions, maxillary sinus, and temporomandibular joint. Teeth constitute approximately 20% of the surface area of mouth, the upper teeth significantly more than the lower teeth. A tooth consists of a crown which is exposed to oral cavity and single or multiple roots, lying in socket of jaw bones. The teeth are composed of the following tissues **(Fig. 1.1)**:

- **Enamel:** It is the hardest tissue in human body, covering the crown of the tooth. It is inert, acellular, and formed from ectoderm. It is supported by underlying dentin.
- **Dentin:** It is less calcified, more resilient, vital, hard tissue forming the main bulk of the tooth. It is formed from and supported by the dental pulp. In crown portion, it is covered by the enamel and in the root portion, it is covered by the cementum. The junction between enamel and dentin is known as dentinoenamel junction.
- **Cementum:** It is less mineralized tissue, covering the radicular portion of the tooth. The junction between enamel and cementum is known as cervical line or cementoenamel junction.
- **Pulp:** It is the soft, connective tissue in the central part of tooth enclosed by dentin. The pulp cavity in crown part is known as pulp chamber and in the root portion, it is known as pulp canal or root canal.
- **Periodontium:** The tissues (periodontal ligament, cementum, and alveolar bone) which support the teeth in jaws are collectively termed periodontium. The tooth is anchored to the socket of bone by periodontal ligament. The part of jaw bone which supports the tooth is known as alveolar bone.

At birth normally, no tooth is visible in the oral cavity. In the postnatal period, teeth of various sizes and shapes are found in the jaws. The human beings are known as diphyodont as human dentition consists of two sets of teeth:

1. Primary, deciduous, or milk dentition:
   - Total 20 in number.
   - 10 in each jaw.
   - 5 in each quadrant.
   - Start erupting in oral cavity at the age of 6 months.
   - Continue to erupt up to 2.5 to 3 years.
2. Secondary, permanent, or succedaneous dentition:
   - Total 32 in number.
   - 16 in each jaw.
   - 8 in each quadrant.

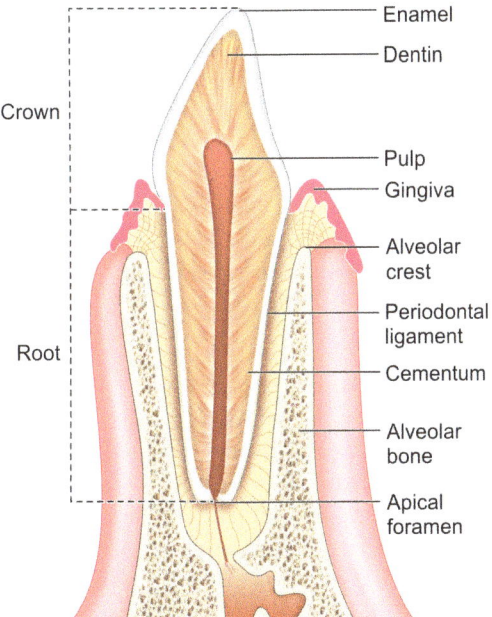

**Fig. 1.1:** Parts of a tooth.

- Start erupting in oral cavity at the age of 6 years.
- 28 teeth erupt by the age of 13 years.
- Remaining four teeth appear between 18 years and 25 years.

The dentition in human can be divided into three stages:
1. Stage of primary dentition:
   a. It lasts for about 6 months–6 years of age.
   b. Only deciduous teeth are present in this phase.
2. Stage of mixed dentition:
   a. It lasts from 6 years to 13 years of age.
   b. Both deciduous and permanent teeth are present in the oral cavity.
3. Stage of permanent dentition:
   a. It lasts from 13 years onward.
   b. Only permanent teeth are present.
   c. The permanent teeth replace deciduous teeth except permanent molars, which do not have any deciduous predecessors.

The teeth are arranged in two dental arches **(Figs. 1.2 and 1.3)**:
1. Maxillary or upper arch
2. Mandibular or lower arch.

The arrangement of teeth is symmetrical in the right and left halves in each arch.

In both dentitions, there are three basic tooth forms—incisiform, caniniform, and molariform.

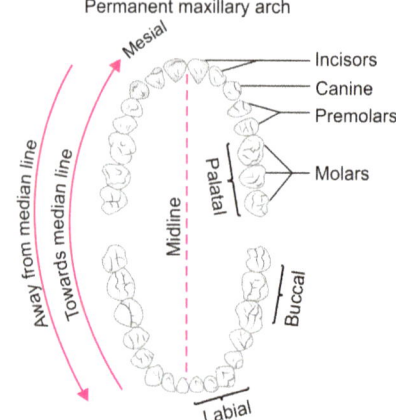

**Fig. 1.3:** Nomenclature used in tooth morphology of permanent tooth.

## INCISORS

- Two in each quadrant of jaws.
- They are flat, have cutting edges, and are delicate.

## CANINES

- One in each quadrant of jaws.
- They have sharp pointed cusp and are strong.
- They are known as cuspids.
- They are meant for piercing or tearing. Eight incisors and four canines together are known as anterior teeth.

## PREMOLARS

- They are two in each quadrant.
- They replace deciduous molars.
- They generally have two cusps and are known as bicuspids.
- They are present only in permanent dentition.

## MOLARS

- There are two deciduous molars and three permanent molars in each quadrant.
- The permanent molars do not have deciduous predecessors.
- They are large and strong.
- They have broad surface designed for grinding.
- They are situated farthest back in the mouth.

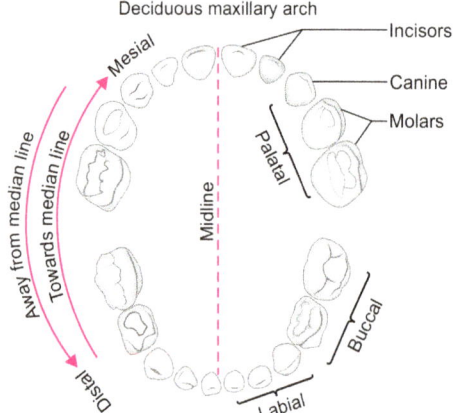

**Fig. 1.2:** Nomenclature used in tooth morphology of deciduous tooth.

# Introduction

The 8 premolars and 12 molars together are known as posterior teeth.

The type of tooth is represented by its initial letter, i.e.
- I for incisors
- C for canines
- P for premolars
- M for molars.

The numbering of teeth is done starting anteriorly at the midline. The incisors closest to midline are called central incisors. The teeth next to the central incisors are known as lateral incisors and the next tooth is canine. The premolars and molars are similarly called first and second premolars and first, second, and third molars.

## FUNCTIONS OF TEETH

1. Helps in mastication (cutting of food by the incisors, tearing by the canines, chopping by the premolars, and grinding by the molars).
2. Helps in articulation and speech.
3. Gives a definite shape and beauty to the face. Vertical height of face is maintained by molars. Helps to maintain the personality of individual.
4. May be used for self-protection.
5. Growth and development of jaws are dependent on tooth.

## DENTAL FORMULA

Dental formula is used in the clinic to simplify tooth identification. The permanent teeth in each quadrant are numbered 1–8 and the deciduous teeth in each quadrant are lettered A to E. The symbols for the quadrants are derived from an imaginary cross, with the horizontal bar placed between the upper and lower jaws and the vertical bar running between the upper and lower central incisors.

| Upper right | Upper left |
|---|---|
| Lower right | Lower left |

Sometimes, it is simplified to denote

| Upper right = ⌟ | Upper left = ⌞ |
|---|---|
| Lower right = ⌐ | Lower left = ⌜ |

There are different systems for recording different teeth. Few important systems are as follows.

## Zsigmondy's Method (Palmer Notation)

- Oldest method.
- Used in most countries.
- Simple method.
- Has many potential sources of errors regarding noting sides.

### For Permanent Teeth

| Upper right | Upper left |
|---|---|
| 8 7 6 5 4 3 2 1 | 1 2 3 4 5 6 7 8 |
| 8 7 6 5 4 3 2 1 | 1 2 3 4 5 6 7 8 |
| Lower right | Lower left |

1. Central incisor
2. Lateral incisor
3. Canine
4. First premolar
5. Second premolar
6. First molar
7. Second molar
8. Third molar

### For Deciduous Teeth

| Upper right | Upper left |
|---|---|
| E D C B A | A B C D E |
| E D C B A | A B C D E |
| Lower right | Lower left |

- A—central incisor
- B—lateral incisor
- C—canine
- D—first molar
- E—second molar

## Universal System

- Less liable to produce mistake.
- Needs more practice for quick and correct notation.

### For Permanent Teeth

R | 1 2 3 4 5 6 7 8 | 9 10 11 12 13 14 15 16 | L
--- | --- | --- | ---
  | 32 31 30 29 28 27 26 25 | 24 23 22 21 20 19 18 17 |

### For Deciduous Teeth

R | A B C D E | F G H I J | L
--- | --- | --- | ---
  | T S R Q P | O N M L K |

## FÉDÉRATION DENTAIRE INTERNATIONALE (FDI) APPROVED SYSTEM

- Two-digit system, suitable for computer handling.
- The first number of the digit indicates the quadrant.
- The second digit indicates the individual tooth within the quadrant.

### For Permanent Teeth

| Upper right | Upper left |
|---|---|
| 18 17 16 15 14 13 12 11 | 21 22 23 24 25 26 27 28 |
| 48 47 46 45 44 43 42 41 | 31 32 33 34 35 36 37 38 |
| Lower right | Lower left |

### For Deciduous Teeth

| Upper right | Upper left |
|---|---|
| 55 54 53 52 51 | 61 62 63 64 65 |
| 85 84 83 82 81 | 71 72 73 74 75 |
| Lower right | Lower left |

## MORPHOLOGY OF TEETH

Morphologically, a tooth is divided into:
a. Crown
b. Root.

For the purpose of description, it is customary to divide the crown and root into thirds (**Figs. 1.4A and B**).

### Crown

I. Occluso-gingivally:
   a. Incisal or occlusal third
   b. Middle third
   c. Cervical third.
II. Facio-lingually:
   a. Facial third (labial or buccal)
   b. Middle third
   c. Lingual third.

### Root

a. Cervical third
b. Middle third
c. Apical third.

## SURFACES OF TOOTH

The crown of each tooth presents five surfaces in case of premolars and molars and four surfaces and an incisal edge in case of anterior teeth.

The surfaces are:
- **Facial** (labial surface of anterior teeth and buccal for posterior teeth)
- **Lingual** (palatal)
- **Occlusal**
- **Proximal**
  - Mesial—surface facing midline
  - Distal—surface away from midline.

## GLOSSARY

### Angle

A line or a point where two or more surfaces or borders meet is called an angle.

### Line Angle

The angle formed by meeting of two surfaces is called a line angle. The name of the angle is

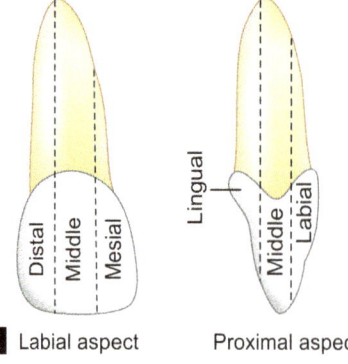
**A** Labial aspect     Proximal aspect

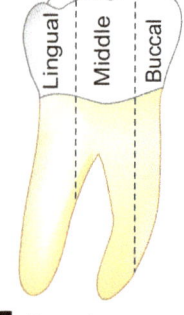 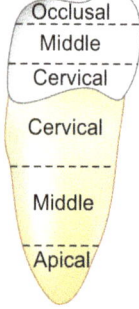
**B** Buccal aspect     Proximal aspect

**Figs. 1.4A and B:** Division of tooth into thirds. (A) Anterior tooth; (B) Posterior tooth.

# Introduction

derived from both the surfaces, e.g. distolingual-angle formed by distal and lingual surfaces.

## Point Angle

The point of junction of three surfaces is called a point angle. The name is derived from all three surfaces, e.g. mesiolinguoincisal angle formed at the junction of mesial and lingual surfaces and incisal edge.

## Apex

The terminal end or tip of the root of a tooth is called an apex.

## Apical

Towards the apex of a root.

## Apical Foramen

It is the opening of the pulp canal at the apical end of the root of a tooth. At this region, pulp is not surrounded by dentin.

## Axial

It is pertaining to the longitudinal axis of the tooth.

## Axial Surface

It is parallel to the long axis of tooth, e.g. labial, buccal, lingual, mesial, and distal.

## Axial Wall

It is any wall of the pulp chamber which is parallel to the long axis of the tooth. The line angles that are parallel to the long axis of the teeth are called axial angles, e.g. distobuccal and mesiolingual angles.

## Axial Root Center

It is an imaginary line passing through the geometric center of a tooth root parallel to its long axis.

## Buccal

It is related to cheek.

## Buccal Surface

It is the surface of posterior tooth, facing the cheek.

## Cementoenamel Junction

It is the junction on the surface of the tooth where enamel meets the cementum.

## Cervix (Neck)

It is a narrow or constricted portion of a tooth in the region of the junction of crown and root.

## Cervical Line

It is a curved line formed by the junction of enamel and cementum of a tooth.

## Cingulum (Latin word for girdle)

It is a bulbous convexity on the cervical third of the lingual surface of an anterior tooth. It is the lingual lobe of an anterior tooth. Its convexity mesiodistally resembles a girdle encircling the lingual surface at the cervical third.

## Contact Point

It is an area on the proximal surfaces of two adjacent teeth on the same arch that come in contact with each other. Every tooth has two contact points, one on mesial side and another on distal side except the third molars which have only one contact point in the mesial side.

Contact area of permanent teeth is given in **Figure 1.5**.

### Upper Arch

| Name of the teeth | Location of contact area |
|---|---|
| a. Two central incisors | Incisal third region |
| b. Central incisor and lateral incisor | Incisal third region, but more apically placed than (a) |
| c. Lateral incisor and canine | At the junction of the middle third and incisal third |
| d. Canine and first premolar | Middle third of the crown |

*Contd...*

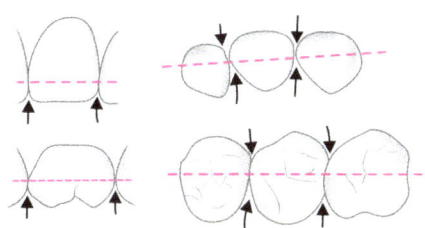

**Fig. 1.5:** Contact area of permanent teeth.

*Contd...*

| Name of the teeth | Location of contact area |
|---|---|
| e. Interpremolar contact area | Above the junction of middle third and occlusal third |
| f. Second premolar and first molar, first molar and second molar, second molar and third molar | Middle third of the crown |

### Lower Arch

| Name of the teeth | Location of contact area |
|---|---|
| a. Two central incisors | Incisal third region |
| b. Central incisor and lateral incisor | Incisal third region |
| c. Lateral incisor and canine | Incisal third region, more apically than (b) |
| d. Canine and first premolar | Middle third |
| e. Interpremolar | Middle third |
| f. Second premolar and first molar, first molar and second molar | Middle third, more apically than (d) and (e) |

### Functions

a. Contact areas keep the food away from being packed between teeth.
b. They help to stabilize dental arches by the combined anchorage of all the teeth in contact with each other.

### Contours

The diameter of the crown of any tooth gradually increases from occlusal or incisal surface to certain points from where it begins to decrease towards the cervical line. This greatest area of circumference of the crown is known as the height of contour **(Fig. 1.6)**. It protects the gingival tissues.

### Crown

- *Clinical crown*: It is the part of the tooth which is visible in the oral cavity.

- *Anatomical crown*: It is the part of the tooth which is covered by enamel.

### Crypt

It is the cavity in the alveolar bone that contains developing tooth germ.

### Cusp

It is a pronounced elevation on the occlusal surface of a tooth terminating in a conical or rounded surface. It is having an independent center of calcification.

### Dentition

It is the type, number, and arrangement of the teeth.

### Diastema

It is the space between two adjacent anterior teeth in the same arch.

### Distal

Away from the median line.

### Distal Surface

The surface of tooth away from the median line following the curve of the dental arch.

### Embrasure

Embrasures or spillway spaces are the triangular-shaped spaces adjacent to the contact points of teeth. When two proximal teeth of the same arch come in contact with each other, their curvatures adjacent to the contact areas form embrasures. Thus, around each contact area, there are four embrasures—facial, lingual, interproximal, and occlusal **(Figs. 1.7A and B)**. The embrasures are continuous and symmetrical. Correct

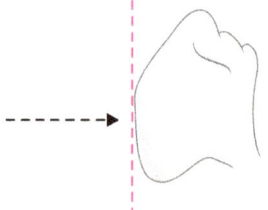

**Fig. 1.6:** Height of contour.

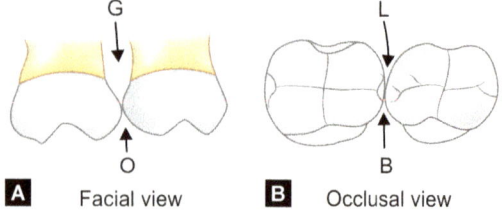

**Figs. 1.7A and B:** Embrasures.

# Introduction

interproximal embrasures result in proper arch alignment.

## Functions

1. The embrasures make a spillway for the escape of food during mastication.
2. It also makes the tooth self-cleansing as the rounded smooth surfaces of the crowns are exposed to the cleansing action of foods and friction of cheeks and lips.
3. The embrasures and contact points protect the gingival tissue from undue trauma.

## Fissure

It is a cleft or crevice in a tooth surface due to imperfect fusion of the enamel of adjoining cusps or lobes.

## Fossa

It is a rounded or angular depression on the surface of a tooth.

## Lingual Fossa

It is a broad and shallow depression on the lingual surface of an incisor or canine **(Fig. 1.8A)**.

## Central Fossa

It is relatively broad, deep, and angular depression in the central portion of the occlusal surface of a molar **(Fig. 1.8B)**.

## Triangular Fossa

It is comparatively shallow pyramid-shaped depression on the occlusal surfaces of posterior teeth located within the confines of the mesial or distal marginal ridges and triangular ridges of adjacent cusps **(Fig. 1.8C)**.

## Groove

It is a shallow linear depression on the surface of a tooth **(Fig. 1.9)**.

## Developmental Groove

It marks the boundaries between adjacent cusps and other divisional parts of a tooth.

## Supplemental Groove

It is an indistinct linear depression, irregular in extent and direction which does not demarcate major divisional portions of a tooth.

## Inclined Plane

It is a sloping area on the occlusal surfaces of premolars and molars. Each cusp has two inclined planes **(Fig. 1.10)**.

## Lobe

It is one of the main morphological divisions of the crown of a tooth. It is one of the primary centers of calcification. Cusps and mamelons are representatives of lobes.

## Mamelons

These are rounded or conical prominences on the incisal ridge of a newly erupted incisor. They are three in number and are separated by two indistinct grooves extending from labial

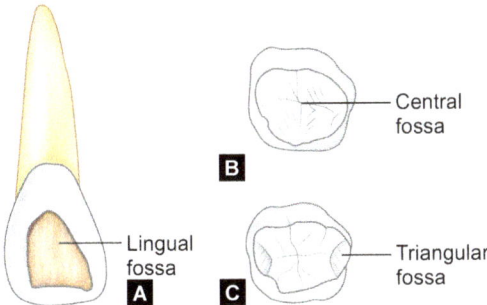

**Figs. 1.8A to C:** (A) Lingual fossa; (B) Central fossa; (C) Triangular fossa.

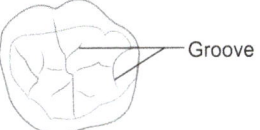

**Fig. 1.9:** Groove.

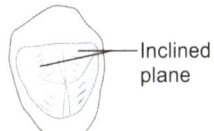

**Fig. 1.10:** Inclined plane.

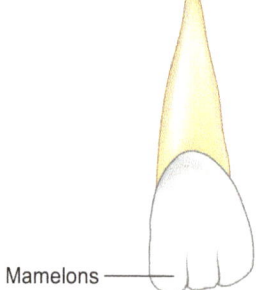

Fig. 1.11: Mamelons.

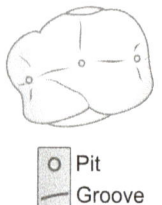

Fig. 1.12: Pit and groove.

surface. They represent three lobes having a separate center of calcification. After eruption gradually, the mamelons are flattened due to attrition **(Fig. 1.11)**.

## Median Line

It is an imaginary line dividing body into right and left equal halves.

## Mesial

Towards the median line.

## Mesial Surface

The surface of a tooth facing towards the median line following the curve of the dental arch.

## Occlusion

Occlusion is defined as the relationship between the occlusal surfaces of the maxillary and mandibular teeth when they are in contact.

## Occlusal

Towards the biting surface of a premolar or molar.

## Occlusal Surface

The surface of a premolar or molar within the marginal ridges and which come in contact (occlusion) with the corresponding surface of opposing jaw during the act of closure is called occlusal surface.

## Pit

It is a sharp pointed depression usually located at the junction of two or more intersecting developmental grooves or at the termination of a single developmental groove **(Fig. 1.12)**.

## Pulp Cavity

It is the central cavity in a tooth which contains tooth pulp.

Pulp chamber is that portion of the pulp cavity which lies in the crown of tooth.

Pulp canal or root canal is that part of pulp cavity which lies in the root portion of tooth.

Pulpal walls are the sides of the pulp chamber.

Pulp horns are extensions of pulp toward occlusal or incisal surface.

## Proximal Surface

The surface of tooth which faces towards an adjoining tooth in the same arch, i.e. both mesial and distal surfaces, is proximal surfaces.

## Proximal Root Concavity

A depression extending long on the mesial and distal surface of the root of an anterior or posterior tooth is known as proximal root concavity.

## Ridge

It is a linear elevation on the surface of tooth. According to location, it is named buccal, incisal, or marginal ridge.

### Marginal Ridges

These are rounded elevations of enamel that form the mesial and distal margins of (a) the occlusal surfaces of the posterior teeth and (b) the lingual surfaces of the anterior teeth **(Fig. 1.13A)**.

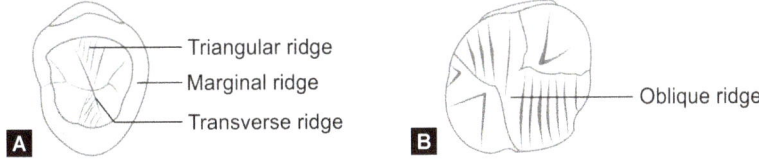

**Figs. 1.13A and B:** (A) Marginal ridge, triangular ridge, and transverse ridge; (B) Oblique ridge.

### Triangular Ridges

These are prominent elevations or ridges, triangular in cross section, and extend from the tip of the cusp towards central portion of the occlusal surface of a tooth. Each triangular ridge has triangular-shaped slope or inclined plane on each side **(Fig. 1.13A)**.

### Transverse Ridge

It is formed by the union of a buccal and lingual triangular ridge on the occlusal surfaces of the posterior teeth and runs transversely **(Fig. 1.13A)**.

### Oblique Ridge

It is formed by the union of two triangular ridges that run obliquely across the occlusal surfaces of maxillary molars and extends from tips of the distobuccal to mesiolingual cusps **(Fig. 1.13B)**.

### Cusp Ridges

These are elevations extending in mesial and distal directions from cusp tips. Cusp ridges form the buccal and lingual margin of the occlusal surfaces of posterior teeth.

### Incisal Ridge

It is the linear elevation at the incisal third of the anterior teeth where labial surface meets with the lingual surface.

### Sulcus

It is an elongated depression on the surface of a tooth formed by the inclines of adjacent cusps or ridges which meet at an angle.

### Trunk

It is the main body of a root of a multirooted tooth from the cervical line to the furcation point.

### Tubercle

It is a small rounded elevation of enamel on the crown of a tooth.

## QUESTIONNAIRE

1. What do you mean by diphyodont?
2. What are the different stages of dentition in human being?
3. Enumerate the functions of teeth.
4. Discuss the different methods of formulation of teeth.
5. Write short notes on:
   a. Line angle and point angle.
   b. Apical foramen.
   c. Cingulum.
   d. Contact point and Contact area.
   e. Diastema.
   f. Embrasure.
   g. Fissure.
   h. Fossa.
   i. Groove.
   j. Mamelons.
   k. Pit.
   l. Ridge.

## BIBLIOGRAPHY

1. Berkovitz BKB, Holland GR, Moxham BJ. A Colour Atlas and Textbook of Oral Anatomy, Histology and Embryology, 4th edition. Mosby: Elsevier; 2009.
2. Biviji AT. Dental Anatomy, 2nd edition. Mumbai: Bhalani Publishing House; 1999.
3. Das AK. Dental Anatomy and Oral Histology, 1st edition. West Bengal: Current Books International; 1972.
4. Kraus BS, Jordon RE, Abrams L. Dental Anatomy and Occlusion. Baltimore: The Williams and Willkin's Company; 1969.
5. Nelson SJ, Ash MJ. Wheeler's Dental Anatomy, Physiology and Occlusion, 9th edition. Philadelphia: Elsevier; 2010.
6. Scott JH, Symons NBB. Introduction to Dental Anatomy, 9th edition. Edinburgh and London: Churchill Livingstone; 1982.

# CHAPTER 2

# The Deciduous (Primary) Teeth

The deciduous (primary) dentition comprises of 20 teeth, 5 in each quadrant of both jaws. These are central incisor, lateral incisor, canine, first molar, and second molar. Premolars are absent in primary set of dentition. The deciduous teeth start erupting at the age of 6 months. Eruption and root completion of all deciduous teeth are completed at about 3 years of age. Permanent teeth start replacing them at the age of 6 years and the replacement is completed by the age of 12 years. The general order of eruption of the primary dentition is central incisor, lateral incisor, first molar, canine, and second molar, with mandibular pairs preceding the maxillary teeth. The second molar in both the arches and the maxillary incisors appears to be the most unstable of the primary teeth.

## IMPORTANCE OF DECIDUOUS TEETH

Though the deciduous teeth are present in the oral cavity for a shorter period of time, they serve a number of purposes. So the maintenance of normal anatomy of deciduous teeth and their supporting structures is as important as their permanent counterpart **(Table 2.1)**.

**TABLE 2.1:** Major contrasts between primary and permanent teeth.

| | | Permanent | Deciduous |
|---|---|---|---|
| 1. | Number | 32 | 20 |
| 2. | Types | Two incisors, one canine, two premolars, and three molars in each quadrant | Two incisors, one canine, and two molars in each quadrant. Premolars are absent |
| 3. | Size | Larger than deciduous teeth | Smaller than permanent teeth. Crowns are relatively short as compared to roots. The mesiodistal width of molar is greater than that of succeeding premolar. The combined width of deciduous canine and first and second deciduous molars is greater than the combined width of permanent canine and first and second premolars. This difference of 1.7 mm in the lower arch and 0.9 mm in the upper arch is known as Leeway space of Nance. This extra space is used in the adjustment of occlusion |
| 4. | Shape | The cusps are blunt. The crowns are not bulbous. The contact areas are broader. | The cusps are more pointed and the crowns are bulbous. The crowns of anterior teeth are wider mesiodistally. The contact areas are smaller |
| 5. | Color | They are bluish-white in color as enamel is more translucent | They are whiter and less pigmented as enamel is less translucent |
| 6. | Cervical margin | The enamel ends gradually. First molars do not have any bulge near cervical margins. Necks are longer and less constricted | The enamel ends abruptly at the neck. First molars show a bulge near the cervical margin at mesiobuccal region, known as cervical ridge. Necks are short and more constricted. The cervical ridges of enamel of the anterior teeth are more prominent |
| 7. | Occlusal surface | Buccal and lingual surfaces of molars are not convergent occlusally. Therefore, buccolingual diameter is wider | Buccal and lingual surfaces of molars are convergent occlusally. Therefore, buccolingual diameter is narrower |

*Contd...*

Contd...

| | Permanent | Deciduous |
|---|---|---|
| 8. Roots | Roots are longer and strong. In multirooted teeth, there is a trunk and roots do not diverge close to crown | Roots are shorter and slender, though compared to crown size they are relatively longer. The roots diverge close to crown. The roots flare widely beyond outlines of crown and allow more room between roots for development of permanent tooth crown |
| 9. Pulp cavity | Dentin is thicker. Pulp chamber is smaller and pulp horns are at lower level | Dentin is less thick. Pulp chamber is larger and pulp horns rise high in the cuspal region |
| 10. Enamel | Enamel is less permeable, more calcified, and shows relatively less attrition. Rods near cervical margin are directed apically | Enamel is relatively thin, more permeable, less calcified, and shows relatively more attrition. Rods near cervical margin are perpendicular to dentinoenamel junction |
| 11. Eruption and shedding | Eruption starts at 6 years and continues till 25 years or more and stays in oral cavity for a long time | Eruption starts at 6 months and continues till 3 years and are exfoliated by 13 years |
| 12. Placement in jaws | They are placed obliquely in jaws | They are set perpendicularly in jaws |
| 13. First upper molar | It has four cusps | It has three cusps |
| Second upper molar | It has four cusps | It has four cusps |
| First lower molar | It has five cusps | It has four cusps |
| Second lower molar | It has four cusps | It has five cusps |

- They help in mastication.
- They are important for development of speech.
- They contribute for growth of jaw bones.
- They maintain the space needed for the development and eruption of the permanent teeth.

## THE DECIDUOUS INCISORS (TABLES 2.2 AND 2.3)

### The Deciduous Maxillary Central Incisor (Figs. 2.1A to E) (Table 2.4)

*Labial Aspect (Fig. 2.1A)*

- In the crown of the deciduous central incisor, the mesiodistal diameter is greater than the cervicoincisal length (the opposite is true of permanent central incisors).
- The labial surface is smooth without any grooves or lobes. It is slightly convex in both directions.
- The incisal edge is nearly straight.
- Developmental lines are usually not seen.
- It has a prominent cervical ridge.
- The root is cone-shaped with even and tapered sides. The root length is greater in comparison with the crown length than that of the permanent central incisor.

*Lingual Aspect (Fig. 2.1B)*

- The lingual aspect of the crown shows well-developed marginal ridges and a highly developed cingulum. The cingulum extends up toward the incisal ridge to

| TABLE 2.2: Chronology of tooth formation and eruption of deciduous incisors. | | | | |
|---|---|---|---|---|
| | Maxillary central | Incisor lateral | Mandibular central | Incisor lateral |
| 1. Initiation of calcification (month in utero) | 3 | 4 | 4 | 4 |
| 2. Crown completion (month) | 4 | 5 | 4 | 4 |
| 3. Eruption (month) | 7 | 8 | 6 | 7 |
| 4. Root completion (year) | 1½–2 | 1½–2 | 1½–2 | 1½–2 |

## The Deciduous (Primary) Teeth

**TABLE 2.3:** Measurement table of the deciduous incisors.

|  | Maxillary central | Incisor lateral | Mandibular central | Incisor lateral |
|---|---|---|---|---|
| 1. Total length (mm) | 16.0 | 15.8 | 14.0 | 15.0 |
| 2. Height of the crown (mm) | 6.0 | 5.6 | 5.0 | 5.2 |
| 3. Length of the root (mm) | 10.0 | 10.2 | 11.0 | 9.8 |
| 4. Mesiodistal crown diameter (mm) | 6.5 | 5.1 | 4.2 | 4.1 |
| 5. Labiolingual crown diameter (mm) | 5.0 | 4.0 | 4.0 | 4.0 |

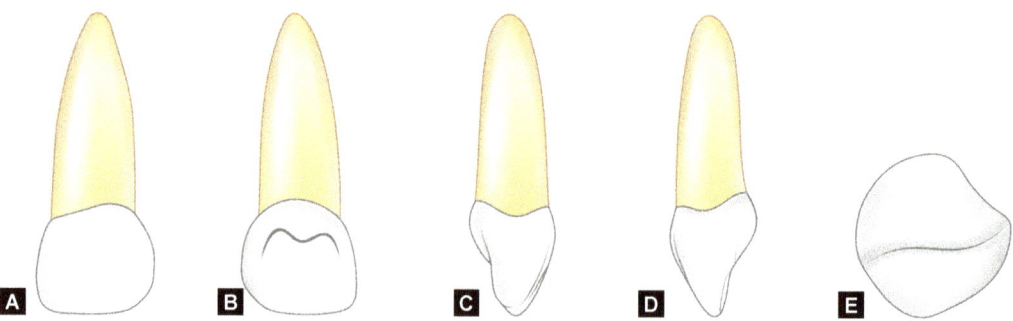

**Figs. 2.1A to E:** Deciduous maxillary left central incisor: (A) Labial aspect; (B) Lingual aspect; (C) Mesial aspect; (D) Distal aspect; (E) Incisal aspect.

**TABLE 2.4:** Differences between deciduous maxillary and mandibular incisors.

| Maxillary | Mandibular |
|---|---|
| 1. Mesiodistal diameter of the crown is greater than cervicoincisal height | 1. Cervicoincisal height of the crown is greater than the mesiodistal |
| 2. Larger than the lower incisors | 2. Smaller than the upper incisors |

make a partial division of the concavity on the lingual surface below the incisal edge, dividing it into a mesial and distal fossa.
- The cervical line appears constricted from all sides.
- The root narrows lingually and presents a ridge for its full length in comparison with a flatter surface labially. A cross section through the root at cervix appears triangular in shape, with the labial surface making one side of the triangle and mesial and distal surfaces making up the other two sides.

### Mesial and Distal Aspects (Figs. 2.1C and D)
- The mesial and distal aspects of the deciduous maxillary central incisors are similar. They are smooth and convex.
- The incisal edge is straight. The mesial angle is well-defined and distal angle is rounded.
- The curvature of cervical line, which represents the cementoenamel junction, is distinct, curving toward the incisal ridge. The cervical curvature distally is less than the amount of curvature mesially.
- The root has an even taper like the shape of a long cone. It is, however, blunt at the apex. Usually, the mesial side of the root will have a developmental groove or concavity, whereas distally the surface is generally convex.

### Incisal Aspect (Fig. 2.1E)
- The incisal edge is centered over the main bulk of the crown and is relatively straight.
- From this aspect, the labial surface is much broader and also smoother than the lingual surface. The lingual surface tapers toward the cingulum.

### The Deciduous Maxillary Lateral Incisor (Figs. 2.2A to E) (Table 2.5)

In general, the maxillary lateral incisor is similar to the central incisor from all

# The Deciduous (Primary) Teeth

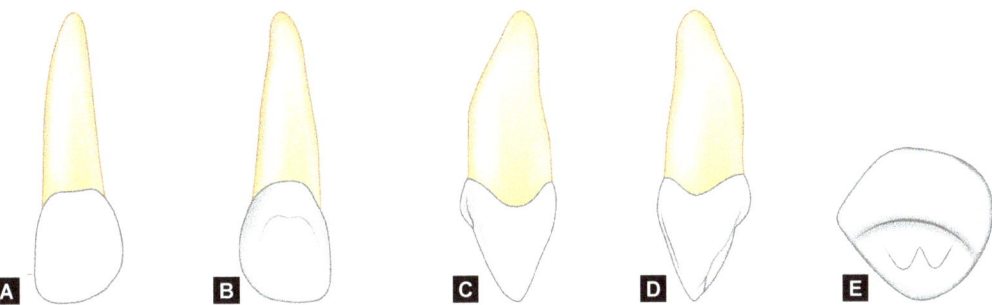

**Figs. 2.2A to E:** Deciduous maxillary left lateral incisor: (A) Labial aspect; (B) Lingual aspect; (C) Mesial aspect; (D) Distal aspect; (E) Incisal aspect.

| TABLE 2.5: Differences between deciduous maxillary central and lateral incisors. | |
|---|---|
| **Maxillary central incisor** | **Maxillary lateral incisor** |
| 1. Larger than lateral incisor | 1. Smaller |
| 2. Cingulum is prominent | 2. Cingulum is not prominent |
| 3. Crown height is smaller than M-D width | 3. Crown height is greater than M-D width |
| 4. Distoincisal angle is less rounded | 4. Distoincisal angle is more rounded |
| 5. Lingual fossa is shallower | 5. Lingual fossa is deeper |

aspects, but it is smaller in all directions. The cervicoincisal length of the lateral crown is greater than its mesiodistal width. The distoincisal angles of the crown are more rounded than those of the central incisor. The cingulum is not prominent. The root has a similar shape, but it is much longer in proportion to its crown.

## The Deciduous Mandibular Central Incisor (Figs. 2.3A to E)

This is the smallest tooth in human dentition.

## Labial Aspect (Fig. 2.3A)

- The labial aspect of this crown is smooth and convex with no developmental groves.
- The mesial and distal sides of the crown are tapered evenly from the contact areas.
- This crown is wide in proportion to its length in comparison with that of its permanent successor.
- The mesial and distal incisal angles are sharp.
- The root of the deciduous central incisor is long and is evenly tapered down to the apex, which is pointed. The root is almost twice the length of the crown.

## Lingual Aspect (Fig. 2.3B)

- The marginal ridges are not well-defined and the cingulum is prominent on the lingual aspect.
- At the middle third and the incisal third of the lingual aspect, there is a shallow concavity, called the lingual fossa.
- The lingual portion of the crown and root converges so that it is narrower towards the lingual than towards the labial surface.

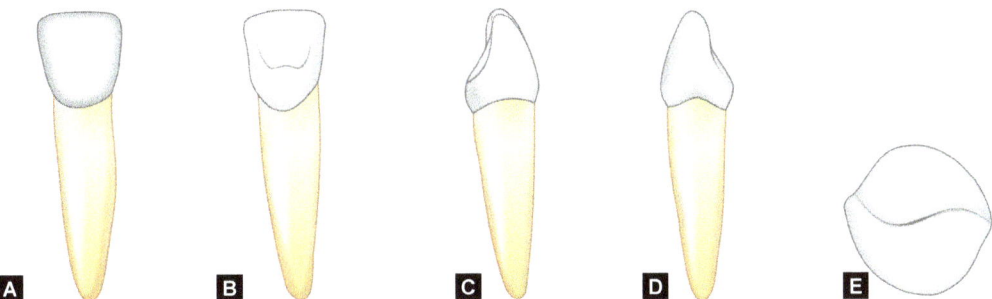

**Figs. 2.3A to E:** Deciduous mandibular left central incisor: (A) Labial aspect; (B) Lingual aspect; (C) Mesial aspect; (D) Distal aspect; (E) Incisal aspect.

## Mesial Aspect (Fig. 2.3C)

- The mesial aspect is triangular, smooth, and convex.
- The incisal ridge is centered over the center of the root and between the crest of curvature of the crown, labially and lingually. The convexity of the cervical contours labially and lingually is present at the cervical third.
- The mesial surface of the root is nearly flat and is evenly tapered.

## Distal Aspect (Fig. 2.3D)

- The cervical line of the crown is less curved toward the incisal ridge than that found on the mesial surface.
- Often there is a developmental depression on the distal side of the root.

## Incisal Aspect (Fig. 2.3E)

- The incisal ridge is straight and bisects the crown labiolingually.
- The mesioincisal angle is sharp and distoincisal angle is rounded. There is a definite taper toward the cingulum on the lingual side.
- The labial surface from this view presents a flat surface slightly convex, whereas the lingual surface presents a flattened surface slightly concave.
- No mamelons are present.

## The Deciduous Mandibular Lateral Incisor (Figs. 2.4A to E) (Table 2.6)

- The fundamental outlines of the deciduous mandibular lateral incisor are similar to those of the deciduous central incisor, but larger in dimension.
- The cingulum of the lateral incisor may be a little more generous than that of the central incisor and the lingual surface of the crown between the marginal ridges may be more concave.
- The incisal ridge slopes downward distally. So the distal contact area is apically positioned to contact with the mesial surface of the deciduous mandibular canine.

**TABLE 2.6:** Differences between deciduous mandibular central and lateral incisor.

| Mandibular central incisor | Mandibular lateral incisor |
|---|---|
| 1. Smallest tooth | 1. Larger than the central incisor but M-D width is narrower |
| 2. Bilaterally symmetrical. Both mesio- and distoincisal angles are sharp | 2. Not symmetrical bilaterally. Incisal margin slopes downward distally. Distoincisal angle is rounded |

## THE DECIDUOUS CANINE (TABLES 2.7 AND 2.8)

The deciduous canines resemble permanent canines. The cervical ridge is well-developed and roots are comparatively larger.

### The Deciduous Maxillary Canine (Figs. 2.5A to E)

#### Labial Aspect (Fig. 2.5A)

- Height of the crown is shorter than the mesiodistal diameter.

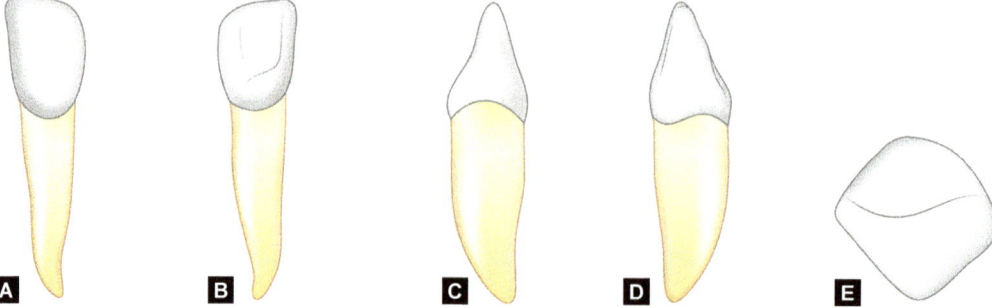

Figs. 2.4A to E: Deciduous mandibular left lateral incisor: (A) Labial aspect; (B) Lingual aspect; (C) Mesial aspect; (D) Distal aspect; (E) Incisal aspect.

## The Deciduous (Primary) Teeth

**TABLE 2.7:** Chronology of tooth formation and eruption of deciduous canines.

|   |   | Maxillary canine | Mandibular canine |
|---|---|---|---|
| 1. | Initiation of calcification (month in utero) | 5 | 5 |
| 2. | Crown completion (month) | 9 | 9 |
| 3. | Eruption (month) | 16–20 | 16–20 |
| 4. | Root completion (year) | 2½–3 | 2½–3 |

**TABLE 2.8:** Measurement table of the deciduous canine.

|   |   | Maxillary canine | Mandibular canine |
|---|---|---|---|
| 1. | Total length (mm) | 19.0 | 17.0 |
| 2. | Height of crown (mm) | 6.5 | 6.0 |
| 3. | Length of root (mm) | 12.5 | 11.0 |
| 4. | Mesiodistal crown diameter (mm) | 7.0 | 5.0 |
| 5. | Labiolingual crown diameter (mm) | 7.0 | 4.8 |

- The crown margins bulge proximally giving the crown a diamond shape. The crown is more constricted at the cervix in relation to its mesiodistal width. Labially, the cervical ridge is prominent.
- Instead of an incisal edge, it has a long, well-developed, and sharp cusp. Compared to the permanent maxillary canine, the cusp on the deciduous canine is much longer and sharper. A line drawn through the contact areas of the deciduous canine would bisect a line drawn from the cervix to the tip of the cusp (in the permanent canine, the contact areas are not at the same level). When the cusp is intact, the mesial slope of the cusp will be longer than the distal slope.
- The root of the deciduous canine is long, slender, and tapering and is more than twice the crown length.

### Lingual Aspect (Fig. 2.5B)

- The lingual aspect shows pronounced enamel ridges that merge with each other. They are the cingulum, mesial, and distal marginal ridges, and incisal ridges, besides a tubercle at the cusp tip, which is a continuation of the lingual ridge connecting the cingulum and the cusp tip. This lingual ridge divides the lingual surface into shallow mesiolingual and distolingual fossae.
- The root of this tooth tapers lingually. It is usually inclined distally.

### Mesial Aspect (Fig. 2.5C)

- The measurement labiolingually at the cervical third is much greater.
- The curvature of the cervical line is more than on distal surface.

### Distal Aspect (Fig. 2.5D)

- The distal outline of this tooth is the reverse of the mesial aspect.
- The curvature of the cervical line toward the cusp ridge is less than on the mesial surface.

### Incisal Aspect (Fig. 2.5E)

- From the incisal aspect, the crown appears diamond-shaped.

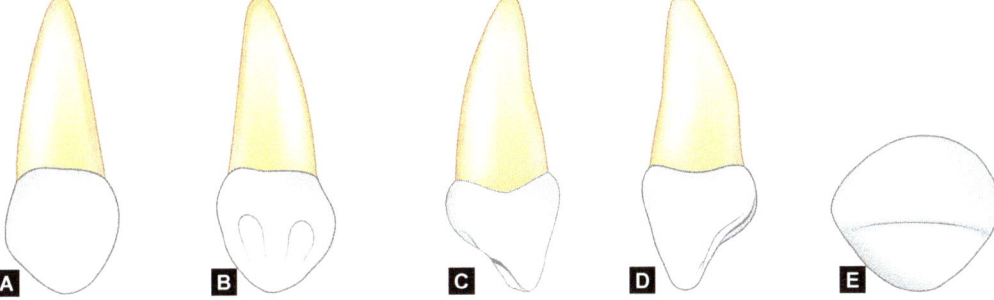

**Figs. 2.5A to E:** Deciduous maxillary left canine: (A) Labial aspect; (B) Lingual aspect; (C) Mesial aspect; (D) Distal aspect; (E) Incisal aspect.

- The tip of the cusp is distal to the center of the crown, and the mesial cusp slope is longer than the distal cusp slope. This allows for intercuspation with the mandibular canine, which has its longest slope distally.

## The Deciduous Mandibular Canine (Figs. 2.6A to E) (Table 2.9)

- The crown is 0.5 mm shorter and the root is at least 2 mm shorter; the mesiodistal measurement of the mandibular canine at the root trunk is greater when compared with its mesiodistal measurement at the contact areas than is the maxillary canine.

**TABLE 2.9:** Differences between maxillary and mandibular deciduous canines.

| Maxillary | Mandibular |
|---|---|
| 1. Total length is more | 1. Total length is less |
| 2. Crown is wider mesiodistally | 2. Crown is narrower mesiodistally |
| 3. Height of crown is shorter than M-D diameter | 3. Height of crown is greater than M-D diameter |
| 4. Wider labiolingually | 4. Narrower labiolingually |
| 5. Crown is blunt | 5. Crown is more pointed |
| 6. Cingulum is prominent | 6. Cingulum is less prominent |

The deciduous maxillary canine is much larger labiolingually.
- The cervical ridges labially and lingually are not as pronounced as the maxillary canine.
- The distal cusp slope is longer than the mesial slope (the opposite arrangement is true of the maxillary canine).

## THE DECIDUOUS MOLARS (TABLES 2.10 AND 2.11)

The deciduous molars are total eight in number, four in each jaw and two in each quadrant. The occlusal surfaces are narrow buccolingually. There is a prominent cervical bulge in the crown and roots are divergent.

### The Deciduous Maxillary First Molar (Figs. 2.7A to E) (Table 2.12)

It is the smallest molar in the oral cavity. It appears as an intermediate between a premolar and a molar.

### Buccal Aspect (Fig. 2.7A)

- The buccal aspect is smooth and convex in both directions. The mesiodistal diameter is greater than the crown height.

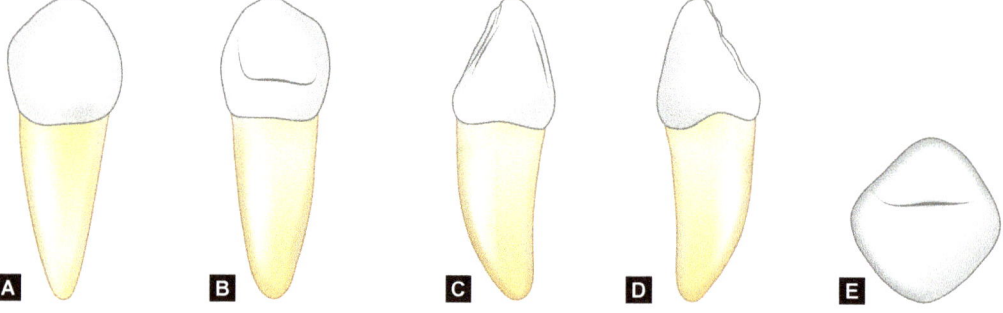

Figs. 2.6A to E: Deciduous mandibular left canine: (A) Labial aspect; (B) Lingual aspect; (C) Mesial aspect; (D) Distal aspect; (E) Incisal aspect.

**TABLE 2.10:** Chronology of tooth formation and eruption of deciduous molars.

| | Maxillary | | Mandibular | |
|---|---|---|---|---|
| | First | Second | First | Second |
| 1. Initiation of calcification (month in utero) | 5 | 6 | 5 | 6 |
| 2. Crown completion (month) | 6 | 12 | 6 | 12 |
| 3. Eruption (month) | 12–16 | 20–30 | 12–16 | 20–30 |
| 4. Root completed (year) | 2–2½ | 3 | 2–2½ | 3 |

| TABLE 2.11: Measurement table of the deciduous molars. | | | | |
|---|---|---|---|---|
| | Maxillary | | Mandibular | |
| | First | Second | First | Second |
| 1. Total length (mm) | 15.2 | 17.5 | 15.8 | 18.8 |
| 2. Height of crown (mm) | 5.1 | 5.7 | 6.0 | 5.5 |
| 3. Length of root (mm) | 10.1 | 11.8 | 9.8 | 13.3 |
| 4. Mesiodistal crown diameter (mm) | 7.3 | 8.2 | 7.7 | 9.9 |
| 5. Labiolingual crown diameter (mm) | 8.5 | 10.0 | 7.0 | 8.7 |

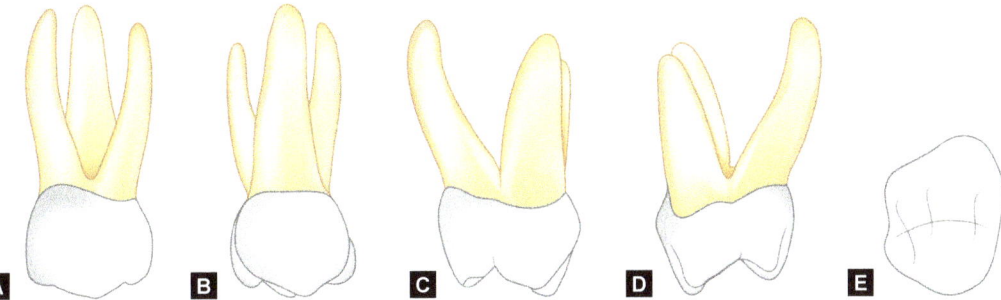

**Figs. 2.7A to E:** Deciduous maxillary left first molar: (A) Buccal aspect; (B) Lingual aspect; (C) Mesial aspect; (D) Distal aspect; (E) Occlusal aspect.

- The widest measurement of the crown is at the contact areas mesially and distally. From these points, the crown converges toward the cervix.
- The occlusal line is slightly scalloped, but there is no definite cusp form.
- The cervical ridge is well-developed and is more prominent mesially and may form a tubercle known as tubercle of Zuckerkandl.
- The cervical line is higher mesially than distally.
- The roots of the maxillary first molar are slender and long and they are divergent. The distal root is considerably shorter than the mesial one. The bifurcation of the roots begins almost immediately at the site of the cervical line (cementoenamel junction).

## Lingual Aspect (Fig. 2.7B)

- The mesiodistal dimension of lingual aspect is less than buccal aspect as the crown converges in a lingual direction.
- The mesiolingual cusp is the longest and sharpest cusp on this tooth and it forms most of the occlusal border. The distolingual cusp is small and rounded.

| TABLE 2.12: Differences between upper and lower deciduous molars. | |
|---|---|
| Deciduous molars | |
| Upper | Lower |
| 1. Three roots | 1. Two roots |
| 2. Two to four cusps are seen on crown | 2. Four to five cusps are seen |

- Some of the deciduous maxillary first molar present one large lingual cusp with no developmental groove lingually. This type is apparently a three-cusped molar.
- All three roots may be seen from this aspect. The lingual root is larger than the others.

## Mesial Aspect (Fig. 2.7C)

- The dimension at the cervical third is greater than the dimension at the occlusal third.
- The buccal outline shows pronounced convexity near cervical third. The lingual outline is evenly convex from cervical to occlusal region.
- The mesiolingual cusp is longer and sharper than the mesiobuccal cusp. There

is a pronounced convexity on the buccal outline in the cervical third.
- The cervical line mesially shows some curvature in the direction of the occlusal surface.
- The mesiobuccal and lingual roots are visible from the mesial side of this tooth. The distobuccal root is hidden behind the mesiobuccal root. The lingual root from this aspect looks long and slender and extends lingually to a marked degree. It curves sharply in a buccal direction above the middle third.

### Distal Aspect (Fig. 2.7D)

- From the distal aspect, the crown is narrower distally than mesially and it tapers markedly toward the distal.
- The distobuccal cusp is long and sharp and the distolingual cusp is poorly developed.
- The prominent bulge seen from the mesial aspect at the cervical third does not continue distally. The cervical line may curve occlusally, or it may extend straight across from the buccal surface to the lingual surface.
- All three roots may be seen from this angle, but the distobuccal root is superimposed on the mesiobuccal root so that only the buccal surface and the apex of the later may be seen. The point of bifurcation of the distobuccal root and the lingual root is near the cementoenamel junction.

### Occlusal Aspect (Fig. 2.7E)

- The surface is trapezoidal in shape with shortest sides represented by marginal ridges. The mesial and distal surfaces are straight and converge lingually. The calibration from the mesiobuccal line angle to the mesiolingual line angle is greater than that found at the distal line angles. Therefore, the crown converges distally also.
- The occlusal surface has a central fossa. There is a mesial triangular fossa, just inside the mesial marginal ridge, with a mesial pit in this fossa and a sulcus with its central groove connecting the two fossae. There is also a well-defined buccal developmental groove dividing the mesiobuccal cusp and the distobuccal cusp occlusally. There are supplemental grooves radiating from the pit in the mesial triangular fossa. These grooves radiate as follows: one buccally, one lingually, and one toward the marginal ridge, the last sometimes extending over the marginal ridge mesially.
- Sometimes the deciduous maxillary first molar has a well-defined triangular ridge connecting the mesiolingual cusp with the distobuccal cusp. When well-developed, it is called the oblique ridge. In some of these teeth, the ridge will be very indefinite and the central development groove will extend from the mesial pit to the distal developmental groove. This distoocclusal groove is always seen and may or may not extend through to the lingual surface, outlining a distolingual cusp. The distal marginal ridge is thin and poorly developed in comparison with the mesial marginal ridge.

## The Deciduous Maxillary Second Molar (Figs. 2.8A to E) (Table 2.13)

### Buccal Aspect (Fig. 2.8A)

- The deciduous maxillary second molar resembles the permanent maxillary first molar, but it is smaller.
- There are two well-defined buccal cusps with a buccal developmental groove between them. The crown is narrow at the cervix in comparison with its mesiodistal measurement at the contact areas. There is a well-developed cervical ridge.
- The roots are much longer and heavier compared to that of the maxillary first molar. The point of bifurcation between the buccal roots is close to the cervical line of the crown.

### Lingual Aspect (Fig. 2.8B)

Lingually, the crown shows three cusps: (1) the mesiolingual cusp, which is large and

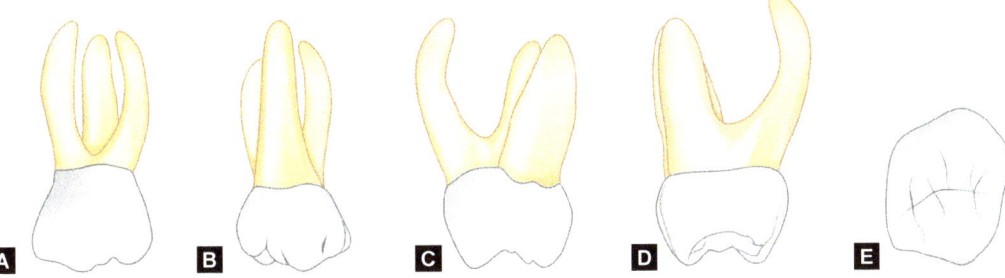

**Figs. 2.8A to E:** Deciduous maxillary left second molar: (A) Buccal aspect; (B) Lingual aspect; (C) Mesial aspect; (D) Distal aspect; (E) Occlusal aspect.

| TABLE 2.13: Differences between maxillary deciduous first and second molars. | |
|---|---|
| **Maxillary deciduous molar** | |
| **First** | **Second** |
| 1. Smaller | 1. Larger |
| 2. It has two to three cusps | 2. It has four cusps |
| 3. It looks like an intermediate between premolar and permanent molar. Basically, it resembles a premolar | 3. It resembles permanent first molar |

well-developed, (2) the distolingual cusp, which is also well-developed, and (3) a third supplemental cusp, which is apical to the mesiolingual cusp and is called the tubercle of Carabelli, or the fifth cusp.

This cusp is poorly developed and merely acts as a supplement to the bulk of the mesiolingual cusp.

- A well-defined developmental groove separates the mesiolingual cusp from the distolingual cusp and connects with the developmental groove, which outlines the fifth cusp.
- All three roots are visible from this aspect; the lingual root is large and thick in comparison with the other two roots.

## Mesial Aspect (Fig. 2.8C)

- The mesiolingual cusp of the crown with its supplementary fifth cusp appears large in comparison with the mesiobuccal cusp. The mesiobuccal cusp from this angle is relatively short and sharp. There is very little curvature to the cervical line. Usually, it is almost straight across from the buccal surface to lingual surface.
- The mesiobuccal root from this aspect is broad and flat. The lingual root has somewhat the same curvature as the lingual root of the maxillary first deciduous molar. The mesiobuccal root extends lingually far out beyond the crown outline. The point of bifurcation between the mesiobuccal root and the lingual root is 2 or 3 mm apical to the cervical line of the crown.

## Distal Aspect (Fig. 2.8D)

- From the distal aspect, the lingual outline is smooth and rounded but the buccal outline is almost straight from the crest of curvature to the tip of the buccal cusp. The distobuccal cusp and the distolingual cusp are about the same in length.
- The cervical line is approximately straight, as was found mesially.
- All three roots are seen from this aspect, although only a part of the outline of the mesiobuccal root may be seen, since the distobuccal root is superimposed over it. The distobuccal root is shorter and narrower than the other roots. The point of bifurcation between the distobuccal root and the lingual root is more apical in location than any of the other points of bifurcation.

## Occlusal Aspect (Fig. 2.8E)

- From the occlusal aspect, this tooth resembles the permanent first molar. It is somewhat rhomboidal and has four well-developed cusps and one supplemental cusp—mesiobuccal, distobuccal, mesiolingual, distolingual, and fifth cusps. The buccal surface is rather flat, with the developmental groove between the cusps less marked than that found on the first permanent molar. Developmental grooves, pits, oblique ridge, and so forth, are almost identical.

- The occlusal surface has a central fossa with a central pit, a well-defined mesial triangular fossa, just distal to the mesial marginal ridge, with a mesial pit at its center. There is a well-defined developmental groove called the central groove at the bottom of a sulcus connecting the mesial triangular fossa with the central fossa. The buccal developmental groove extends buccally from the central pit, separating the triangular ridges, which are occlusal continuations of the mesio- and distobuccal cusps. Supplemental grooves often radiate from these developmental grooves.
- The oblique ridge is prominent and connects the mesiolingual cusp with the distobuccal cusp. Distal to the oblique ridge, there is the distal fossa, which harbors the distal developmental groove. The distal groove has branches of supplemental grooves within the distal triangular fossa.
- The distal groove acts as a line of demarcation between the mesiolingual and distolingual cusps and continues on to the lingual surface as the lingual developmental groove. The distal marginal ridge is as well-developed as the mesial marginal ridge.

## The Deciduous Mandibular First Molar (Figs. 2.9A to E)

### Buccal Aspect (Fig. 2.9A)

- From the buccal aspect, the mesial outline of the crown of the deciduous mandibular first molar is almost straight from the contact area to the cervix. The distal outline converges more toward the cervix, making the contact area extend distally to a marked degree.
- The distal portion of the crown is shorter than the mesial portion, the cervical line dipping apically where it joins the mesial root.
- The two buccal cusps are rather distinct and there is no developmental groove between them. The mesial cusp is larger than the distal cusp. There is a developmental depression dividing them (not a groove), which extends over to the buccal surface.
- The roots are long and slender and they spread greatly at the apical third beyond the outline of the crown. From the buccal aspect, if a line is drawn from the bifurcation of the roots to the occlusal surface, the tooth will be evenly divided mesiodistally.

### Lingual Aspect (Fig. 2.9B)

- The crown and root converge lingually to a marked degree on the mesial surface. The distolingual cusp is rounded and suggests a developmental groove between this cusp and the mesiolingual cusp.

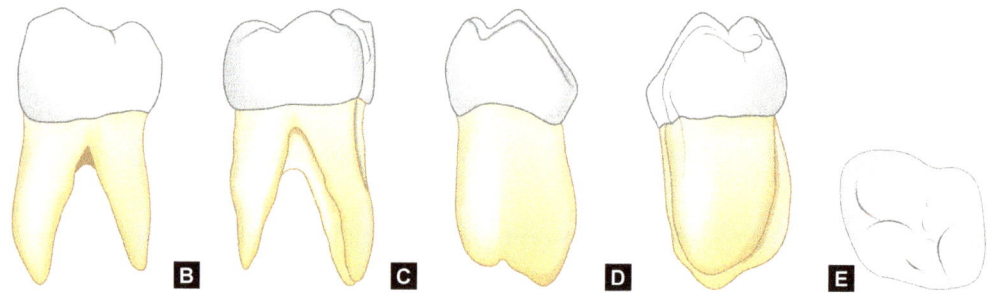

**Figs. 2.9A to E:** Deciduous mandibular left first molar: (A) Buccal aspect; (B) Lingual aspect; (C) Mesial aspect; (D) Distal aspect; (E) Occlusal aspect.

- The mesiolingual cusp is long and sharp at the tip. The sharp and prominent mesiolingual cusp (almost centered lingually but in line with the mesial root) is an outstanding characteristic found occlusally on the deciduous first mandibular molar.
- The mesial marginal ridge is well-developed.

## Mesial Aspect (Fig. 2.9C)

- The buccal cusps are placed over the root base, and the lingual outline of the crown extends out lingually beyond the confines of the root base.
- Both the mesiobuccal cusp and the mesiolingual cusp are visible from this aspect. The mesial marginal ridge is well-developed. All of the deciduous molars have flattened buccal surfaces above this cervical ridge.
- The buccal and lingual outlines of the root drop straight down from the crown and are approximately parallel for over half their length, tapering only slightly at the apical third. A developmental depression usually extends almost the full length of the root on the mesial side.

## Distal Aspect (Fig. 2.9D)

- The length of the crown buccally and lingually is more uniform and the cervical line extends almost straight across buccolingually.
- The distobuccal cusp and the distolingual cusp are not as long or as sharp as the two mesial cusps.
- The distal marginal ridge is not as straight and well-defined as the mesial marginal ridge.
- The distal root is rounder and shorter and tapers more apically.

## Occlusal Aspect (Fig. 2.9E)

- The general outline of this tooth from the occlusal aspect is rhomboidal.
- The mesiolingual cusp is the largest and the best developed of all the cusps and it has a broad flattened surface lingually.
- The *buccal developmental groove* of the occlusal surface divides the two buccal cusps evenly and extends to the center of the crown at a central pit. The central developmental groove joins it at this point and extends mesially, separating the mesiobuccal cusp and the mesiolingual cusp. The central groove ends in a mesial pit in the mesial triangular fossa, which is immediately distal to the mesial marginal ridge.
- The mesiobuccal cusp exhibits a well-defined triangular ridge on the occlusal surface, which terminates in the center of the occlusal surface buccolingually at the central developmental groove. The lingual developmental groove extends lingually from this point, separating the mesiolingual cusp and the distolingual cusp.

## The Deciduous Mandibular Second Molar (Figs. 2.10A to E) (Table 2.14)

The deciduous mandibular second molar resembles the permanent mandibular first molar.

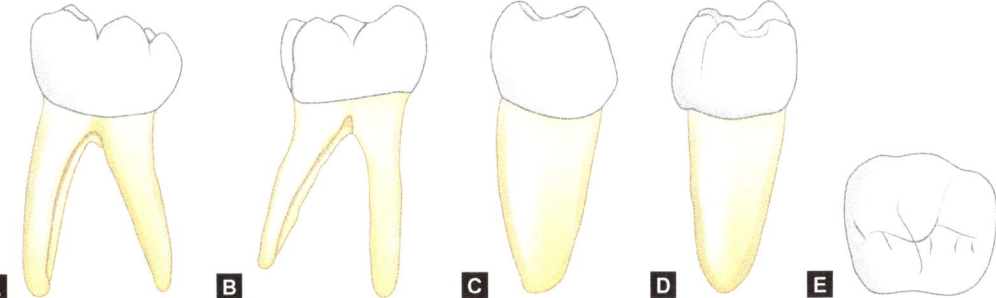

**Figs. 2.10A to E:** Deciduous mandibular left second molar: (A) Buccal aspect; (B) Lingual aspect; (C) Mesial aspect; (D) Distal aspect; (E) Occlusal aspect.

| TABLE 2.14: Differences between mandibular deciduous first and second molars. ||
|---|---|
| Mandibular deciduous molar ||
| First | Second |
| 1. Smaller | 1. Larger |
| 2. Has four cusps | 2. Has five cusps |
| 3. Does not resemble any permanent tooth | 3. Resembles permanent first molar |

## Buccal Aspect (Fig. 2.10A)

- From the buccal aspect, the mesiobuccal and distobuccal developmental grooves divide the buccal surface of the crown occlusally into a mesiobuccal, a buccal, and a distobuccal cusp.
- The roots of the deciduous second molar from this angle are slender and long. They have a characteristic flare mesiodistally at the middle and apical thirds. The roots of this tooth may be twice as long as the crown.
- The point of bifurcation of the roots starts immediately below the cementoenamel junction of crown and root.

## Lingual Aspect (Fig. 2.10B)

- From the lingual aspect, two cusps are of almost equal dimensions. Between them, there is a short lingual groove. The two lingual cusps are not quite as wide as the three buccal cusps and thus narrow the crown lingually.
- The cervical line is relatively straight.
- The mesial portion of the crown appears little higher than the distal portion of the crown when viewed from the lingual aspect.
- The roots from this aspect give somewhat the same appearance as from the buccal aspect.

## Mesial Aspect (Fig. 2.10C)

- The crest of contour buccally is more prominent on the deciduous molar, and the tooth seems to be more constricted occlusally because of the flattened buccal surface above this cervical ridge.
- The marginal ridge is high, a characteristic that makes the mesiobuccal cusp and the mesiolingual cusp appear rather short. The lingual cusp is longer or extends higher at any rate than the buccal cusp.
- The cervical line is regular, although it extends upward buccolingually.
- The mesial root is unusually broad and flat with a blunt apex.

## Distal Aspect (Fig. 2.10D)

- The crown is not as wide distally as it is mesially.
- The distolingual cusp appears well developed and the triangular ridge from the tip of this cusp extending down into the occlusal surface is seen over the distal marginal ridge.
- The distal marginal ridge dips down more sharply and is shorter buccolingually than the mesial marginal ridge. The cervical line of the crown is regular, although it has the same upward incline buccolingually on the distal as on the mesial.
- The distal root is almost as broad as the mesial root and it is flattened on the distal surface. The distal root tapers more at the apical end than does the mesial root.

## Occlusal Aspect (Fig. 2.10E)

- The occlusal aspect of the deciduous mandibular second molar is somewhat rectangular. The three buccal cusps are similar in size. The two lingual cusps are also equally matched.
- There are well-defined triangular ridges extending occlusally from the cusp tips. The triangular ridges end in the center of the crown buccolingually in a central developmental groove that extends from the mesial triangular fossa, just inside the mesial marginal ridge, to the distal triangular fossa, just mesial to the distal marginal ridge. The two buccal grooves are confluent with the buccal developmental grooves of the buccal surface, one mesial and one distal, and the single lingual developmental groove is confluent with

the lingual groove on the lingual surface of the crown.
- The mesial marginal ridge is better developed and more pronounced than the distal marginal ridge. The outline of the crown converges distally.

## QUESTIONNAIRE

1. What is deciduous dentition? What are the functions of deciduous dentition?
2. How do you differentiate between deciduous and permanent dentition?
3. Discuss the morphology of deciduous maxillary central incisor with diagram. How do you differentiate between deciduous maxillary and mandibular central incisor?
4. Discuss the morphology of deciduous maxillary canine with diagram. How do you differentiate between the features of deciduous maxillary and mandibular canine?
5. Discuss the morphology of deciduous maxillary first molar with diagram. How do you differentiate between the morphological features of deciduous maxillary first and second molar?
6. Discuss the morphology of deciduous mandibular first molar with diagram. How do you differentiate between the features of deciduous mandibular first and second molar?
7. Write short notes on:
   a. Leeway space of Nance.
   b. Tubercle of Zuckerkandl.
   c. Tubercle of Carabelli.

## BIBLIOGRAPHY

1. Berkovitz BKB, Holland GR, Moxham BJ. A Colour Atlas and Textbook of Oral Anatomy, Histology and Embryology, 4th edition. Mosby: Elsevier; 2009.
2. Biviji AT. Dental Anatomy, 2nd edition. Mumbai: Bhalani Publishing House; 1999.
3. Das AK. Dental Anatomy and Oral Histology, 1st edition. West Bengal: Current Books International; 1972.
4. Kraus BS, Jordon RE, Abrams L. Dental Anatomy and Occlusion. Baltimore: Williams and Willkin's Company; 1969.
5. Nelson SJ, Ash MJ. Wheeler's Dental Anatomy, Physiology and Occlusion, 9th edition. Philadelphia: Elsevier; 2010.

# CHAPTER 3

# The Permanent Teeth

## THE PERMANENT INCISORS

- There are eight incisor teeth, four in maxillary arch and four in mandibular arch **(Tables 3.1 and 3.2)**.
- Four incisors teeth one on each side of midline in both the jaws are central incisors. The incisors on the distal aspects of each central incisor are called lateral incisors.
- The incisors of upper jaw are called maxillary incisors and that of lower jaw are called mandibular incisors.
- The incisors have convex labial surface and concave lingual surface. The crowns are triangular when viewed from proximal aspect. The incisal edges of newly erupted teeth show mamelons.
- The incisors have thin blade-like incisal edges in their crown which are adapted for the cutting and shearing of the food preparatory to grinding.
- The incisors with canine form anterior group of teeth. Their presence, proper form, and arrangement are highly important esthetically.
- Phonetically, they play a major role in the proper enunciation of certain speech sounds.

### The Permanent Maxillary Central Incisor (Figs. 3.1A to E) (Tables 3.3 and 3.4)

The maxillary permanent central incisors are the most prominent teeth in the mouth. It is widest mesiodistally of any of the anterior teeth.

### Labial Aspect (Fig. 3.1A)

- The labial surface is convex cervically and flattened incisally.
- The mesial outline of the crown is slightly convex, with the crest of curvature (representing the contact area) approaching

**TABLE 3.1:** Chronology of tooth formation and eruption of the incisors.

|   |   | Maxillary incisor | | Mandibular incisor | |
|---|---|---|---|---|---|
|   |   | Central | Lateral | Central | Lateral |
| 1. | Initiation of calcification | 3–4 months | 10–12 months | 3–4 months | 3–4 months |
| 2. | Crown completion | 4–5 years | 4–5 years | 4–5 years | 4–5 years |
| 3. | Eruption | 7–8 years | 8–9 years | 6–7 years | 7–8 years |
| 4. | Root completion | 10–11 years | 10–11 years | 9–10 years | 10–11 years |

**TABLE 3.2:** Measurement of the incisors.

|   |   | Maxillary incisor | | Mandibular incisor | |
|---|---|---|---|---|---|
|   |   | Central | Lateral | Central | Lateral |
| 1. | Total length | 23.5 mm | 22.0 mm | 21.5 mm | 23.5 mm |
| 2. | Height of crown | 10.5 mm | 9.0 mm | 9.0 mm | 9.5 mm |
| 3. | Length of root | 13.0 mm | 13.0 mm | 12.5 mm | 14 mm |
| 4. | Mesiodistal crown diameter | 8.5 mm | 6.5 mm | 5.0 mm | 5.5 mm |
| 5. | Labiolingual crown diameter | 7.0 mm | 6.0 mm | 6.0 mm | 6.5 mm |

# The Permanent Teeth

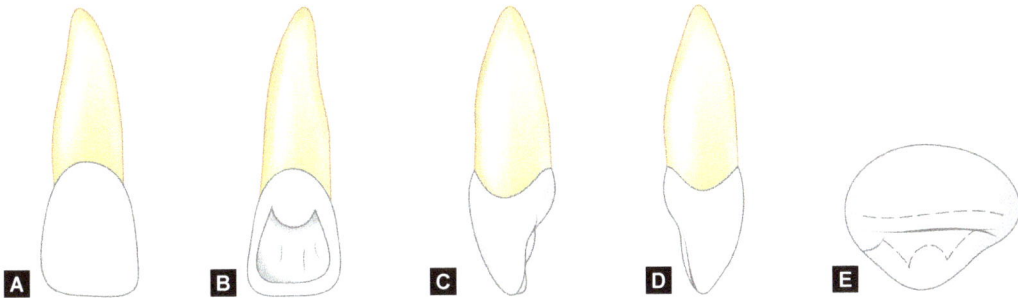

**Figs. 3.1A to E:** Permanent maxillary left central incisor: (A) Labial aspect; (B) Lingual aspect; (C) Mesial aspect; (D) Distal aspect; (E) Incisal aspect.

**TABLE 3.3:** Differences between permanent maxillary and mandibular incisors.

| Maxillary incisors | Mandibular incisors |
|---|---|
| 1. Four upper incisors form the fixed cutting edge | 1. Four lower incisors form the moving cutting edge |
| 2. They are wider | 2. They are narrower |
| 3. The central incisor is wider and larger than lateral incisor | 3. The lateral incisor is larger and wider than central incisor |
| 4. Marginal ridges and cinguli are prominent | 4. Marginal ridges and cinguli are less prominent |
| 5. Lingual fossa is deeper | 5. Lingual fossa is shallower |
| 6. Labial surfaces are more convex | 6. Labial surfaces are less convex |
| 7. Crowns are wider mesiodistally than labiolingually | 7. Crowns are wider labiolingually than mesiodistally |
| 8. Roots are triangular in cross section. No depressions are present on mesial and distal surfaces of root | 8. Roots are oval. Depressions are present on mesial and distal surfaces of roots |
| 9. Incisal surfaces are inclined lingually | 9. Incisal surfaces are perpendicular to the tooth axis |

**TABLE 3.4:** Differences between permanent maxillary central and lateral incisors.

| Maxillary central incisors | Maxillary lateral incisors |
|---|---|
| 1. The crown is larger | 1. The crown is smaller and slender |
| 2. Wider mesiodistally | 2. Narrower mesiodistally |
| 3. Mesioincisal angle is sharp and is a right angle | 3. Mesioincisal angle is rounded |
| 4. Distoincisal angle is slightly rounded | 4. Distoincisal angle is more rounded |
| 5. Cingulum is wide but less prominent. Marginal ridges are prominent. Lingual fossa is moderately deep | 5. Cingulum and marginal ridges are less prominent. Lingual fossa is deep |

the mesioincisal angle. The distal outline of the crown is more convex than the mesial outline, the crest of curvature being higher toward the cervical line.
- The incisal edge is nearly straight and mamelons are present in the newly erupted teeth, the central one being the smallest. Close to incisal ridge, mesiolabial and distolabial grooves mark the border of the lobes forming mamelons.
- The mesioincisal angle is relatively sharp and the distoincisal angle is more or less rounded.
- Both mesial and distal margins converge cervically and form cervical line which is semicircular and convex cervically.
- The root of the central incisor from the labial aspect is cone-shaped, in most instances with a relatively blunt apex, the outline mesially and distally being regular.

## Lingual Aspect (Fig. 3.1B)

- The lingual aspect has convexities and a concavity. Immediately below the cervical line, there is a smooth convexity, called the cingulum. Mesially and distally confluent with the cingulum are the marginal ridges.

- Between the marginal ridges and below the cingulum, the shallow concavity is known as the lingual fossa.
- The lingual fossa is bordered mesially by the mesial marginal ridge, incisally by the lingual portion of the incisal ridge, distally by the distal marginal ridge, and cervically by the cingulum. Developmental grooves may be present extending from the cingulum into the lingual fossa.
- A central ridge may divide lingual fossa into two shallow depressions.
- The cervical line is convex cervically.
- The crown and root taper lingually. A cross section of the root at the cervix shows the root to be triangular with rounded angles; one side of the triangle is labial, with the mesial and distal sides pointing lingually.

*Mesial Aspect (Fig. 3.1C)*

- The mesial aspect of this tooth is roughly triangular, with the base of the triangle at the cervix and the apex at the incisal ridge.
- Labially and lingually, immediately coronal to the cervical line are the crests of curvature of these surfaces.
- The labial outline of the crown from the crest of curvature to the incisal ridge curves smoothly and is slightly convex.
- The lingual outline is "S"-shaped with convexities near cingulum and at the incisal region.
- The cervical line is curved with a pronounced convexity pointing incisally.
- The root of this tooth from the mesial aspect is cone-shaped and the apex of the root is usually bluntly rounded.

*Distal Aspect (Fig. 3.1D)*

- This surface is similar to mesial surface.
- From distal aspect, the crown appears thicker toward the incisal third.
- The cervical line is less convex.

*Incisal Aspect (Fig. 3.1E)*

- Labial surface meets with the lingual surface on incisal aspect.
- It extends from mesial to distal angle of tooth.
- The incisal edge is centered over the root.
- It is inclined lingually.

## The Permanent Maxillary Lateral Incisor (Figs. 3.2A to E)

*Labial Aspect (Fig. 3.2A)*

- The permanent maxillary lateral incisor has a more convex labial surface. The tooth is narrow mesiodistally with rounded incisal ridge. Although the crown is smaller in all dimensions, its proportions usually correspond to those of the central incisor.
- The mesial outline of the crown from the labial aspect is straight with a more rounded mesioincisal angle compared to central incisor (mesioincisal angle is sharper compared to distoincisal angle of the same tooth). The crest of contour mesially is usually at the point of junction of the middle and incisal thirds.
- The distal outline is more rounded and shorter than mesial outline. The crest of contour is more cervical, usually in the center of the middle third. The distoincisal angle is rounded.

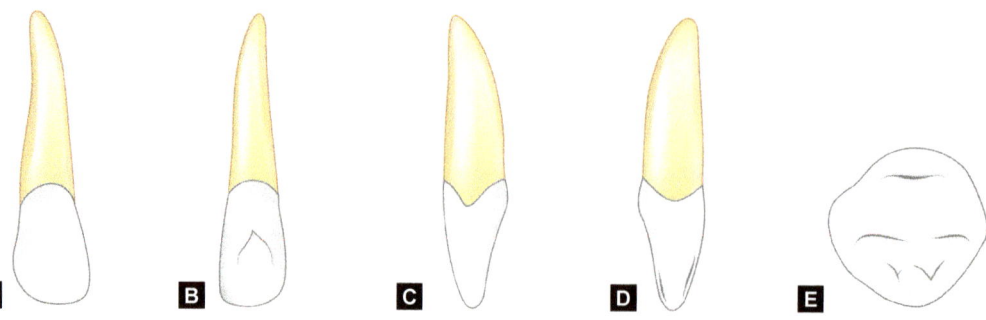

**Figs. 3.2A to E:** Permanent maxillary left lateral incisor: (A) Labial aspect; (B) Lingual aspect; (C) Mesial aspect; (D) Distal aspect; (E) Incisal aspect.

- The root length is greater in proportion to its crown length than that of the central incisor. The root tapers evenly from the cervical line to a point approximately two-thirds of its length apically.

## Lingual Aspect (Fig. 3.2B)
- The tooth tapers toward lingual aspect. The mesial and distal marginal ridges and cingulum are more prominent.
- The lingual fossa is more concave, compared to the central incisor.

## Mesial Aspect (Fig. 3.2C)
- It is triangular in shape. The crown is shorter and the root is relatively longer.
- The incisal ridge is thicker and cingulum is more convex.
- The curvature of the cervical line is marked in the direction of the incisal ridge.
- The root appears as a tapered cone from this aspect, with a bluntly rounded, apical end.

## Distal Aspect (Fig. 3.2D)
- The distal surface is convex.
- The curvature of the cervical line is slightly less in depth than on the mesial side.
- There is a developmental groove on this surface extending to root.

## Incisal Aspect (Fig. 3.2E)
- It is shorter than the central incisor.
- The mamelons are indistinct.
- The lateral incisors exhibit more convexity labially and lingually from incisal aspect than central incisor.

# The Permanent Mandibular Central Incisor (Figs. 3.3A to E)
- This is the smallest of all permanent tooth.
- It is bilaterally symmetrical and narrowest mesiodistally of all incisors.

## Labial Aspect (Fig. 3.3A)
- The labial aspect of the crown of mandibular central incisor is convex in the cervical third and flat in the incisal region.
- The mesial and distal margins are straight and converge evenly toward narrow cervical margin.
- The incisal ridge is straight and is approximately at a right angle to the long axis of the tooth. It shows three mamelons. Both the mesioincisal and distoincisal angles are sharp and at right angles.
- The contact areas are incisal to the junction of incisal and middle thirds of the crown.
- The mesial and distal root outlines are straight with the mesial and distal outlines of the crown down to the apical portion. The apical third of the root terminates in a small pointed taper.

## Lingual Aspect (Fig. 3.3B)
- The lingual surface of the crown is smooth with very slight concavity at the incisal half and convexity cervically. The outlines and surfaces of the mandibular incisors are regular and symmetrical.
- The marginal ridges and the cingulum are inconspicuous.
- Lingual fossa is shallow between marginal ridges and cingulum.

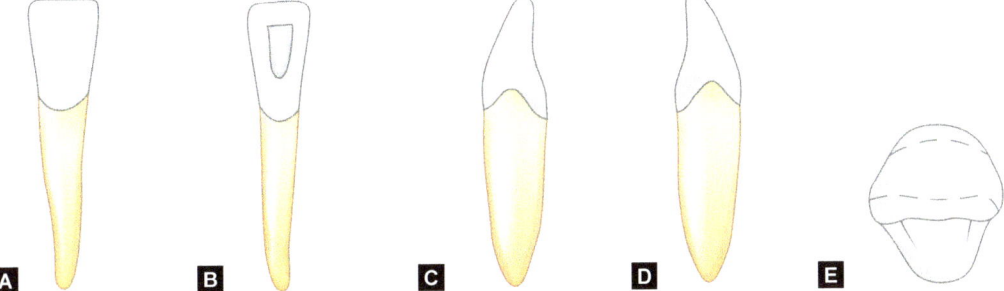

**Figs. 3.3A to E:** Permanent mandibular left central incisor: (A) Labial aspect; (B) Lingual aspect; (C) Mesial aspect; (D) Distal aspect; (E) Incisal aspect.

## Mesial Aspect (Fig. 3.3C)

- The crown in roughly triangular on mesial aspect. It is convex and smooth at the incisal third and broader and flatter at the middle and cervical third.
- The labial outline is straight above cervical curvature, sloping rapidly from the crest of curvature to the incisal ridge. The lingual outline is "S"-shaped, convex in the cingulum region and concave incisally.
- The cervical line is curving incisally approximately one-third the length of the crown.
- The root outlines from the mesial aspect are straight with the crown outline from the cervical line.

The outline of the root begins to taper in the middle third area, tapering rapidly in the apical third to either a bluntly rounded or a pointed root end.

## Distal Aspect (Fig. 3.3D)

- This surface is similar to that of the mesial surface, except the cervical line which curves incisally about 1 mm less than on the mesial.
- The developmental depression on the distal surface of the root may be more marked, with a deeper and more well-defined developmental groove at its center.

## Incisal Aspect (Fig. 3.3E)

- The incisal edge is straight and is almost at right angles to the line bisecting the crown labiolingually.
- The incisal angles are sharp.

## The Permanent Mandibular Lateral Incisor (Figs. 3.4A to E) (Table 3.5)

- It is very similar to mandibular central incisor but is slightly larger.
- The mesial side of the crown is often longer than the distal side, causing straight incisal edge to slope downward in a distal direction. The distal contact area is more toward the cervical than the mesial contact area to contact properly the mesial contact area of the mandibular canine.
- The distoincisal angle is rounded.
- The incisal edge is not approximately at right angle to the line bisecting the crown and root labiolingually. The edge follows

**TABLE 3.5:** Differences between permanent mandibular central and lateral incisors.

| Mandibular central incisors | Mandibular lateral incisors |
|---|---|
| 1. Mesiodistally narrower and smallest tooth | 1. Mesiodistally wider |
| 2. Bilaterally symmetrical. Mesial and distal surfaces are parallel | 2. Bilaterally asymmetrical. Mesial surface is longer than distal |
| 3. Incisal ridge is straight. Mesioincisal and distoincisal angles are sharp and at right angle | 3. Incisal ridge is inclined toward distal. Mesioincisal angle is sharp and distoincisal angle is rounded |
| 4. Marginal ridges and cingulum are less prominent. Lingual fossa is shallow | 4. Marginal ridges, cingulum, and lingual fossa are prominent |
| 5. Incisal edge is at right angle to the labiolingual bisecting line | 5. Incisal edge is twisted on the crown. Distoincisal angle is projected lingually |

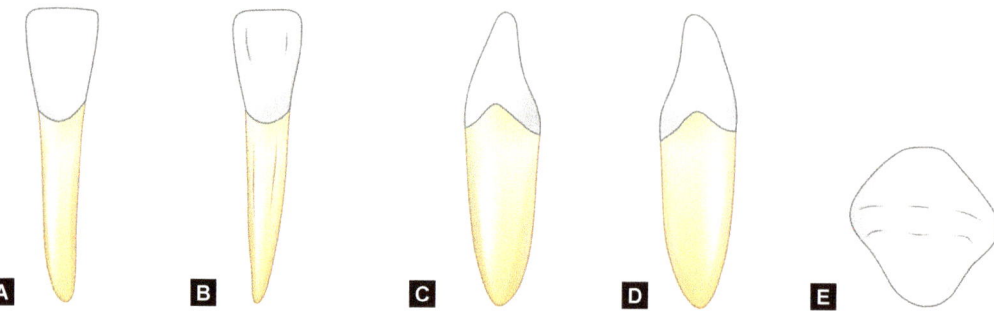

**Figs. 3.4A to E:** Permanent mandibular left lateral incisor: (A) Labial aspect; (B) Lingual aspect; (C) Mesial aspect; (D) Distal aspect; (E) Incisal aspect.

the curvature of mandibular dental arch, giving the crown the appearance of being twisted slightly on its root base.
- Root is similar to that of central incisor having grooves both on mesial and distal surfaces.

## THE PERMANENT CANINES

- There are four canine teeth, one on each quadrant (right and left) of both maxilla and mandible **(Tables 3.6 and 3.7)**.
- They are placed at the "corners" of the mouth, each one the third tooth from the median line.
- They are the longest teeth in the mouth. They have single conical cusp. The middle lobes have been highly developed incisally into strong well-formed cusps.
- Their roots are thickest and longest and they are the most stable teeth in the dental arch.
- They are only cusped tooth with a functional lingual surface.
- The single conical cusp, location in the mouth, and anchorage furnished by long, strongly developed roots, make these canines resemble those of the carnivora, hence they are named as canine.
- The shape of the crown promotes self-cleansing quality and helps to maintain natural facial expression.
- The efficient anchorage in jawbone gives their stability and they are able to withstand masticatory stress.
- They support both incisors and premolars and they are important "guideposts" in occlusion for their firm anchorage and strategic position in the dental arch.

**TABLE 3.6:** Chronology of tooth formation and eruption of canines.

|   |   | Maxillary canine | Mandibular canine |
|---|---|---|---|
| 1. | Initiation of calcification | 4–5 months | 4–5 months |
| 2. | Crown completion | 6–7 years | 6–7 years |
| 3. | Eruption | 11–12 years | 9–10 years |
| 4. | Root completion | 13–15 years | 12–14 years |

**TABLE 3.7:** Measurement of the canines.

|   |   | Maxillary canine | Mandibular canine |
|---|---|---|---|
| 1. | Total length | 27.0 mm | 26.0 mm |
| 2. | Height of crown | 10.0 mm | 11.0 mm |
| 3. | Length of root | 17.0 mm | 15.0 mm |
| 4. | Mesiodistal crown diameter | 7.5 mm | 7.0 mm |
| 5. | Labiolingual crown diameter | 8.0 mm | 7.5 mm |

### The Permanent Maxillary Canine (Figs. 3.5A to E)

#### Labial Aspect (Fig. 3.5A)

- Labial surface is convex and smooth in both directions.
- Crown and root are narrower mesiodistally than those of the maxillary central incisor.
- The cervical line labially is convex, with convexity toward root portion.
- Mesially, the outline of the crown is slightly convex from the cervix to the center of the mesial contact area with slight concavity above the contact area. The center of the contact area mesially is approximately at

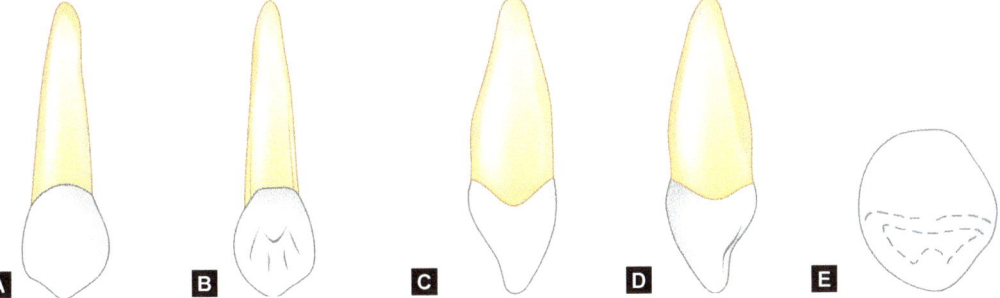

**Figs. 3.5A to E:** Permanent maxillary left canine: (A) Labial aspect; (B) Lingual aspect; (C) Mesial aspect; (D) Distal aspect; (E) Incisal aspect.

the junction of the middle and incisal third of the crown.
- Distally, the outline of the crown is usually concave between the cervical line and distal contact area and strongly convex in incisal half. The distal contact area is usually at the center of the middle third of the crown.
- The incisal margin is divided into two slopes which meet approximately in the midline of the tooth. The distal incisal margin slopes more and is longer. The mesial incisal margin is smaller and the mesioincisal angle is more incisally situated than the distoincisal angle.
- The labial ridge runs from the tip of cusp toward the cervical margin and divides the surface into smaller mesial and larger distal portion. Two depressions or developmental grooves are present on either side of labial ridge. The greatest mesiodistal dimension of this surface is between mesioincisal and distoincisal angles.
- The root of the maxillary canine appears slender, conical in form with a bluntly pointed apex.

*Lingual Aspect (Fig. 3.5B)*

- The crown and root are narrower lingually than labially.
- The mesial and distal marginal ridges are prominent and converge to form cervical margin which shows a more even curvature. The cervical line is convex toward root. The cingulum is large and well developed.
- A well-developed lingual ridge may be present from cusp tip toward cingulum. There are two shallow concavities between lingual ridge and marginal ridges. They are called mesial and distal lingual fossae.
- The lingual portion of the root of the maxillary canine is narrower than the labial portion. Developmental depressions may be present on mesial and distal aspects of the roots.

*Mesial Aspect (Fig. 3.5C)*

- The crown is wedge-shaped or triangular from this aspect, with base at cervical region and apex at incisal edge.
- Labially and lingually, immediately coronal to the cervical line are the crests of curvature of these surfaces. The labial outline of the crown from the crest of curvature to the incisal ridge is very slightly convex.
- The lingual profile shows pronounced convexity of cingulum, a shallow concavity in the middle third, and then convexity incisally.
- The cervical outline shows convexity toward crown, approximately 2.5 mm from cementoenamel junction.
- Incisal third is convex in all directions while cervical third is flatter. The contact point is in incisal third region.
- The root of this tooth from the mesial aspect is cone-shaped and the apex of the root is usually bluntly rounded.

*Distal Aspect (Fig. 3.5D)*

- Both labiolingually and incisogingivally, the incisal half is more convex and cervical area is more concave.
- The distoincisal angle is situated more cervically. The contact point is in middle third region.
- The cervical outline shows less curvature toward the crown.

*Incisal Aspect (Fig. 3.5E)*

- From this aspect, the tip of the cusp is labial to the center of the crown labiolingually and mesial to the center mesiodistally.
- The incisal edge is divided into mesial and distal cusp ridge which ends in a mesioincisal and distoincisal angle.
- The distal cusp ridge is slightly longer than the mesial cusp ridge.

## The Permanent Mandibular Canine (Figs. 3.6A to E) (Table 3.8)

*Labial Aspect (Fig. 3.6A)*

- The mesiodistal dimensions of the mandibular canine are about 1 mm less than those of the maxillary canine. The crowns of the mandibular canines appear longer.
- The mesial outline of the crown is nearly straight with the mesial outline of the root,

# The Permanent Teeth

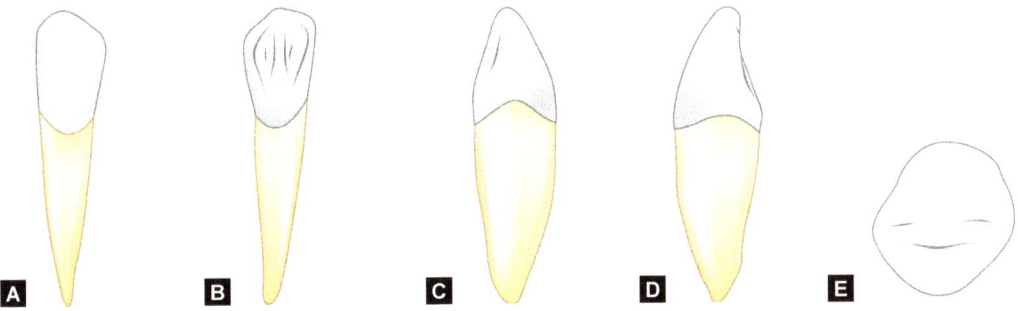

**Figs. 3.6A to E:** Permanent mandibular left canine: (A) Labial aspect; (B) Lingual aspect; (C) Mesial aspect; (D) Distal aspect; (E) Incisal aspect.

| TABLE 3.8: Differences between permanent maxillary and mandibular canine. | |
|---|---|
| *Maxillary canine* | *Mandibular canine* |
| 1. The crown is larger and stronger | 1. The crown is smaller and slender |
| 2. The crown is wider mesiodistally | 2. The crown is narrower mesiodistally |
| 3. The mesial and distal margins converge cervically when viewed from labial aspect | 3. The mesial and distal margins are parallel when viewed from labial aspect |
| 4. Incisal margin occupies about half of crown height | 4. Incisal margin occupies one-fourth of crown height |
| 5. Labial ridge and mesial/distal marginal ridges are more prominent | 5. Labial ridge and mesial/distal marginal ridges are less prominent |
| 6. Lingual ridge and cingulum are much more prominent. Lingual fossa is deeper | 6. Lingual surface is flatter. Marginal ridges and cingulum are not so prominent |
| 7. Incisal profile shows asymmetry of mesial and distal halves of crown | 7. Incisal profile shows symmetry of mesial and distal halves of crown |

the mesial contact area being near the mesioincisal angle.
- The distal outline is convex. The distal contact area is in middle third region.
- The mesial cusp ridge is shorter than distal cusp ridge. The mesioincisal angle is more incisally placed than distoincisal angle. The cusp angle (where the cuspal ridges meet) is on a line with the center of the root.
- The mesial and distal margins converge cervically to form cervical line which is convex rootward.
- The mandibular canine root is shorter by 1–2 mm on an average than that of the maxillary canine. Its apical end is more sharply pointed and often curves in a mesial direction.

## Lingual Aspect (Fig. 3.6B)

- The lingual aspect of the crown is flatter and smooth.
- The cingulum is smooth and poorly developed. The marginal ridges are less distinct.

- Mesial and distal margins converge cervically to form cervical margin which is convex rootward.
- The lingual portion of the root is narrower than that of the maxillary canine.

## Mesial Aspect (Fig. 3.6C)

- The labial outline is convex. The lingual outline shows convexity in the cingulum region, concavity in the middle third region, and convexity incisally. The cingulum is not pronounced and incisal part is thinner.
- The cervical line curves more toward incisal region than maxillary canine.
- The root appears to be tilted mesially in relation to long axis of crown.

## Distal Aspect (Fig. 3.6D)

- This surface resembles mesial surface.
- The labial surface is inclined lingually.
- This surface is convex incisally and is flatter cervically.

**TABLE 3.9:** Chronology of tooth formation and eruption of the premolars.

|  | Maxillary | | Mandibular | |
|---|---|---|---|---|
|  | First premolar | Second premolar | First premolar | Second premolar |
| Initiation of calcification | 1½–1¾ years | 2–2¼ years | 1¾–2 years | 2¼–2½ years |
| Crown completion | 5–6 years | 6–7 years | 5–6 years | 6–7 years |
| Eruption | 10–11 years | 10–12 years | 10–12 years | 11–12 years |
| Root completion | 2–13 years | 12–14 years | 12–13 years | 13–14 years |

**TABLE 3.10:** Measurement of the premolars.

|  | Maxillary | | Mandibular | |
|---|---|---|---|---|
|  | First | Second | First | Second |
| 1. Total length | 22.5 mm | 22.5 mm | 22.5 mm | 22.5 mm |
| 2. Height of crown | 8.5 mm | 8.5 mm | 8.5 mm | 8 mm |
| 3. Length of root | 14.0 mm | 14.0 mm | 14.0 mm | 14.5 mm |
| 4. Mesiodistal crown diameter | 7.0 mm | 7.0 mm | 7.0 mm | 7.0 mm |
| 5. Labiolingual crown diameter | 9.0 mm | 9.0 mm | 7.5 mm | 8.0 mm |

*Incisal Aspect (Fig. 3.6E)*

- The mesiodistal dimension of the mandibular canine is less than the labiolingual dimension.
- The outline of the mesial surface is less curved.
- The cusp tip and mesial cusp ridge are more inclined in a lingual direction.
- The incisal edge is divided into mesial and distal cusp ridge which ends in a mesioincisal and distoincisal angle. The distal cusp ridge is slightly longer than the mesial cusp ridge.

## THE PREMOLARS

- There are eight premolars in the human permanent dentition, two in each quadrant of the maxillary and mandibular arches **(Tables 3.9 and 3.10)**.
- Premolars occupy a position in the dental arch between the canines and molars.
- The premolars succeed the deciduous molars and erupt earlier than canines and second molars.
- They generally have two cusps and are called bicuspids but mandibular premolars may show a variation in the number of cusps from one to three.
- The premolars along with molars are called "posterior teeth."

Maxillary First Premolar (Figs. 3.7A to E) (Table 3.11)

- The maxillary first premolar has two sharply defined cusps, a buccal and a

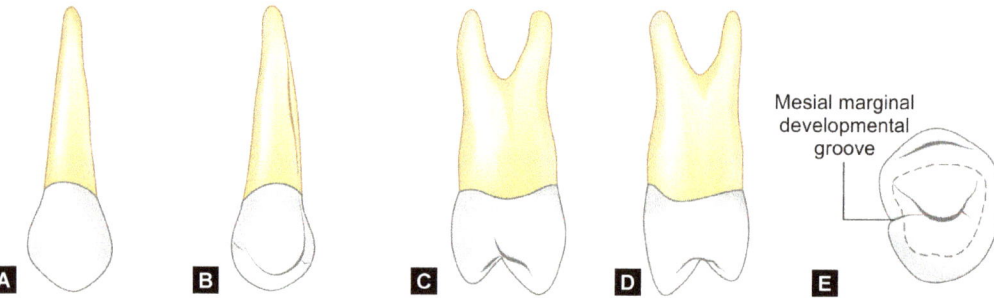

**Figs. 3.7A to E:** Maxillary left first premolar: (A) Buccal aspect; (B) Lingual aspect; (C) Mesial aspect; (D) Distal aspect; (E) Occlusal aspect.

# The Permanent Teeth

**TABLE 3.11: Differences between maxillary and mandibular premolars.**

| Maxillary premolars | Mandibular premolars |
|---|---|
| 1. They have two major cusps—a buccal and a lingual. Both are of almost equal size and prominence | 1. They have one major cusp and one or more minor cusps |
| 2. Crown is wider buccolingually than it is mesiodistally | 2. Buccolingual and mesiodistal diameter of crown is almost the same |
| 3. Buccal surface is inclined slightly lingually | 3. Buccal surface has a strong lingual inclination |
| 4. First and second premolars are very similar | 4. First and second premolars are widely different |

lingual. The buccal cusp is about 1 mm longer than the lingual cusp.
- The maxillary first premolars have usually two roots, a buccal and a lingual and two pulp canals.

## Buccal Aspect (Fig. 3.7A)

- From this aspect, the crown is roughly trapezoidal. The buccal surface of the crown is convex. The greatest diameter of this surface is near the angles of the tooth. It is bounded by four margins—occlusal, cervical, mesial, and distal.
- The occlusal margin is formed by mesial and distal cuspal ridges. The mesial ridge is straight and longer than the distal ridge, which is shorter and more curved. As the mesial ridge is longer, the tip of the buccal cusp is distal to a line bisecting the buccal surface of the crown.
- From the tip of the buccal cusp, the buccal ridge is present toward the cervical line. The ridge is prominent occlusally.
- The mesial and distal margins taper slightly cervically to form a convex cervical margin (the width of the crown mesiodistally is about 2 mm less at the cervix than its width at the points of its greatest mesiodistal measurement). The convexity of the cervical margin is toward root and the crest of curvature is near the center of the root.
- The mesial outline is slightly concave from the cervical line to the mesial contact area which lies immediately occlusal to the midpoint between the cervical line and the tip of the buccal cusp.
- The distal outline is straighter than that of the mesial. The contact area is slightly more occlusally placed.

## Lingual Aspect (Fig. 3.7B)

- The crown tapers toward the lingual aspect, as the lingual cusp is narrower mesiodistally than the buccal cusp. The lingual cusp is smooth, convex, and is at a lower level than buccal cusp.
- The mesial and distal outlines of the crown are convex and these outlines are continuous with the mesial and distal slopes of the lingual cusp. The mesial and distal sides are straight as they join the lingual root at the cervical line.
- The cervical line is regular, with slight curvature toward the root and the crest of curvature is centered on the root.
- The lingual root is smooth and convex at all points. The apex of the lingual root is more blunt than the buccal root apex.

## Mesial Aspect (Fig. 3.7C)

- The mesial aspect of the crown is also roughly trapezoidal. The longest of the uneven sides is toward the cervical portion and shortest is toward the occlusal portion.
- The measurement from the tip of the buccal cusp to the tip of the lingual cusp is less than the buccolingual measurement of the root at its cervical portion. So the tips of the cusps are well within the confines of the root trunk.
- The buccal outline of the crown is well defined and curves outward below the cervical line. The crest of curvature is often located approximately at the junction of cervical and middle thirds.
- The lingual outline of the crown is smoothly curved and rounded and the crest of curvature is at the center of the middle third.

- The occlusal margin is concave; the deepest part of concavity is midway between the cusps. The lingual cusp is about 1 mm shorter than buccal cusp. There is a well-defined developmental groove on the mesial marginal ridge. The groove is continuous with the central groove of the occlusal surface of the crown and crossing the marginal ridge, it terminates at a short distance cervical to mesial marginal ridge. This groove is in alignment with the developmental depression on the mesial surface of the root but is not connected with it.
- The cervical margin is almost straight, though mildly convex occlusally. There is mesial developmental depression immediately cervical to mesial contact area. This mesial concavity continues apically beyond the cervical line, joins a deep developmental depression between the roots, and ends at the root of bifurcation.
- The buccal outline of the buccal root, above the cervical line, is straight, with a tendency toward a lingual inclination. The lingual outline of the lingual root is rather straight above the cervical line.

### Distal Aspect (Fig. 3.7D)

- The crown surface is convex at all points except for a small flattened area just cervical to the contact area and buccal to the center of the distal surface.
- The curvature of the cervical line is less on the distal than on the mesial surface, often showing a line straight across from buccal to lingual aspect.
- There is no evidence of a deep developmental groove crossing the distal marginal ridge of the crown.
- The root trunk is flattened on the distal surface above the cervical line. The bifurcation of the roots is abrupt near the apical third, with no developmental groove.

### Occlusal Aspect (Fig. 3.7E)

- The occlusal aspect of the maxillary first premolar is roughly hexagonal and is circumscribed by the cusp ridges and marginal ridges. They are mesiobuccal, distobuccal, mesiolingual, and distolingual cusp ridges and mesial and distal marginal ridges. The two buccal cusp ridges are nearly equal, the mesial marginal ridge is shorter than the distal marginal ridge, and the mesiolingual cusp ridge is shorter than the distolingual.
- A well-defined central developmental groove divides the surface evenly buccolingually. It is located at the bottom of the central sulcus of the occlusal surface, extending from distal pit (a point just mesial to the distal marginal ridge) to the mesial marginal ridge, where it joins the mesial marginal developmental groove, which crosses the mesial marginal ridge and ends on the mesial surface of the crown.
- The collateral developmental grooves join the central groove inside the mesial and distal marginal ridges. These grooves are called the mesiobuccal developmental groove and the distobuccal developmental groove. The grooves are deeply pointed and are named the mesial and distal developmental pits.
- The triangular depression distal to the mesial marginal ridge and harboring the mesiobuccal developmental groove is called the mesial triangular fossa. The depression in the occlusal surface, just mesial to the distal marginal ridge, is called the distal triangular fossa.
- The buccal triangular ridge of the buccal cusp is prominent, arising near the center of the central groove, and converging with the tip of the buccal cusp. The lingual triangular ridge is less prominent. It also arises near the center of the central groove and converges with the tip of the lingual cusp. The lingual cusp is pointed more sharply than the buccal cusp.

## Maxillary Second Premolar (Figs. 3.8A to E) (Table 3.12)

### Buccal Aspect (Fig. 3.8A)

- The buccal cusp of the second premolar is smaller and less pointed than that of the first premolar. The mesial slope of the

# The Permanent Teeth

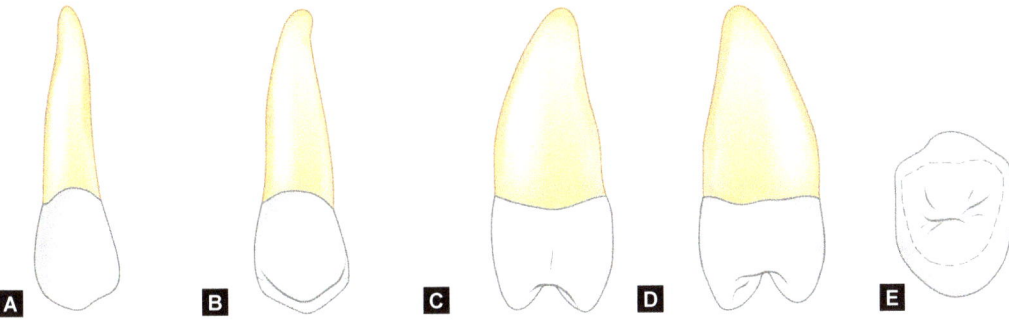

**Figs. 3.8A to E:** Left maxillary second premolar: (A) Buccal aspect; (B) Lingual aspect; (C) Mesial aspect; (D) Distal aspect; (E) Occlusal aspect.

| TABLE 3.12: Differences between maxillary first and second premolars. | |
|---|---|
| *First premolar* | *Second premolar* |
| 1. Relatively a less stronger tooth | 1. Stronger and more rugged |
| 2. Two roots—a buccal and a lingual | 2. One root only |
| 3. Occlusal crown outline is hexagonal | 3. Occlusal crown outline is ovoid or rectangular |
| 4. Mesial and distal sides converge lingually | 4. Mesial and distal sides are parallel |
| 5. Buccal cusp is higher and bulkier than lingual | 5. Both cusps are almost equal in height. The lingual cusp is bulkier |
| 6. Two root canals | 6. Single root canal |
| 7. Crown and occlusal pit groove pattern presents less variation | 7. More variation in crown and occlusal pit groove pattern is seen |
| 8. Marginal ridges are narrower and not so strong | 8. Marginal ridges are wider and strong |
| 9. Mesial and distal pits are placed wider apart. Central groove longer | 9. Mesial and distal pits are closer. Central groove shorter |
| 10. Mesial marginal groove interrupts mesial marginal ridge | 10. There is no mesial marginal groove |

buccal cusp ridge is usually shorter than the distal slope (the opposite is true for the first premolar).
- The buccal ridge of the crown is not as prominent as first premolar.

## Lingual Aspect (Fig. 3.8B)

The lingual surface is larger and more convex compared to that of maxillary first premolar.

## Mesial Aspect (Fig. 3.8C)

- The cusps of the second premolar are shorter than first premolars. The buccal and lingual cusps have more nearly the same length. The greater distance between the tips of buccal and lingual cusps widens the occlusal surface buccolingually.
- There is no deep developmental groove crossing the mesial marginal ridge.

## Distal Aspect (Fig. 3.8D)

The depression on distal aspect of the root is deeper than on mesial aspect (in maxillary first premolar, depression on mesial aspect of root is more prominent).

## Occlusal Aspect (Fig. 3.8E)

- The occlusal outline of the crown is more rounded or oval.
- The buccal triangular ridge meets the lingual triangular ridge and forms a transverse ridge.
- The central developmental groove is shorter and irregular. It terminates in mesial and distal pits. Multiple supplemental grooves radiate from central groove, giving the surface a wrinkled appearance. The mesial and distal pits are closer to the center of the crown (in case

of first premolar, the mesial and distal pits are closer to the marginal ridges).

### Mandibular First Premolar (Figs. 3.9A to E)

The mandibular first premolar is the fourth tooth from the median line and the first posterior tooth in the mandible. This tooth is situated between the canine and second premolar and has some characteristics common to each of them.

### Buccal Aspect (Fig. 3.9A)

- From this aspect, the crown appears roughly trapezoidal and the buccal surface is inclined lingually. The middle lobe is well developed and the buccal cusp is large and pointed. The mesial cusp ridge is shorter than the distal cusp ridge.
- The contact areas are broad and at a level little more than half the distance from cervical line to cusp tip. The contact points are almost at the same level mesially and distally.
- The mesial outline of the crown is straight above the cervical line to the contact area. The outline of the mesial slope of the buccal cusp usually shows some concavity.
- The distal outline of the crown is slightly concave above the cervical line to the distal contact area. The distal slope of the buccal cusp usually exhibits some concavity.
- The cervix of the mandibular first premolar crown is narrow mesiodistally when compared with the crown width at the contact areas. The cervical line is convex toward root. The ridge from the cervical margin to the cusp tip is called the buccal ridge.
- The root of this tooth is 3–4 mm shorter than that of the mandibular canine.

### Lingual Aspect (Fig. 3.9B)

- The lingual surface is narrower than buccal and is uniformly convex on both directions. It is unmarked by any lobes or ridges.
- The contact areas and marginal ridges are pronounced and extend out above the narrow cervical portion of the crown.
- The lingual cusp is always small with a pointed cusp tip in alignment with the buccal triangular ridge of the occlusal surface. The mesial and distal occlusal fossae are on each side of the triangular ridge.
- There is the mesiolingual developmental groove which acts as a line of demarcation between the mesiobuccal lobe and the lingual lobe and extends into the mesial fossa of the occlusal surface.
- The root of this tooth tapers evenly from the cervix to a pointed apex and is much narrower on lingual side. There is a narrow ridge, smooth and convex along the full length of the root.

### Mesial Aspect (Fig. 3.9C)

- From the mesial aspect, the crown outline is roughly rhomboidal and the tip of the buccal cusp is nearly centered over the root. The occlusal plane is tilted in a lingual direction.

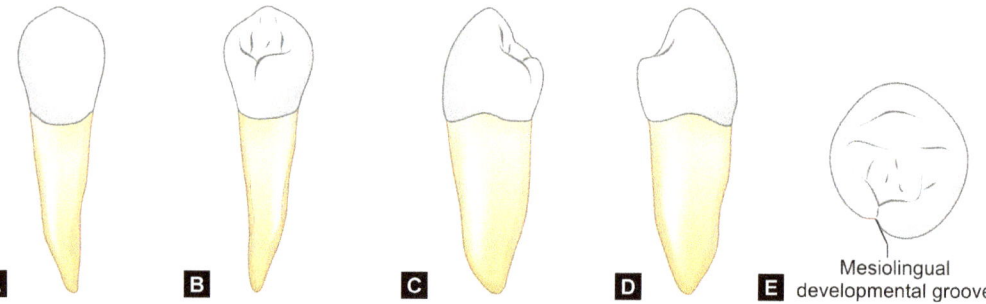

**Figs. 3.9A to E:** Mandibular right first premolar: (A) Buccal aspect; (B) Lingual aspect; (C) Mesial aspect; (D) Distal aspect; (E) Occlusal aspect.

- The buccal outline of the crown from this aspect is prominently curved from the cervical line to the tip of the buccal cusp. The crest of the curvature is near the middle third of the crown.
- The lingual outline of the crown is not very prominent. The crest of curvature lingually approaches the middle third of the crown.
- The cervical line on the mesial surface is regular, curving occlusally.
- The surface of the crown mesially is smooth except for the mesiolingual groove. The mesial contact area is centered on a line with the tip of the buccal cusp.
- The root outline from the mesial aspect is tapered from the cervix, ending in a relatively pointed apex in line with the tip of the buccal cusp. The lingual outline may be straight, the buccal outline more curved. Often, there is a deep developmental groove on the mesial aspect of root.

## Distal Aspect (Fig. 3.9D)

- The major portion of the distal surface of the crown is smoothly convex.
- The distal marginal ridge is higher above the cervix. The marginal ridge is confluent with the lingual cusp ridge. It has no developmental groove on the distal marginal ridge.
- The surface of the root shows more convexity than was found mesially. A shallow developmental depression is centered on the root.

## Occlusal Aspect (Fig. 3.9E)

- The occlusal outline is roughly diamond-shaped and similar to the incisal aspect of mandibular canines. Some of these teeth have a circular form similar to that of some mandibular second premolars; others conform to the gross outlines of the more common second premolars.
- When viewed from the occlusal aspect, the middle buccal lobe makes up the major bulk of the tooth crown and the buccal ridge is prominent.
- The crown converges sharply to the center of the lingual surface, starting from points approximating the mesial and distal contact areas. This formation makes that part of the crown represented by buccal cusp ridges, marginal ridges, and lingual lobe triangular in form, with the base of the triangle at the buccal cusp ridges and the point of the triangle at the lingual cusp.
- The marginal ridges are well developed and lingual cusp is small.
- The buccal triangular ridge is prominent and lingual triangular ridge is small.
- The occlusal surface presents the mesial and distal fossae. The mesial fossa is more linear in form and contains the mesial developmental groove, which extends buccolingually. This groove is confluent with its extension, which becomes the mesiolingual developmental groove as it passes over the mesiolingual surface.
- The distal fossa is more circular and is circumscribed by the distobuccal cusp ridge, the distal marginal ridge, the buccal triangular ridge, and the distolingual cusp ridge. The distal fossa may contain a distal developmental groove.
- Because of the position of the crown over the root, most of the buccal surface may be seen from the occlusal aspect, whereas very little of the lingual surface is in view.

## Mandibular Second Premolar (Figs. 3.10A to E) (Table 3.13)

The mandibular second premolar is larger and well-developed of the two mandibular premolars. It has two common forms. The first form is the three-cusp type, which appears more angular from occlusal aspect. The second form is two-cusp type, which appears more rounded from occlusal aspect.

## Buccal Aspect (Fig. 3.10A)

- From the buccal aspect, the mandibular second premolar presents a shorter buccal cusp than the first premolar, with mesiobuccal and distobuccal cusp ridges presenting angulation of less degree.
- The contact areas, both mesial and distal, are broad. The contact areas appear to be higher because of the short buccal cusp.

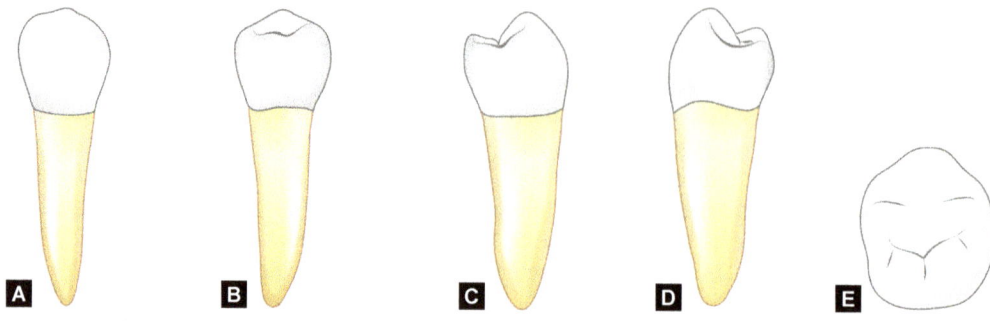

**Figs. 3.10A to E:** Mandibular left second premolar: (A) Buccal aspect; (B) Lingual aspect; (C) Mesial aspect; (D) Distal aspect; (E) Occlusal aspect.

| TABLE 3.13: Differences between mandibular premolars. | |
|---|---|
| **First premolar** | **Second premolar** |
| 1. Occlusal outline is diamond-shaped | 1. Occlusal outline is squarish or triangular |
| 2. Mesial and distal margins converge lingually | 2. Mesial and distal margins are parallel |
| 3. Buccal cusp is prominent and lingual cusp is rudimentary | 3. Both cusps are equal in size |
| 4. Mesial marginal ridge is shorter and less prominent | 4. Both the marginal ridges are equally prominent |
| 5. Central pit is never present | 5. Central pit may be present (in three-cusp type) |
| 6. Transverse ridge is common linking buccal and lingual cusps | 6. No transverse ridge is seen |
| 7. Mesial marginal ridge inclines cervically | 7. Mesial marginal ridge horizontal |
| 8. Occlusal surface slopes lingually | 8. Occlusal surface is horizontal |
| 9. Mesiolingual groove is present | 9. Mesiolingual groove is generally absent |
| 10. Lingual surface is narrower than that of buccal | 10. Lingual surface is not much narrower than that of buccal |
| 11. Buccally crown is bilaterally asymmetrical | 11. Buccally crown is bilaterally symmetrical |

- The root is broader mesiodistally than that of the first premolar.

### Lingual Aspect (Fig. 3.10B)

- The mesial and distal surfaces converge to form lingual surface. From the lingual aspect, the lingual lobes are well developed, making the cusp or cusps longer. Since the lingual cusps are not as long as the buccal cusp, part of the buccal portion of the occlusal surface that is visible from this aspect may be seen.
- In the three-cusp type, there are a mesiolingual and a distolingual cusp, the former being the larger and the longer one in most cases. There is a groove between them, extending a very short distance on the lingual surface and usually centered over the root.
- In the two-cusp type, the single lingual cusp attains equal height with the three- cusp. The two-cusp type has no groove, but it shows a developmental depression distolingually where the lingual cusp ridge joins the distal marginal ridge.
- The lingual surface of the crown of all mandibular second premolars is smooth and spheroidal, having a bulbous form above the constricted cervical portion.
- From lingual aspect, the root is wide and smoothly convex for most of its length.

### Mesial Aspect (Fig. 3.10C)

- From the mesial aspect, the crown and root are wider buccolingually.
- The buccal cusp is not centered over the root trunk and the lingual lobe is well developed.
- The marginal ridge is at right angles to the long axis of the tooth.
- The root is longer and slightly convex on the mesial surface. The apex of the

root is usually more blunt on the second premolar.

## Distal Aspect (Fig. 3.10D)

- This surface is similar to mesial surface. From this aspect, more of the occlusal surface is visible as the distal marginal ridge is at a lower level than the mesial marginal ridge.
- The crown of the tooth is tipped distally to the long axes of the roots.

## Occlusal Aspect (Fig. 3.10E)

- The three-cusp type appears square lingual to the buccal cusp ridges when highly developed. The round or two-cusp type appears round lingual to the buccal cusp ridges.
- The square type has three cusps that are distinct; the buccal cusp is the largest, the mesiolingual cusp is next, and the distolingual cusp is the smallest.
- Each cusp has well-formed triangular ridges separated by deep developmental grooves. These grooves converge in a central pit and form a Y on the occlusal surface. The central pit is located midway between the buccal cusp ridge and the lingual margin of the occlusal surface and slightly distal to the central point between mesial and distal marginal ridges.
- The mesial developmental groove travels from central pit in a mesiobuccal direction and ends in the mesial triangular fossa just distal to the mesial marginal ridge. The distal developmental groove travels in a distobuccal direction. It is shorter than the mesial groove and ends in the distal triangular fossa mesial to the distal marginal side. The lingual developmental groove extends lingually between the two lingual cusps and ends on the lingual surface of the crown just below the convergence of the lingual cusp ridges.
- A central developmental groove on the occlusal surface travels in a mesiodistal direction. The central groove has its terminals centered in mesial and distal fossae, which are roughly circular depressions having mesial and distal developmental pits centered in them.

## THE PERMANENT MOLARS (TABLES 3.14 AND 3.15)

There are three permanent molars in each quadrant of each jaw. They occupy the posterior part of the dentition. They are the largest and strongest teeth. They are not succedaneous (do not replace deciduous teeth) but erupt distal to the deciduous dentition. The strong crown matched with

**TABLE 3.14:** Chronology of tooth formation and eruption of the molars.

|  | Maxillary | | | Mandibular | | |
| --- | --- | --- | --- | --- | --- | --- |
|  | First | Second | Third | First | Second | Third |
| Initiation of calcification | At birth | 2½–3 years | 8–10 years | At birth | 2½–3 years | 8–10 years |
| Crown completion | 2½–3 years | 8–9 years | 12–16 years | 2½–3 years | 8–9 years | 12–16 years |
| Eruption | 6 years | 12 years | 18+ years | 6 years | 12 years | 18+ years |
| Root completion | 9–10 years | 14–16 years | 18–25 years | 9–10 years | 14–16 years | 18–25 years |

**TABLE 3.15:** Measurement table of the molars.

|  | Maxillary | | | Mandibular | | |
| --- | --- | --- | --- | --- | --- | --- |
|  | First | Second | Third | First | Second | Third |
| 1. Total length (mm) | 19.5 | 18.0 | 17.5 | 21.5 | 20.0 | 18.0 |
| 2. Height of crown (mm) | 7.5 | 7.0 | 6.5 | 7.5 | 7.0 | 7.0 |
| 3. Length of root (mm) | 12.0 | 11.0 | 11.0 | 14.0 | 13.0 | 11.0 |
| 4. Mesiodistal crown diameter (mm) | 10.0 | 9.0 | 8.5 | 11.0 | 10.5 | 10.0 |
| 5. Labiolingual crown diameter (mm) | 11.0 | 11.0 | 10.0 | 10.5 | 10.5 | 9.5 |

**TABLE 3.16: Differences between permanent maxillary and mandibular molars.**

| Maxillary molars | Mandibular molars |
|---|---|
| 1. They have three roots, two buccal and one lingual | 1. They have two roots, one mesial and other distal |
| 2. They have four cusps and sometimes a rudimentary cusp | 2. They have four large cusps and a fifth small cusp |
| 3. Mesiobuccal cusp is larger than distobuccal cusp. Distolingual cusp is small | 3. Two major buccal and two major lingual cusps are of almost equal sizes |
| 4. Distobuccal cusp is joined to mesiolingual cusp by an oblique ridge | 4. All cusps are separated by grooves |
| 5. Crown is broader buccolingually | 5. Crown is broader mesiodistally |

well-formed roots is ideal for withstanding grinding stress. The first permanent molars erupt at the age of 6 years and are called 6-year molars. The second permanent molars erupt at the age of 12 years and are called 12-year molars. The third molar is called wisdom tooth and is the last tooth to erupt.

Besides mastication, they are vital in maintaining vertical height of face. They have four to five cusps and two to three roots **(Table 3.16)**.

### The Permanent Maxillary First Molar (Figs. 3.11A to E)

#### Buccal Aspect (Fig. 3.11A)

- The buccal surface is made by the union of mesiobuccal and distobuccal cusps which are separated by buccal developmental groove.
- The crown is roughly trapezoidal, with cervical and occlusal outlines representing the uneven sides. The cervical line is the shorter of the uneven sides.
- The mesiobuccal cusp is broader than the distobuccal cusp and its mesial slope meets its distal slope at an obtuse angle. The mesial slope of the distobuccal cusp meets its distal slope at approximately a right angle.
- The cervical line of the crown does not have much curvature from mesial to distal. The line is generally convex with the convexity toward the roots.
- The mesial outline of the crown from this aspect follows a nearly straight path downward and mesially, curving occlusally as it reaches the crest of contour of the mesial surface. The crest is approximately two-thirds the distance from cervical line to tip of mesiobuccal cusp.
- The distal outline of the crown is convex. The crest of curvature on the distal side of the crown is located at a level approximately half the distance from cervical line to tip of cusp.
- All three of the roots may be seen from the buccal aspect. The common root base is called the root trunk. The point of bifurcation of the two buccal roots is located approximately 4 mm above the cervical line. There is a deep developmental groove buccally on the root trunk of the maxillary first molar, which starts at the bifurcation and progresses downward, becoming more shallow until it terminates in a shallow depression at the cervical line.

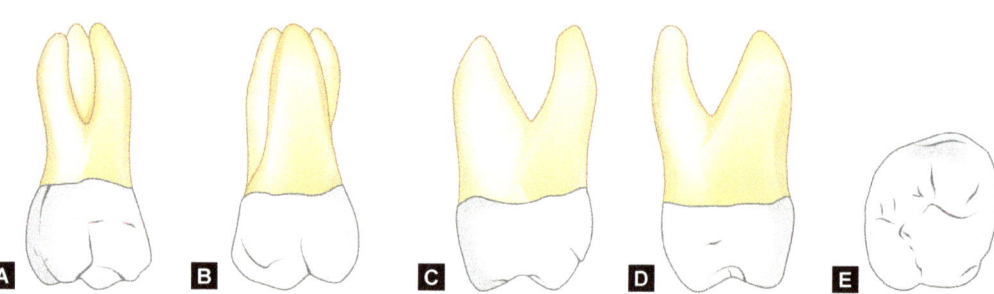

**Figs. 3.11A to E:** Permanent maxillary right first molar: (A) Buccal aspect; (B) Lingual aspect; (C) Mesial aspect; (D) Distal aspect; (E) Occlusal aspect.

- Usually, the lingual root is the longest and the two buccal roots approximately are equal in length. On the average, the roots are about twice as long as the crown.

## Lingual Aspect (Fig. 3.11B)
- Mesiolingual and distolingual cusps join to form lingual surface. The cusps are inequal in size. Mesiolingual cusp is blunt, prominent, and constitutes three-fifth of the mesiodistal width. The distolingual cusp is shorter and narrower and has a rounded outline.
- The lingual developmental groove starts approximately in the center of the lingual surface mesiodistally, curves sharply to the distal as it crosses between the cusps, and continues onto the occlusal surface.
- The fifth cusp appears attached to the mesiolingual surface of the mesiolingual cusp. It is known as the tubercle or cusp of Carabelli. It is outlined occlusally by an irregular developmental groove. The cusp ridge of the fifth cusp is approximately 2 mm cervical to the cusp ridge of the mesiolingual cusp.
- All three of the roots are visible from the lingual aspect, the largest being the lingual root. The lingual portion of the root trunk is continuous with the entire cervical portion of the crown lingually. The lingual root is conical, terminating in a bluntly rounded apex.

## Mesial Aspect (Fig. 3.11C)
- The mesiobuccal and mesiolingual margins converge from cervical area to the tip of the mesiobuccal and mesiolingual cusps, respectively.
- The buccal outline is convex at cervical third, up to crest of curvature, and then shows shallow concavity. Then the outline is slightly convex as it progresses downward and inward to circumscribe the mesiobuccal cusp, ending at the tip of the cusp.
- The lingual outline of the crown curves outward and lingually. The level of the crest of curvature is near the middle third of the crown. If the fifth cusp is well developed, the lingual outline dips inward to reveal it. The mesiolingual cusp is on a line with the long axis of the lingual root.
- The mesial marginal ridge, which is confluent with the mesiobuccal and mesiolingual cusp ridges, is irregular, the outline curving cervically about one-fifth the crown length and centering its curvature below the center of the crown buccolingually.
- The cervical line of the crown is irregular, curving occlusally but as a rule not more than 1 mm at any one point.
- The mesiobuccal root is broad and flattened on its mesial surface; this flattened surface often exhibits smooth flutings for part of its length. The buccal outline of the root extends upward and outward from the crown, ending at the blunt apex. The lingual outline of the root is relatively straight from the bluntly rounded apex down to the bifurcation with the lingual root. The level of the bifurcation is a little closer to the cervical line than is found between the roots buccally. The lingual root is longer than the mesial root but is narrower from this aspect. It is banana-shaped, extending lingually with its convex outline to the lingual and its concave outline to the buccal.

## Distal Aspect (Fig. 3.11D)
- Distal aspect is similar to that of the mesial aspect. Certain variations must be noted when the tooth is viewed from the distal aspect.
- The distal marginal ridge dips sharply in a cervical direction, exposing triangular ridges on the distal portion of the occlusal surface of the crown.
- The cervical line is almost straight across from buccal to lingual. Occasionally, it curves apically 0.5 mm or so.
- The distal surface of the crown is generally convex, with a smoothly rounded surface except for a small area near the distobuccal root at the cervical third.

- The distobuccal root is narrower at its base than either of the others. The lingual outline of the root from the apex to the bifurcation is slightly concave. There is no concavity between the bifurcation of the roots and the cervical line. The bifurcation here is more apical than either of the other two areas on this tooth. The area from cervical line to bifurcation is 5 mm or more in extent.

### Occlusal Aspect (Fig. 3.11E)

- From the occlusal aspect, the maxillary first molar is somewhat rhomboidal. The maxillary first molar crown is wider mesially than distally and wider lingually than buccally.
- The four major cusps are well developed, with the small minor, or fifth, cusp appearing on the lingual surface of the mesiolingual cusp near the mesiolingual line angle of the crown. The fifth cusp may be indistinct, or absent. The mesiolingual cusp is the largest cusp; it is followed in point of size by the mesiobuccal, distolingual, distobuccal, and fifth cusps.
- The occlusal surface of the maxillary first molar is within the confines of the cusp ridges and marginal ridges. There are two major fossae and two minor fossae. The major fossae are the central fossa, which is roughly triangular and mesial to the oblique ridge, and the distal fossa, which is roughly linear and distal to the oblique ridge. The two minor fossae are the mesial triangular fossa, immediately distal to the mesial marginal ridge, and the distal triangular fossa, immediately mesial to the distal marginal ridge.
- The oblique ridge is a ridge that crosses the occlusal surface obliquely. It is formed by the union of the triangular ridge of the distobuccal cusp and the distal ridge of the mesiolingual cusp. Sometimes, it is crossed by a developmental groove that partially joins the two major fossae by means of its shallow sulcate groove.
- The mesial marginal ridge and the distal marginal ridge are irregular ridges confluent with the mesial and distal cusp ridges of the mesial and distal major cusps.
- The central fossa of the occlusal surface is a concave area bounded by the distal slope of the mesiobuccal cusp, the mesial slope of the distobuccal cusp, the crest of the oblique ridge, and the crests of the two triangular ridges of the mesiobuccal and mesiolingual cusps.

  The central fossa has connecting sulci, developmental grooves, and the central developmental pit. From this pit, the buccal developmental groove radiates buccally at the bottom of the buccal sulcus of the central fossa, continuing on to the buccal surface of the crown between the buccal cusps. The central developmental groove starts at central pit and progresses in a mesial direction to the buccal sulcate groove. The central groove usually terminates at the apex of the mesial triangular fossa.
- The mesial triangular fossa is rather indistinct in outline, but it is generally triangular in shape with its base at the mesial marginal ridge and its apex at the point where the supplemental grooves join the central groove.
- An additional short developmental groove may cross the oblique ridge transversely, joining the central and distal fossae with a shallow groove. It is called the transverse groove of the oblique ridge.
- The distal fossa of the maxillary first molar is roughly linear in form and is located immediately distal to the oblique ridge. An irregular developmental groove transverses its deepest portion. This developmental groove is called the distal oblique groove. Any part of the developmental groove that outlines a fifth cusp is called the fifth cusp groove.

## The Permanent Maxillary Second Molar (Figs. 3.12A to E)

The maxillary second molar supplements the first molar in function. The roots of this tooth are as long as those of the first molar. The distobuccal cusp is not as well developed

# The Permanent Teeth

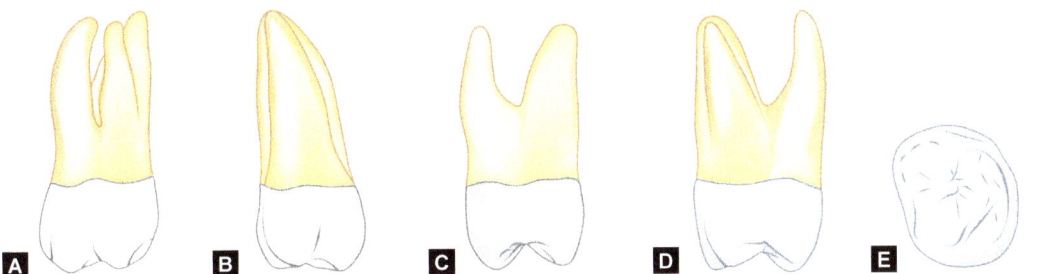

**Figs. 3.12A to E:** Permanent maxillary left second molar: (A) Buccal aspect; (B) Lingual aspect; (C) Mesial aspect; (D) Distal aspect; (E) Occlusal aspect.

and the distolingual cusp is smaller. No fifth cusp is evident.

## Buccal Aspect (Fig. 3.12A)

- The surface is convex. The crown is a little shorter cervico-occlusally and narrower mesiodistally than the maxillary first molar. The distobuccal cusp is smaller and allows part of the distal marginal ridge and part of the distolingual cusp to be seen.
- The buccal roots are about the same length. These roots are more nearly parallel and are inclined distally more than those of the maxillary first molar so that the end of the distobuccal root is slightly distal to the distal extremity of the crown. The apex of the mesiobuccal root is on a line with the buccal groove of the crown instead of the tip of the mesiobuccal cusp, as was found on the first molar.

## Lingual Aspect (Fig. 3.12B)

- The distolingual cusp of the crown is smaller.
- The distobuccal cusp may be seen through the sulcus between the mesiolingual and distolingual cusp.
- No fifth cusp is evident.
- The apex of the lingual root is in line with the distolingual cusp tip instead of the lingual groove as was found on the first molar.

## Mesial Aspect (Fig. 3.12C)

- The buccolingual dimension is about the same as that of the first molar, but the crown length is less.
- The roots do not spread as far buccolingually, being within the confines of the buccolingual crown outline.

## Distal Aspect (Fig. 3.12D)

Because the distobuccal cusp is smaller than in the maxillary first molar, more of the mesiobuccal cusp may be seen from this angle. The mesiolingual cusp cannot be seen. The apex of the lingual root is in line with the distolingual cusp.

## Occlusal Aspect (Fig. 3.12E)

- The outline of this surface is rhomboidal. The buccolingual diameter of the crown is about equal, but the mesiodistal diameter is approximately 1 mm less than that of maxillary first molar. The mesiobuccal and mesiolingual cusps are just as large and well developed as in the first molar, but the distobuccal and distolingual cusps are smaller and less well developed.
- Mesiobuccal and distolingual angles are more acute and mesiolingual and distobuccal angles are more obtuse.
- The oblique ridge is not very prominent. There is a more variable pit groove pattern and supplemental grooves are more numerous.
- The crown is generally constricted mesiodistally.

## The Permanent Maxillary Third Molar (Figs. 3.13A to E)

The maxillary third molar often appears as a developmental anomaly. It can vary

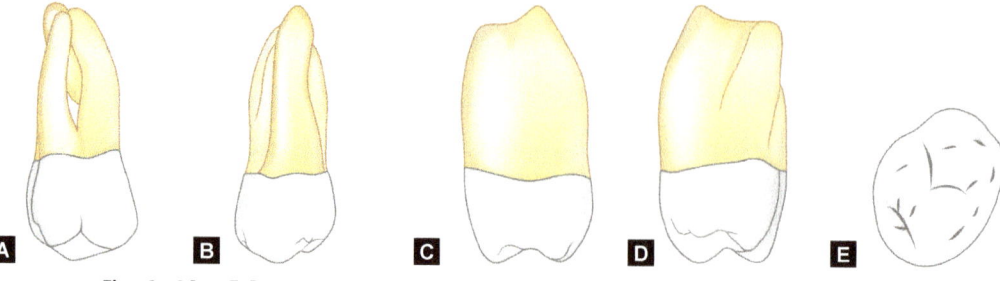

**Figs. 3.13A to E:** Permanent maxillary right third molar: (A) Buccal aspect; (B) Lingual aspect; (C) Mesial aspect; (D) Distal aspect; (E) Occlusal aspect.

considerably in size, contour, and relative position to the other teeth.

### Buccal Aspect (Fig. 3.13A)

- The crown is shorter cervico-occlusally and narrower mesiodistally than that of the second molar.
- The roots are usually fused, functioning as one large root, and they are shorter cervicoapically. The fused roots end in a taper at the apex. The roots have a distinct slant to the distal, giving the apices of the fused root a more distal relation to the center of the crown.

### Lingual Aspect (Fig. 3.13B)

The distolingual cusp is usually missing and there is usually just one large lingual cusp and therefore no lingual groove. However, in many cases, a third molar with the same essential features has a poorly developed distolingual cusp with a developmental groove lingually.

### Mesial Aspect (Fig. 3.13C)

- The occlusal one-third is round and convex and gingival two-thirds are flat. The contact area is in the middle third.
- There is fusion of mesiobuccal and lingual roots which taper and there may be bifurcation in the region of apical third.
- The roots are invariably short and the crown profiles may be irregular.

### Distal Aspect (Fig. 3.13D)

- The distolingual cusp is absent and distobuccal cusp is reduced in size.
- From this aspect, most of the buccal surface of the crown is in view. More of the occlusal surface may be seen than can be seen on the second molar from this aspect because of the more acute angulation of the occlusal surface in relation to the long axis of the root.
- The measurement from the cervical line to the marginal ridge is short.

### Occlusal Aspect (Fig. 3.13E)

- The occlusal aspect of a typical maxillary third molar presents a heart-shaped outline. The lingual cusp is large and well developed, and there is little or no distolingual cusp.
- The occlusal aspect of this tooth usually presents many supplemental grooves and many accidental grooves unless the tooth is very much worn.
- The third molar may show four distinct cusps. This type may have a strong oblique ridge, a central fossa, and a distal fossa, with a lingual developmental groove similar to that of the rhomboidal type of second molar.
- In most instances, the crown converges more lingually from the buccal areas than the second molar does, losing its rhomboidal outline **(Table 3.17)**.

### The Permanent Mandibular First Molar (Figs. 3.14A to E)

Normally, the mandibular first molar is the largest tooth in the mandibular arch. It has five well-developed cusps: two buccal, two lingual, and a distal cusp. It has two well-developed roots, one mesial and one distal,

# The Permanent Teeth

| TABLE 3.17: Differences between permanent maxillary first, second, and third molars. | | |
|---|---|---|
| **First molar** | **Second molar** | **Third molar** |
| 1. Buccal cusps are equal in height | 1. Distobuccal cusp is smaller | 1. Distobuccal cusp is much shorter |
| 2. Distolingual cusp is large | 2. Distolingual cusp is smaller | 2. Distolingual cusp is often missing |
| 3. Cusp of Carabelli may be present | 3. Cusp of Carabelli is absent | 3. Cusp of Carabelli is absent |
| 4. Occlusal outline is rhomboid | 4. Occlusal outline is rhomboid | 4. Occlusal outline is triangular |
| 5. Oblique ridge is prominent | 5. Oblique ridge is smaller | 5. Oblique ridge is barely visible |

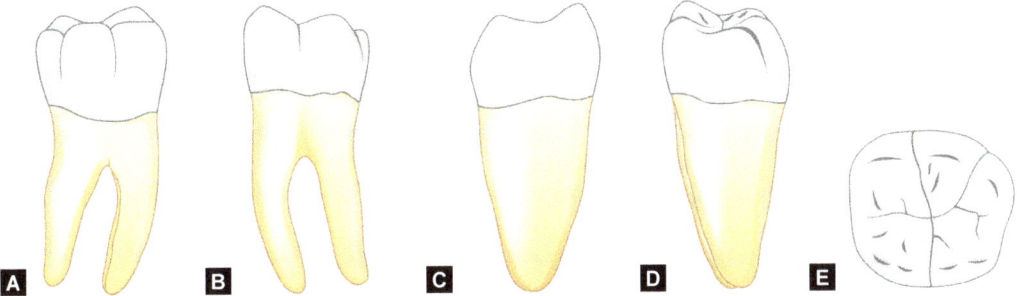

**Figs. 3.14A to E:** Permanent mandibular right first molar: (A) Buccal aspect; (B) Lingual aspect; (C) Mesial aspect; (D) Distal aspect; (E) Occlusal aspect.

which are very broad buccolingually. These roots are widely separated at the apices.

The dimension of the crown mesiodistally is greater by about 1 mm than the dimension buccolingually. Although the crown is relatively short cervico-occlusally, it has mesiodistal and buccolingual measurements that provide a broad occlusal form.

The mesial root is broad and curved distally. The distal root is rounder, broad at the cervical portion, and pointed in a distal direction.

## Buccal Aspect (Fig. 3.14A)

- From the buccal aspect, the crown of the mandibular first molar is roughly trapezoidal, with cervical and occlusal outlines representing the uneven sides of the trapezoid. The occlusal side is the longer.
- The buccal cusps are mesiobuccal, distobuccal, and distal. Two developmental grooves are called the mesiobuccal developmental groove and the distobuccal developmental groove. The first named groove acts as a line of demarcation between the mesiobuccal lobe and the distobuccal lobe. The latter groove separates the distobuccal lobe from the distal lobe.
- The mesiobuccal, distobuccal, and distal cusps are relatively flat. The distal cusp, which is small, is more pointed than either of the buccal cusps. The mesiobuccal cusp is usually the widest mesiodistally of the three cusps. The distobuccal cusp is almost as wide, with a cusp ridge of somewhat greater curvature.

The two buccal cusps make up the major portion of the buccal surface of the crown. The distal cusp provides a very small part of the buccal surface, since the major portion of the cusp makes up the distal portion of the crown.

- The cervical line of the mandibular first molar is commonly regular in outline, dipping apically toward the root bifurcation.
- The mesial outline of the crown is somewhat concave at the cervical third up to its junction with the convex outline of the broad contact area. The distal outline of the crown is straight above the cervical line to its junction with the convex outline

of the distal contact area, which is also the outline of the distal portion of the distal cusp.
- The roots of this tooth are, in most instances, well formed. The mesial root is curved mesially from a point shortly below the cervical line to the middle third portion. From this point, it curves distally to the tapered apex, which is located directly below the mesiobuccal cusp. The crest of curvature of the root mesially is mesial to the crown cervix.
- The distal root is less curved than the mesial root, and its axis is in a distal direction from cervix to apex. The root may show some curvature at its apical third in either a mesial or a distal direction.
- Developmental depressions are present on the mesial and distal sides of both roots. The point of bifurcation of the two roots is located approximately 3 mm below the cervical line. There is a deep developmental depression buccally on the root trunk, which starts at the bifurcation and progresses cervically, becoming more shallow until it terminates at or immediately above the cervical line. This depression is smooth with no developmental groove or fold.

### Lingual Aspect (Fig. 3.14B)
- From the lingual aspect, three cusps may be seen: two lingual cusps and the lingual portion of the distal cusp. The two lingual cusps are pointed, and the cusp ridges are high. The mesiolingual cusp is the widest mesiodistally, with its cusp tip somewhat higher than the distolingual cusp. The distolingual cusp is almost as wide mesiodistally as the mesiolingual cusp. The mesiolingual and distolingual cusp ridges are inclined at angles that are similar on both lingual cusps.
- The lingual developmental groove serves as a line of demarcation between the lingual cusps, extending downward on the lingual surface of the crown for a short distance only. The angle formed by the distolingual cusp ridge of the mesiolingual cusp and the mesiolingual cusp ridge of the distolingual cusp is more obtuse than the angulation of the cusp ridges at the tips of the lingual cusps.
- The distal cusp is at a lower level than the mesiolingual cusp.
- The mesial outline of the crown from this aspect is convex from the cervical line to the marginal ridge. The crest of contour mesially, which represents the contact area, is somewhat higher than the crest of contour distally.
- The distal outline of the crown is straight immediately above the cervical line to a point immediately below the distal contact area; this area is represented by a convex curvature that also outlines the distal surface of the distal cusp. The cervical line lingually is irregular and tends to point sharply toward the root bifurcation and immediately above it.
- The roots of the mandibular first molar measure about 1 mm longer lingually than buccally. The root bifurcation lingually starts at a point approximately 4 mm below the cervical line. This developmental depression is quite deep at this point, although it is smooth throughout and progresses cervically and becomes more shallow until it fades out entirely immediately below the cervical line. This bifurcation groove of the root trunk is located almost in line with the lingual developmental groove of the crown.

### Mesial Aspect (Fig. 3.14C)
- From the mesial aspect, two cusps and one root only are to be seen: the mesiobuccal and mesiolingual cusps and the mesial root. The buccolingual measurement of the crown is greater at the mesial portion than it is at the distal portion. The buccolingual measurement of the mesial root is also greater than the same measurement of the distal root. Therefore, since the mesial portions of the tooth are broader and the mesial cusps are higher, the distal portions of the tooth cannot be seen from this angle.

- The crown from the mesial or distal aspect is roughly rhomboidal and the entire crown has a lingual tilt in relation to the root axis. It should be remembered that the crowns of maxillary posterior teeth have the center of the occlusal surfaces between the cusps in line with the root axes.
- From the mesial aspect, the buccal outline of the crown of the mandibular first molar is convex immediately above the cervical line. This curvature is over the cervical third of the crown buccally, outlining the buccal cervical ridge. The mesiobuccal cusp is located directly above the buccal third of the mesial root.
- The lingual outline of the crown is straight in a lingual direction, starting at the cervical line and joining the lingual curvature at the middle third, the lingual curvature being pronounced between this point and the tip of the mesiolingual cusp. The crest of the lingual contour is located at the center of the middle third of the crown.
- The mesial marginal ridge is confluent with the mesial ridges of the mesiobuccal and mesiolingual cusps. The marginal ridge is placed about 1 mm below the level of the cusp tips.
- The cervical line mesially is rather irregular and tends to curve occlusally about 1 mm toward the center of the mesial surface of the tooth instances; the cervical line is at a higher level lingually than buccally, usually about 1 mm higher. The difference in level may be greater. This relation depends upon the assumption that the tooth is posed vertically. When the first molar is in its normal position in the lower jaw, leaning to the lingual, the cervical line is nearly level buccolingually.
- The lingual outline of the mesial root is slanted in a buccal direction. The mesial surface of the mesial root is convex at the buccal and lingual borders, with a broad concavity between these convexities the full length of the root from cervical line to apex. The mesial surface of the distal root is smooth, with no deep developmental depressions.

## Distal Aspect (Fig. 3.14D)

- The gross outline of the distal aspect of crown and root of the mandibular first molar is similar to the mesial aspect. The crown is shorter distally than mesially, and the buccal and lingual surfaces of the crown converge distally. The buccal surface shows more convergence than the lingual surface.
- The distal root is narrower buccolingually than the mesial root.
- From the distal aspect, the distal cusp is in the foreground on the crown portion. The distal cusp is placed a little buccal to center buccolingually, the distal contact area appearing on its distal contour. The distal contact area is placed just below the distal cusp ridge of the distal cusp and at a slightly higher level above the cervical line than was found mesially when comparing the location of the mesial contact area.
- The distal marginal ridge is short and is made up of the distal cusp ridge of the distal cusp and the distolingual cusp ridge of the distolingual cusp.
- The surface of the distal portion of the crown is convex on the distal cusp and the distolingual cusp.
- The cervical line distally usually extends straight across buccolingually. It may be irregular, dipping root-wise just below the distal contact area.

## Occlusal Aspect (Fig. 3.14E)

- The mandibular first molar is somewhat hexagonal from the occlusal aspect. The crown measurement is 1 mm or more mesiodistally than buccolingually. The buccolingual measurement of the crown is greater on the mesial than on the distal. The crown converges lingually from the contact areas. The mesiobuccal cusp is slightly larger than the two lingual cusps, which are almost equal to each other in size; the distobuccal cusp is smaller than

anyone of the other three mentioned, and the distal cusp is the smallest of all.
- The occlusal surface of the mandibular first molar shows a major fossa and there are two minor fossae. The major fossa is the central fossa. It is roughly circular, and it is centrally placed on the occlusal surface between buccal and lingual cusp ridges. The two minor fossae are the mesial triangular fossae, immediately distal to the mesial marginal ridge, and the distal triangular fossae, placed immediately mesial to the distal marginal ridge.
- The developmental grooves on the occlusal surface are the central developmental groove, the mesiobuccal developmental groove, the distobuccal developmental groove, and the lingual developmental groove. Supplemental grooves and developmental pits are also found.
- The central fossa of the occlusal surface is a concave area bounded by the distal slope of the mesiobuccal cusp, both mesial and distal slopes of the distobuccal cusp, the mesial slope of the distal cusp, the distal slope of the mesiolingual cusp, and the mesial slope of the distolingual cusp. All of the developmental grooves converge in the center of the central fossa at the central pit.
- The mesial triangular fossa of the occlusal surface is a smaller concave area than the central fossa, and it is bounded by the mesial slope of the mesiobuccal cusp, the mesial marginal ridge, and the mesial slope of the mesiolingual cusp. The mesial portion of the central developmental groove terminates in this fossa. Usually, a buccal and a lingual supplemental groove join it at a mesial pit within the boundary of the mesial marginal ridge. Sometimes, a supplemental groove crosses the mesial marginal ridge lingual to the contact area.
- The distal triangular fossa is less distinct than the mesial fossa. It is bounded by the distal slope of the distal cusp, the distal marginal ridge, and the distal slope of the distolingual cusp. The central groove has its other terminal in this fossa.
- Starting at the central pit in the central fossa, the central developmental groove travels an irregular course mesially, terminating in the mesial triangular fossa. A short distance mesially from the central pit, it joins the mesiobuccal developmental groove. Again starting at the central pit, the central groove may be followed in a distobuccal direction to a point where it is joined by the distobuccal developmental groove of the occlusal surface. From this point, the central groove courses in a distolingual direction, terminating in the distal triangular fossa.

## The Permanent Mandibular Second Molar (Figs. 3.15A to E)

### Buccal Aspect (Fig. 3.15A)

- The crown is somewhat shorter cervico-occlusally and narrower mesiodistally than in the first molar.
- The buccal developmental groove acts as a line of demarcation between the mesiobuccal and the distobuccal cusps,

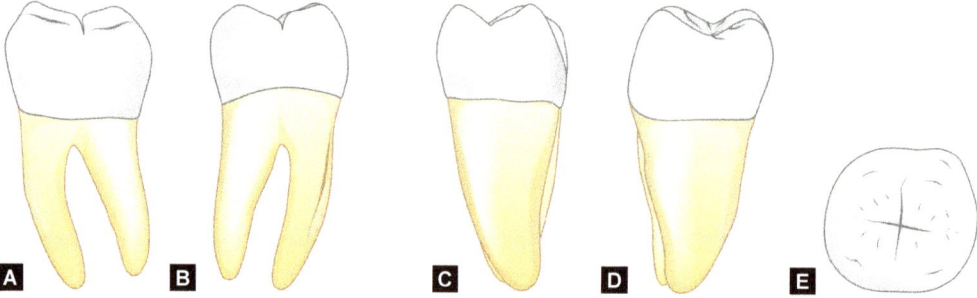

**Figs. 3.15A to E:** Permanent mandibular left second molar: (A) Buccal aspect; (B) Lingual aspect; (C) Mesial aspect; (D) Distal aspect; (E) Occlusal aspect.

which are about equal in their mesiodistal measurements.
- The cervical line buccally points sharply toward the root bifurcation.
- The roots may be shorter than those of the first molar, they are usually closer together, and their axes are nearly parallel.
- The roots are inclined distally in relation to the occlusal plane of the crown, their axes forming more of an acute angle with the occlusal plane than is found on the first molar.

## Lingual Aspect (Fig. 3.15B)

- The surface is similar to mandibular first molar but is smaller. The two cusps are of equal prominence and are separated by lingual groove.
- The crown and root of the mandibular second molar converge lingually but to a slight degree.
- The mesiodistal calibration at the cervix lingually is always greater accordingly than that of the first molar.
- The curvatures mesially and distally on the crown that describe the contact areas are more noticeable from the lingual aspect.

## Mesial Aspect (Fig. 3.15C)

- Except for the differences in measurement from the mesial aspect, the second molar closely resembles that of the first molar.
- The cervical ridge buccally on the crown portion is less pronounced and the occlusal surface may be more constricted buccolingually.
- The cervical line shows less curvature, being straight and regular in outline buccolingually.
- The mesial root is pointed apically.

## Distal Aspect (Fig. 3.15D)

- From the distal aspect, the second molar is similar into the first molar except for the absence of a distal cusp and a distobuccal groove.
- The contact area is centered on the distal surface buccolingually and is placed equidistant from cervical line and marginal ridge.

## Occlusal Aspect (Fig. 3.15E)

- The occlusal aspect is usually rectangular.
- The occlusal aspect of the mandibular second molar differs considerably from the first molar. The small distal cusp of the first molar is not present. There is no distobuccal developmental groove occlusally or buccally. The buccal and lingual developmental grooves meet the central developmental groove at right angles at the central pit on the occlusal surface. These grooves form a cross, dividing the occlusal portion of the crown into four parts that are nearly equal.
- The cusp slopes on the occlusal surface are not as smooth as those found on first molars, since they are roughened by many supplemental grooves radiating from the developmental grooves.
- Mesiobuccal cusp shows cervical prominence.

## The Permanent Mandibular Third Molar (Figs. 3.16A to E)

The mandibular third molar varies considerably in different individuals and presents many anomalies both in form and in position. It may be of four-cusp type resembling lower second molar or five-cusp type resembling lower first molar.

## Buccal Aspect (Fig. 3.16A)

- From the buccal aspect, mandibular third molars vary considerably in outline. The crown is wider at contact areas mesiodistally than at the cervix, the buccal cusps are short and rounded, and the crest of contour mesially and distally is located a little more than half the distance from the cervical line to tips of cusps.
- The average third molar also shows two roots, one mesial and one distal. These roots are usually shorter than other molars. The roots may be separated with a

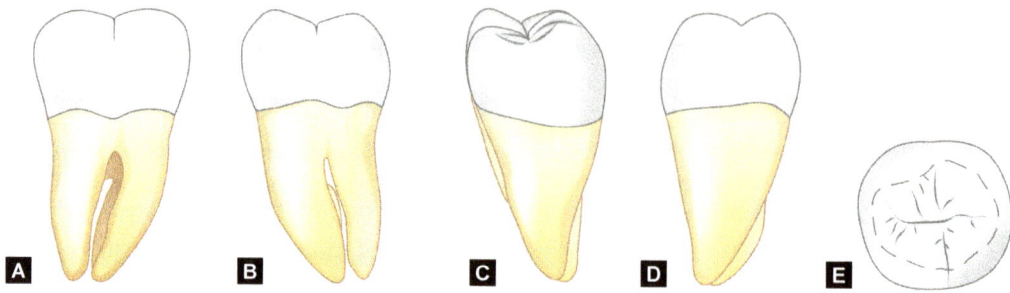

**Figs. 3.16A to E:** Permanent mandibular right third molar: (A) Buccal aspect; (B) Lingual aspect; (C) Mesial aspect; (D) Distal aspect; (E) Occlusal aspect.

**TABLE 3.18:** Differences between permanent mandibular first, second, and third molars.

| First molar | Second molar | Third molar |
| --- | --- | --- |
| 1. Occlusal outline is hexagonal | 1. Occlusal outline is rectangular | 1. Occlusal outline is ovoid |
| 2. Five cusps are present | 2. Four cusps are present | 2. Four cusps are present |
| 3. Mesial and distal marginal ridges are straight and converge lingually | 3. Mesial and distal marginal ridges are curved and do not converge lingually | 3. Mesial and distal marginal ridges are highly curved and do not converge lingually |
| 4. Roots are divergent | 4. Roots are more or less parallel | 4. Roots are often fused |

definite point of bifurcation or they may be fused for all or part of their length.

### Lingual Aspect (Fig. 3.16B)

- The mandibular third molar, when well developed, corresponds closely to the form of the second molar except for size and root development.
- The crown is short with highly bulbous outline. Cusps are rounded.
- Roots are short. They are close together or fused with a distal inclination.

### Mesial Aspect (Fig. 3.16C)

- The crowns are highly bulbous in outline. Both buccal and lingual crown profiles may be highly convex with their respective heights of contour located in the middle third of the crown.
- The mesial root is short but relatively broad buccolingually.

### Distal Aspect (Fig. 3.16D)

- The distal outline of the crown may be bulbous.
- The distal root appears small, both in length and in buccolingual measurement, when compared with the large crown portion.

### Occlusal Aspect (Fig. 3.16E)

- The occlusal aspect of the crown is ovoid in outline. The mesial part of the crown is wider buccolingually than the distal portion.
- The entire occlusal surface is marked by numerous supplemental grooves and irregularity of the pit groove pattern **(Table 3.18)**.

### QUESTIONNAIRE

1. Describe the morphology of permanent maxillary central incisor with diagram. Differentiate between characteristic features of permanent maxillary and mandibular incisors.
2. Describe the morphology of permanent maxillary canine with diagram. Differentiate between the morphological features of permanent maxillary and mandibular canine.
3. Describe the morphology of maxillary first premolar with diagram. Differentiate between the characteristic features of

maxillary first premolar and second premolar.
4. Describe the morphology of mandibular first premolar with diagram. Differentiate between the features of mandibular first premolar and second premolar.
5. Describe the morphology of occlusal surface of permanent maxillary first molar with diagram. Differentiate between the characteristic features of permanent maxillary first, second and third molars.
6. Describe the morphology of occlusal surface of permanent mandibular first molar with diagram. Differentiate between the features of permanent mandibular first, second and third molars.

## BIBLIOGRAPHY

1. Berkovitz BKB, Holland GR, Moxham BJ. A Colour Atlas and Textbook of Oral Anatomy, Histology and Embryology, 4th edition. Mosby: Elsevier; 2009.
2. Biviji AT. Dental Anatomy, 2nd edition. Mumbai: Bhalani Publishing House; 1999.
3. Das AK. Dental Anatomy and Oral Histology, 1st edition. West Bengal: Current Books International; 1972.
4. Kraus BS, Jordon RE, Abrams L. Dental Anatomy and Occlusion. Baltimore: Williams and Willkin's Company; 1969.
5. Nelson SJ, Ash MJ. Wheeler's Dental Anatomy, Physiology and Occlusion, 9th edition. Philadelphia: Elsevier; 2010.

# CHAPTER 4

# Method of Tooth Carving

Comprehensive knowledge of tooth morphology is very much essential for a good clinician. To gain thorough knowledge about the morphology of tooth, one should study the detailed description of individual tooth and should gain the skill of drawing perfect diagram of all surfaces of tooth. Whatever perfection is attained with the diagram, it is only two dimensional. The carving of individual tooth renders three-dimensional knowledge of morphology of a tooth and it is the best way to understand anatomy of tooth.

## EQUIPMENT (FIG. 4.1)

1. Wax block
2. Diagram of all surfaces of tooth
3. Scale
4. Lacron carver and carving knife
5. Cotton wool and smooth cotton cloth
6. Glass slab or piece of rubber cloth.

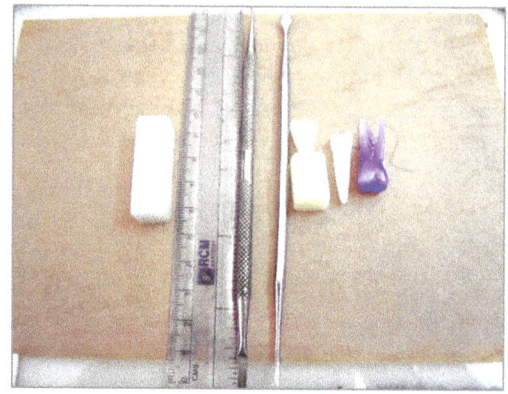

Fig. 4.1: Equipment for tooth carving.

## CARVING OF PERMANENT MAXILLARY CENTRAL INCISOR

- A standard size wax block is taken. Center line and border lines are drawn and four sides are marked as M (mesial), D (distal), La (labial), and L (lingual). Crown heights and root heights are marked on all four sides (**Figs. 4.2A and B**).
- The labial and lingual outlines are drawn both for crown and root (**Fig. 4.2C**). Wax outside the drawn lines is removed from mesial and distal surfaces (**Fig. 4.2D**). Similarly, mesial and distal surfaces are drawn and wax is removed (**Fig. 4.2E**). Cervical line is marked all around and carved according to the curvature (**Fig. 4.2F**).
- Final finishing is done with proper carving of cingulum, ridges, and fossa (**Figs. 4.2G and H**). Finishing and polishing are done with cotton wool and smooth cloth very delicately.

## CARVING OF PERMANENT MAXILLARY CANINE

- Central lines and border lines are drawn on a wax block. Surfaces are marked with initial letter. Crown height and root lengths are measured and marked. Labial and lingual surfaces are drawn (**Figs. 4.3A and B**). Wax is removed from mesial and distal surfaces (**Fig. 4.3C**).
- Mesial and distal outlines are carved and wax is removed (**Fig. 4.3D**).
- The cervical line is marked and carved with proper curvature (**Fig. 4.3E**). Final finishing is done with mesial and distal slopes at incisal edge, cingulum, fossa, and marginal ridges. Polishing is done with cotton wool and cloth (**Fig. 4.3F**).

# Method of Tooth Carving

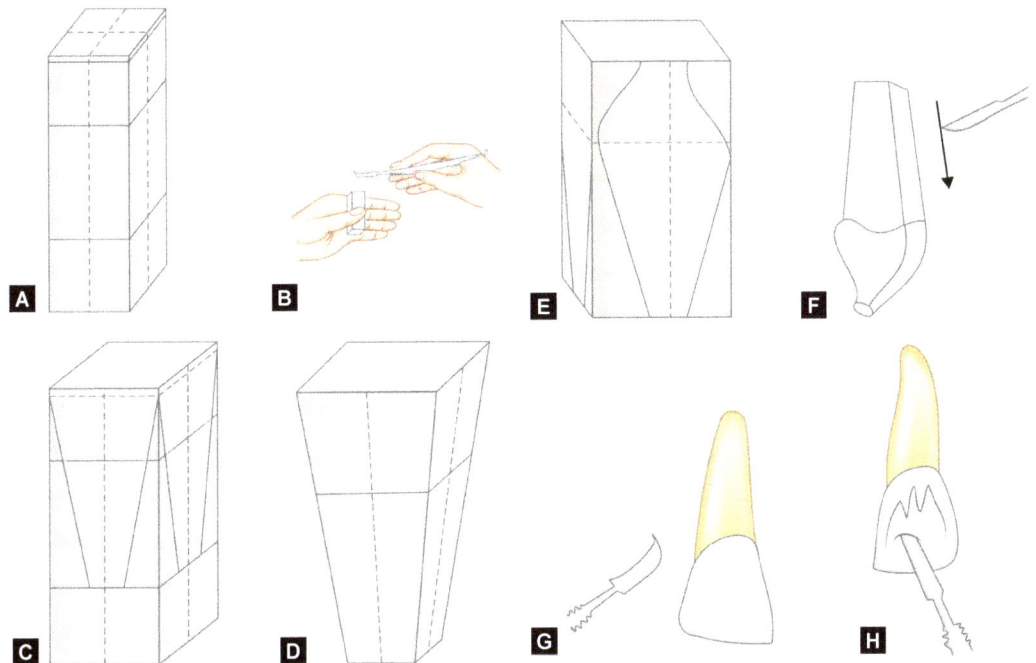

**Figs. 4.2A to H:** Steps for carving permanent maxillary central incisor.

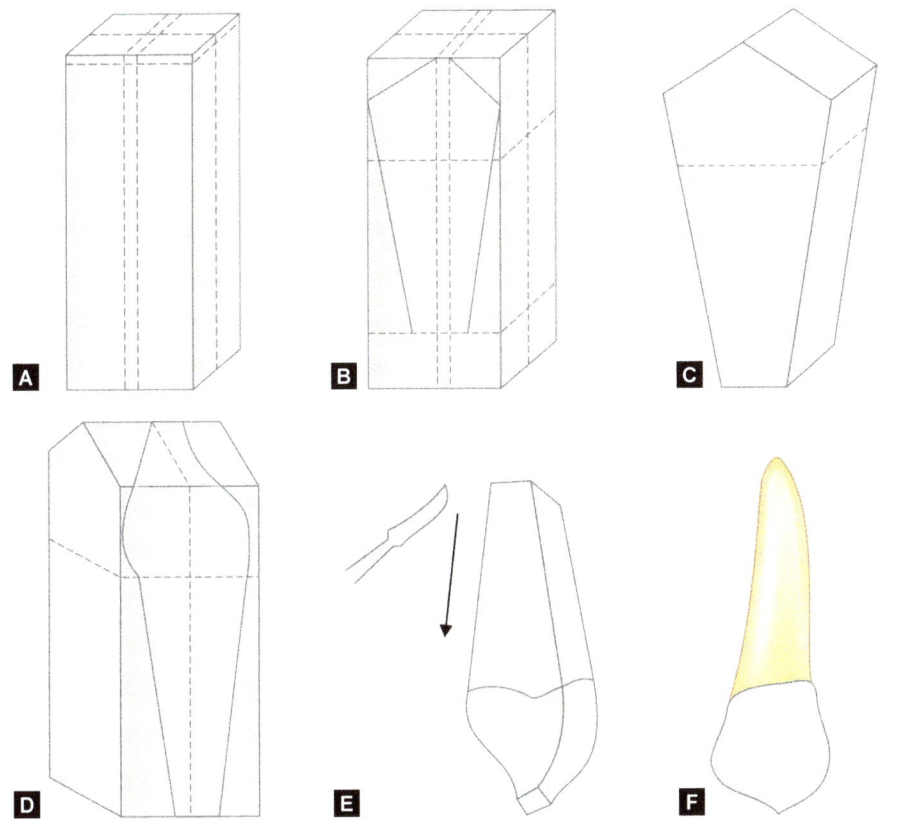

**Figs. 4.3A to F:** Steps for carving permanent maxillary canine.

## CARVING OF MAXILLARY PREMOLAR

- Central lines and border lines are drawn on a wax block. Surfaces are marked with initial letter. Crown height and root lengths are measured and marked. First occlusal outline is drawn on top of wax block and wax is removed up to the cervical line **(Fig. 4.4A)**.
- Root outline is drawn and gross carving of root is done **(Fig. 4.4B)**.
- Buccal and lingual surfaces are drawn and carved. Height of lingual cusp is reduced. Mesial and distal surfaces are drawn and carved **(Fig. 4.4C)**.
- Convexities of buccal and lingual surfaces, cervical line, mesial and distal pits on occlusal surface, triangular ridges,

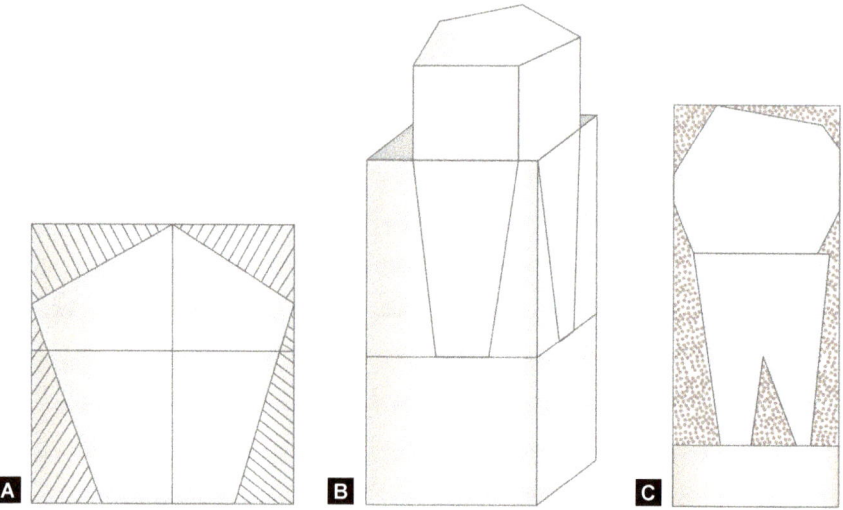

**Figs. 4.4A to C:** Steps of carving maxillary first premolar.

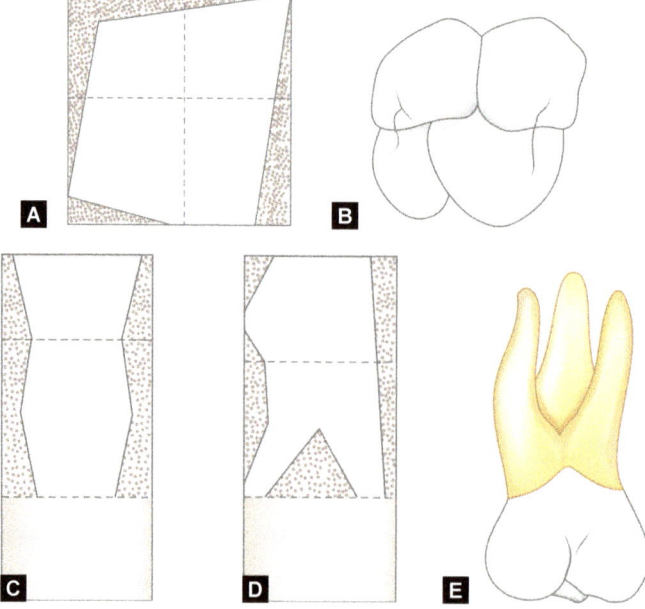

**Figs. 4.5A to E:** Steps of carving maxillary first molar.

and cuspal margins are prominently carved.

## CARVING OF MAXILLARY FIRST MOLAR

- Central lines and border lines are drawn on a wax block. Surfaces are marked with initial letter. Crown height and root lengths are measured and marked. First occlusal outline is drawn on top of wax block, wax is removed up to the cervical line, and gross carving of occlusal surface is done **(Figs. 4.5A and B)**.
- Buccal and lingual surfaces are drawn and carved **(Fig. 4.5C)**. Mesial and distal surfaces are drawn and carved **(Fig. 4.5D)**. Pits, grooves, and ridges are carved on tooth.

Four cusps and roots are carved. Finally, tooth surface is finished and polished **(Fig. 4.5E)**.

Every curve and segment of a normal tooth has some functional basis. A successful clinician should have adequate knowledge of tooth anatomy and he must be able to reproduce them accurately at the time of dental restoration.

## BIBLIOGRAPHY

1. Berkovitz BKB, Holland GR, Moxham BJ. A Colour Atlas and Textbook of Oral Anatomy Histology and Embryology, 4th edition. Mosby: Elsevier; 2009.
2. Biviji AT. Dental Anatomy, 2nd edition. Mumbai: Bhalani Publishing House; 1999.
3. Das AK. Dental Anatomy and Oral Histology, 1st edition. West Bengal: Current Books International; 1972.
4. Kraus BS, Jordon RE, Abrams L. Dental Anatomy and Occlusion. Baltimore: The Williams and Willkin's Company; 1969.
5. Nelson SJ, Ash MJ. Wheeler's Dental Anatomy, Physiology and Occlusion, 9th edition. Philadelphia: Elsevier; 2010.
6. Scott JH, Symons NBB. Introduction to Dental Anatomy, 9th edition. Edinburgh and London: Churchill Livingstone; 1982.

# CHAPTER 5

# Vasculature and Innervations of the Teeth and Associated Structures

The arteries and nerve branches to the teeth are mere terminals of the central systems.

## ARTERIAL SUPPLY OF THE TEETH AND ASSOCIATED STRUCTURES

Orofacial structures are supplied by different branches of external carotid artery which gives off lingual, facial, maxillary, and several other branches. The lingual artery supplies the tongue, floor of the mouth, and the sublingual salivary gland. The facial artery supplies tonsils, submandibular salivary gland, and muscles of face and lips.

### Blood Supply of the Face

The face is supplied through the facial artery **(Fig. 5.1)**, a branch of external carotid artery in the neck. The facial artery first appears on the face as it hooks round the lower border of mandible, at the anterior edge of the masseter. It then runs a tortuous course between the facial muscles toward the medial angle of the eye.

### Blood Supply of the Teeth and the Jaw

The arteries to the teeth and jaws are derived from maxillary artery, a terminal branch of the external carotid artery.

It begins opposite to the neck of the mandible, crosses the inferior alveolar nerve, passes between two heads of lateral pterygoid muscle, and enters pterygopalatine fossa where it divides into terminal branches **(Fig. 5.2)**.

### Blood Supply of the Lower Jaw and Periodontium

The inferior alveolar artery, which supplies the mandibular teeth, is derived from the maxillary artery before it crosses the lateral

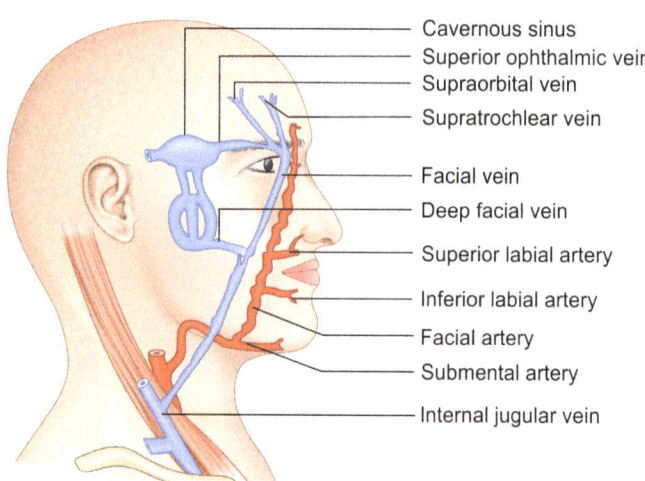

**Fig. 5.1:** Arteries and veins of face.

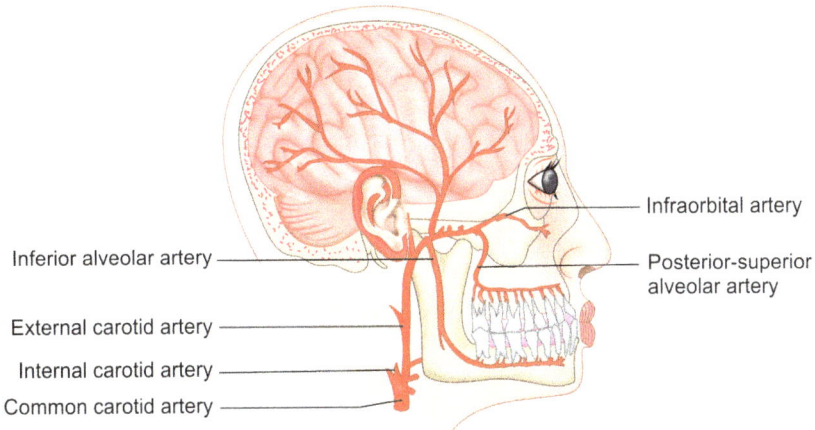

Fig. 5.2: Maxillary artery and its branches to maxilla, mandible, and teeth.

pterygoid muscle in the infratemporal fossa. It descends on the medial aspect of ramus of the mandible to the mandibular foramen. It gives off a mylohyoid branch before it passes through the mandibular foramen to enter the mandibular canal. As it enters the mandibular canal, it is accompanied by inferior alveolar nerve and at the level of first premolar tooth, it bifurcates into incisive and mental branch.

Posteriorly, the buccal gingiva is supplied by the buccal artery (branch of maxillary artery) as well as branches from inferior alveolar artery. Anteriorly, the labial gingiva is supplied by the mental artery and branches of incisive artery. The lingual gingiva is supplied by the branches from inferior alveolar artery and lingual artery, a branch of the external carotid artery.

## Blood Supply of the Upper Jaw and Periodontium

The posterior-superior alveolar artery arises from the maxillary artery in the pterygopalatine fossa. It courses tortuously over the maxillary tuberosity to enter the alveolar canals along with the posterior superior alveolar nerves and supplies the maxillary molar and premolar teeth, alveolar bone, and maxillary sinus. A branch of variable size runs forward on the periosteum at the junction of the alveolar process and maxillary body supplying the gingiva, alveolar mucosa, and cheek.

A middle superior alveolar branch is usually given off by the infraorbital artery, a branch of maxillary artery. It runs downward in the lateral wall of the maxillary sinus, terminating near the canine tooth where it anastomoses with the posterior and anterior-superior alveolar arteries. Its main distribution is to the maxillary premolar teeth.

Anterior-superior alveolar branches arise from the infraorbital artery just before this vessel leaves its foramen. They course down the anterior aspect of the maxilla in bony canals to supply the maxillary anterior teeth and their supporting tissues and to join the middle and posterior-superior alveolar branches in completing an anastomotic plexus.

Branches to the teeth, periodontal ligament, and bone are derived from the superior alveolar artery. The palatal gingiva around the maxillary teeth is supplied by the branches of the greater palatine artery, a branch of maxillary artery.

## Blood Supply of the Palate, Cheek, Tongue, and Lips

The palate derives its blood supply from the greater and lesser palatine branches of the maxillary artery. The greater palatine artery passes through the incisive fossa, where it anastomoses with the nasopalatine artery. The cheek is supplied by the buccal branch of the maxillary artery and the floor of the mouth and the tongue by the lingual arteries. The lips are mainly supplied by the superior and inferior labial branches of the facial arteries.

## VENOUS DRAINAGE OF ORODENTAL TISSUES

The venous drainage of this region is extremely variable. The facial vein is the main vein draining the face. It begins at the medial corner of the eye by confluence of the supraorbital and supratrochlear veins and passes across the face behind the facial artery **(Fig. 5.1)**. Below the mandible, it receives the anterior branch of retromandibular vein before draining into the internal jugular vein. The facial vein communicates with the cavernous sinus through superior ophthalmic vein, deep facial vein, and pterygoid venous plexus **(Fig. 5.1)**. Small veins from the teeth and alveolar bone pass into larger veins surrounding the apex of each tooth or into veins running in the interdental septa. In the mandible, the veins are then collected into one or more inferior alveolar veins, which may drain anteriorly through the mental foramen to join the facial vein or posteriorly through the mandibular foramen to join the pterygoid plexus of veins in the infratemporal fossa. In the maxilla, the veins may drain anteriorly into the facial vein or posteriorly into the pterygoid plexus.

## INNERVATION OF ORODENTAL TISSUES

The sensory nerve supply to the jaws and teeth is derived from the maxillary and mandibular branches of the fifth cranial or trigeminal nerve, whose ganglion, the trigeminal, is located at the apex of the petrous portion of the temporal bone. Both the major and minor salivary glands are supplied by secretomotor parasympathetic fibers from the facial and glossopharyngeal nerves. The motor innervation of the muscles of the jaws and oral cavity is from the trigeminal, facial, accessory, and hypoglossal nerve.

### Nerve Supply of Maxilla and Maxillary Teeth

The maxillary teeth and gingiva are supplied by the maxillary division of trigeminal nerve. It arises from trigeminal ganglion. The maxillary nerve has a posterior superior alveolar branch from its pterygopalatine part. The nerve enters the alveolar canals on the infratemporal surface of the maxilla, forms a plexus, and is distributed to the molar teeth and supporting tissues **(Fig. 5.3)**. Maxillary nerve enters the orbit as the infraorbital nerve, runs in infraorbital canal, and terminates at the infraorbital foramen in branches distributed to the upper face. A middle superior alveolar

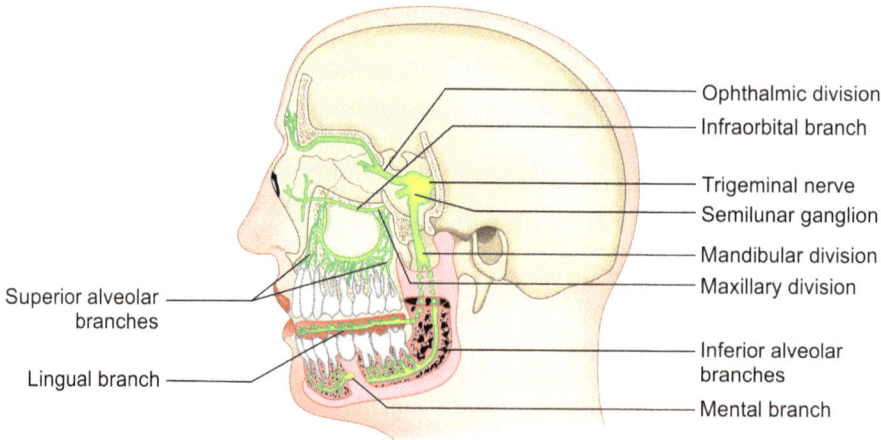

**Fig. 5.3:** Distribution of trigeminal nerve.

# Vasculature and Innervations of the Teeth and Associated Structures

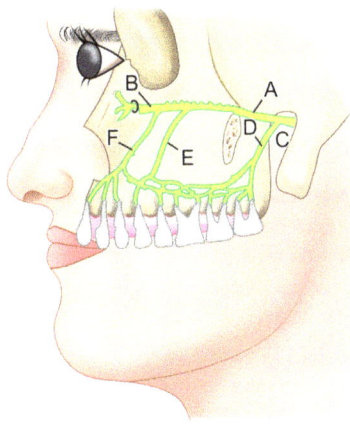

**Fig. 5.4:** The superior alveolar nerve. A. Trunk of maxillary division of trigeminal nerve, B. Infraorbital nerve, C. Pterygopalatine fossa, D. Posterior-superior alveolar nerve, E. Middle superior alveolar nerve, and F. Anterior-superior alveolar nerve.

branch arises from the infraorbital nerve and runs through the lateral wall of the maxillary sinus. It is distributed to the premolar teeth and surrounding tissues. An anterior-superior alveolar branch leaves the infraorbital nerve just inside the infraorbital foramen and is distributed through bony canals to the incisor and canine teeth. All three superior alveolar nerves join in a plexus above the process. From the plexus, dental branches are given off to each tooth root and interdental branches to the bone, periodontal membrane, and gingiva **(Fig. 5.4)**.

The branches of clinical significance include a greater palatine branch that enters the hard palate through the greater palatine foramen and is distributed to the hard palate and palatal gingival as far forward as the canine tooth, a lesser palatine branch from the ganglion that enters the soft palate through the lesser palatine foramina, and a nasopalatine branch of the posterior or superior lateral nasal branch of the ganglion that runs downward and forward on the nasal septum.

Entering the palate through the incisive canal, it is distributed to the incisive papilla and to the palate anterior to the anterior palatine nerve **(Fig. 5.5)**.

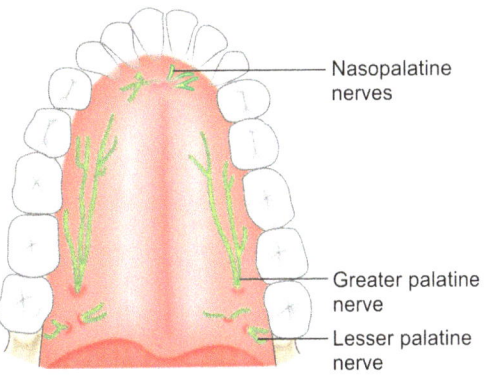

**Fig. 5.5:** The sensory nerve supply to the palate.

## Nerve Supply of Mandible and Mandibular Teeth

The inferior alveolar nerve, branch of mandibular nerve runs directly downward across the medial surface of the lateral pterygoid muscle. It is directed laterally and downward across the outer surface of the medial pterygoid muscle to reach the mandibular foramen. Just before entering the foramen, it releases the mylohyoid branch, a motor branch to the mylohyoid muscle and anterior belly of the digastric.

The inferior alveolar nerve continues forward through the mandibular canal beneath the roots of the molar teeth to the level of the mental foramen. During this part of its course, it gives off branches to the molar and premolar teeth, and their supporting bone and soft tissues.

At the mental foramen, the nerve divides and a smaller incisive branch continues forward to supply the anterior teeth and bone and a larger mental branch emerges through the foramen to supply the skin of the lower lip and chin **(Figs. 5.3 and 5.6)**.

Other branches of the mandibular nerve contribute in some degree to the innervation of the mandible and its investing membranes. The buccal nerve, although chiefly distributed to the mucosa of the cheek, has a branch that is usually distributed to a small area of the buccal gingival in the first molar area, but in some cases, its distribution may extend from

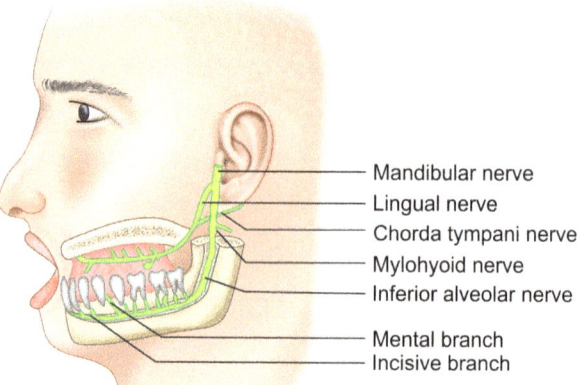

Fig. 5.6: Branches of mandibular division of trigeminal nerve.

canine to the third molar. The lingual nerve, as it enters the floor of the mouth, lies against the body of the mandible and has mucosal branches to a variable area of lingual mucosa and gingiva.

## Sensory Nerve Supply of Face (Fig. 5.7)

All three divisions of trigeminal nerve are involved in the cutaneous innervations of the face. The ophthalmic division supplies the upper part of face, forehead, and scalp.

The maxillary and mandibular divisions supply the upper and lower jaw regions.

**Knowledge of innervations is important:**
1. To assess the effects of nerve damage.
2. Successful anesthetizing of the buccal, infraorbital, and inferior alveolar nerves during dental treatment.
3. Cutaneous innervations of face are also related to development of face.

## QUESTIONNAIRE

1. Describe the arterial supply of teeth and associated structure.
2. Discuss the innervation of orodental tissues.

## BIBLIOGRAPHY

1. Berkovitz BKB, Holland GR, Moxham BJ. A Colour Atlas and Textbook of Oral Anatomy, Histology and Embryology, 4th edition. Mosby: Elsevier; 2009.
2. Das AK. Dental Anatomy and Oral Histology, 1st edition. West Bengal: Current Books International; 1972.
3. Dutta AK. Essentials of Human Anatomy, Head and Neck, 5th edition. West Bengal: Current Books International; 2010.
4. Nelson SJ, Ash MJ. Wheeler's Dental Anatomy, Physiology and Occlusion, 9th edition. Philadelphia: Elsevier; 2010.
5. Romanes GJ. Cunningham's Manual of Practical Anatomy, 15th edition. London: Oxford University Press; 2002. p. 3.

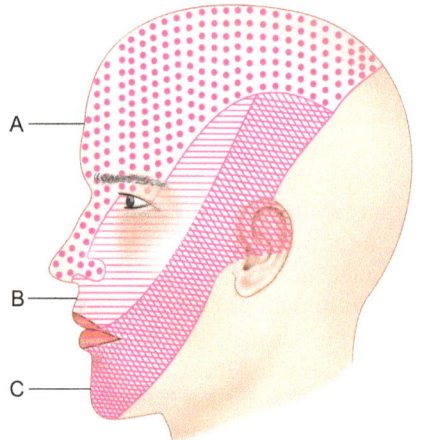

Fig. 5.7: Sensory nerve supply of face. A. Ophthalmic division of trigeminal nerve, B. Maxillary division of trigeminal nerve, and C. Mandibular division of trigeminal nerve.

# CHAPTER 6
# The Temporomandibular Joint and Muscles of Mastication

The temporomandibular joint (TMJ) is unique in its anatomy, histology, and function. The right and left joints function as one unit. It is the synovial articulation between the mandible and cranium. The joint is formed by mandibular fossa and articular eminence of temporal bone and mandibular condyle with articular disk interposed in between **(Fig. 6.1)**. The TMJ, although basically a hinge joint, also allows for some gliding movements. The condylar head undertakes translatory as well as rotary movements within the mandibular fossa and down a bony prominence immediately anterior to the mandibular fossa, the articular eminence of the temporal bone. Therefore, the human TMJ is described as a synovial sliding ginglymoid joint.

**The TMJ has some unusual features:**
- The joint space is divided into two joint cavities (upper and lower) by an intra-articular disk—upper joint space allows for gliding movements and lower joint space for hinge movements.
- The articular surfaces are not composed of hyaline cartilage but of fibrous tissue.
- A secondary condylar cartilage is present in the head of the condyle until adolescence.
- Movement of the joint is influenced by the teeth.
- There are two TMJs associated with a single mandible—has considerable functional significance as movement at one joint is accompanied by movement at the other.

## ANATOMY IN BRIEF

### Mandibular Fossa

The mandibular fossa is an oval depression in the temporal bone lying immediately anterior to the external acoustic meatus. Its mediolateral dimension is greater than its anteroposterior one in order to accommodate the mandibular condyle, and it is wider laterally than medially. The mandibular fossa is bounded anteriorly by the articular eminence, laterally by the zygomatic process, and posteriorly by the tympanic plate. The shape of the mandibular fossa does not exactly conform to the shape of mandibular condyle, the intra-articular disk molding together the joint surfaces.

### Mandibular Condyle

The convex anterior and superior surfaces of the head of the condyle are the articular surfaces. The nonarticular posterior surface of the condyle is broad and flat. The articular surface is separated from nonarticular surface by a ridge, indicating the site of attachment of the joint capsule.

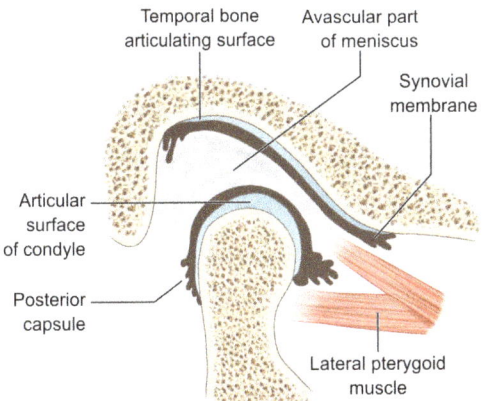

**Fig. 6.1:** Schematic representation of the temporomandibular joint.

## Joint Capsule

The articular capsule is a fibrous sac that attaches anteriorly to the articular tubercle, posteriorly to the lips of the squamotympanic fissure and between the two attachments to the margins of the mandibular fossa, and to the neck of the mandible below. It is strengthened laterally by the temporomandibular ligament.

## Synovial Membrane

The inner aspect of the capsule and margins of the intra-articular disk are lined by a synovial membrane, which is especially well developed behind the disk. It lines the capsule in each of the two cavities but does not extend over the surfaces of the disks, the articular tubercle, or the condyle. The synovial membrane secretes the synovial fluid that occupies the joint cavities, lubricates the joint, and has nutritive function.

## Temporomandibular Ligament

The joint capsule is strengthened by temporomandibular ligament. It takes origin from the lateral surface of the articular eminence of the temporal bone and inserts onto the posterior surface of the condyle. The ligament provides main support for the joint, restricting backward and inferior movements of the mandible and resisting dislocation during functional movements.

## Intra-articular Disk

The articular disk is interposed between the articular surfaces of the two bones. It is an oval, fibrous plate. At anterior margin, fuses with the fibrous capsule, posterior border is connected to capsule by loose connective tissue and medial and lateral corners are directly attached to the poles of the condyle (Figs. 6.2 and 6.3).

The articular space is divided into two compartments. The lower is in between the condyle and the disk and an upper in between the disk and temporal bone. The disk is biconcave with a thin intermediate zone, a thick anterior band, and a thick posterior band. The latter is continuous with a loose fibroelastic portion called the bilaminar zone, which is highly vascular and highly innervated. The superior stratum or lamina of the bilaminar zone is attached to the posterior wall of the mandibular or glenoid fossa and the squamotympanic suture, while the inferior stratum attaches to the back of the mandibular condyle.

Some fibers of the lateral pterygoid muscle are attached to the anterior border of the disk. The disk produces a movable articulation for the condyle. In the inferior portion of the joint, rotational movement about an axis through the heads of the condyles permits opening of the jaws.

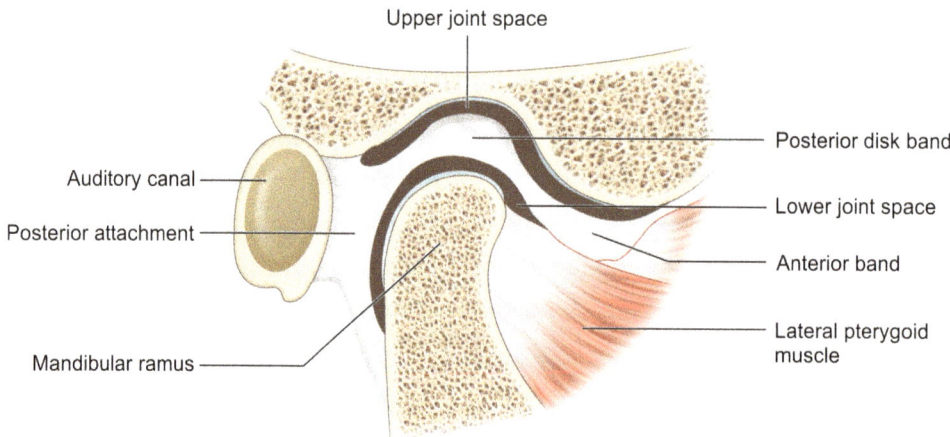

**Fig. 6.2:** Articular disk and associated structure.

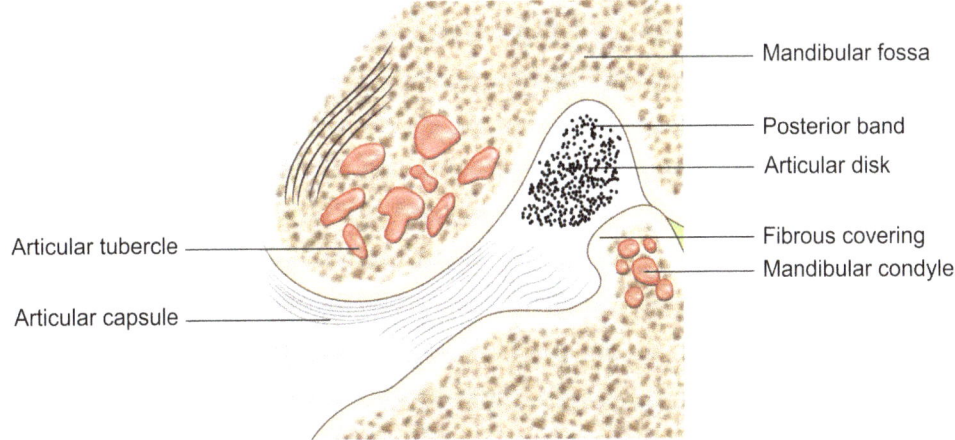

**Fig. 6.3:** Sagittal section through temporomandibular joint.

This is designated as hinge movement. The superior portion of the joint permits a translatory movement as the disks and the condyles traverse anteriorly along the inclines of the articular tubercles to provide an anterior and inferior movement of the mandibular head.

## Arterial Supply

1. Superficial temporal branch of the external carotid artery.
2. Masseteric branch of the maxillary artery.

## Nerve Supply

**Auriculotemporal nerve**: Branch of posterior division of the mandibular nerve.

**Masseteric**: Branch of the anterior division of the mandibular nerve.

Sensations from the joint structures have usually been considered proprioceptive in nature. It has been suggested that there exist a number of free, complex, and encapsulated receptors among the synovial villi of the joint capsule.

## Movements

Movements permitted at the temporomandibular joints are protrusion and retraction, depression and elevation, and side-to-side chewing movements of the mandible. The superior compartment permits translatory or gliding movements in protrusion, retraction, and in chewing. The lower compartment allows rotation around two independent axes:
1. A transverse axis for hinge movement during depression and elevation of the mandible.
2. A vertical axis for side-to-side movements.

### Muscles Producing Movements

**Protrusion (Protraction):** It is done by simultaneous action of lateral and medial pterygoid muscles of both sides.

**Retraction:** This is done by the posterior fibers of the temporalis muscle, which brings the joint in resting position.

**Depression:** The mandible is depressed during opening of the mouth and the muscles concerned are:
a. Lateral pterygoid.
b. Geniohyoid, mylohyoid, and digastrics, at the same time the hyoid bone is kept fixed by the infrahyoid muscles. Gravity also assists depression. During depression, the head of the mandible and the articular disk together glide forward in the upper compartment by the contraction of lateral pterygoid muscles. At the same time, the head rotates forward below the articular disk by the contraction of suprahyoid muscles. The movement is initiated in the lower compartment by forward rotation of the mandibular head below the disk.

Thereafter, the movement appears in the upper compartment by forward gliding of the disk carrying the mandibular head with it. Subsequently, the forward gliding is prevented by the tension of the posterior fibers of temporalis muscle and upper lamella of articular disk. Thus, the depression is completed in the lower compartment.

**Elevation:** Masseter, temporalis, and medial pterygoid act as elevators of the mandible to close the mouth.

**Side-to-side movement:** It takes place in chewing by the contraction of lateral and medial pterygoid muscles of one side, acting alternately with the other side. The mandibular head of one side glides forward in the upper compartment and rotates below the disk around a vertical axis which passes through the posterior border of the opposite ramus of mandible. The head then returns to its former position so that other head can move forward in its turn.

## Histology

**Bony component:** The condyle of the mandible is composed of cancellous bone covered by a thin layer of compact bone (**Fig. 6.4**). The trabeculae are grouped in such a way that they radiate from the neck of the mandible and reach the cortex at right angles, thus giving maximal strength to the condyle. The large marrow spaces decrease in size with progressing age. During the period of growth, a layer of hyaline cartilage lies underneath the fibrous covering of the condyle.

This cartilaginous plate grows by apposition from the deepest layers of the covering connective tissue. At the same time, its deep surface is replaced by bone. Remnants of this cartilage may persist into old age. The roof of the mandibular fossa consists of a thin, compact layer of bone. The articular tubercle is composed of spongy bone covered with a thin layer of compact bone. In rare cases, islands of hyaline cartilage are found in the articular tubercle.

## ARTICULAR FIBROUS COVERING

The condyle as well as the articular tubercle is covered by a thick layer of fibrous tissue containing a variable number of chondrocytes. The fibrous covering of the mandibular condyle is of fairly even thickness (**Fig. 6.5**). Its superficial layers consist of a network of strong collagenous fibers. Chondrocytes may be present and they have a tendency to increase in number with age. The fibrous layer covering the articulating surface of the temporal bone is thin in the articular fossa and thickens rapidly on the posterior slope of the articular tubercle. In this region, the fibrous tissue shows a definite arrangement in two layers, with a small transitional zone between them. The two layers are characterized by the different course of the constituent fibrous bundles. In the inner zone, the fibers are at right angles to the bony surface. In the outer

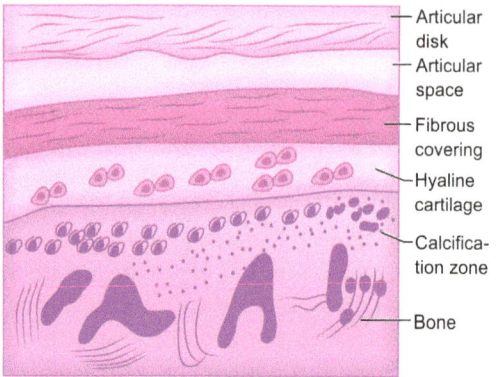

**Fig. 6.4:** Histology of mandibular condyle.

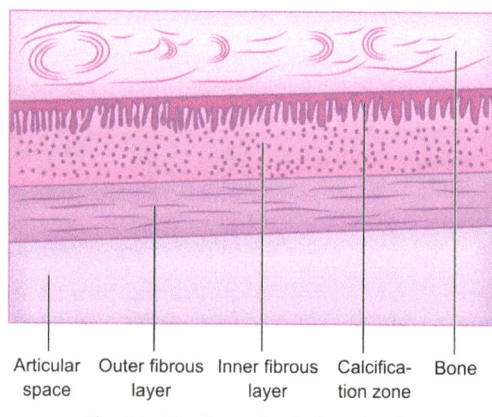

**Fig. 6.5:** Histology of articular tubercle.

zone, they run parallel to that surface. As in the fibrous covering of the mandibular condyle, a variable number of chondrocytes are found in the tissue on the temporal surface. In adults, the deepest layer shows a thin zone of calcification.

## ARTICULAR DISK

In young individuals, the articular disk is composed of dense fibrous tissue. The interlacing fibers are straight and tightly packed **(Fig. 6.6)**. Elastic fibers are found only in relatively small numbers. The fibroblasts in the disk are elongated and send flat cytoplasmic wig-like processes into the interstices between the adjacent bundles. With advancing age, some of the fibroblasts develop into chondroid cells, which later may differentiate into true chondrocytes. The presence of chondrocytes may increase the resistance and resilience of the fibrous tissue.

The fibrous tissue covering the articular eminence and mandibular condyle, as well as the large central area of the disk, is devoid of blood vessels and nerves and has limited reparative ability.

## ARTICULAR CAPSULE

The articular capsule consists of an outer fibrous layer that is strengthened on the lateral surface to form the temporomandibular ligament. The articular capsule is lined with synovial membrane which folds into synovial villi and project into the joint spaces **(Fig. 6.7)**. The synovial membrane consists of internal cells which do not form a continuous layer but show gaps between the cells and the subintimal connective tissue layer, rich in blood capillaries. The internal cells are of three types. The first is rich in rough endoplasmic reticulum and is called the fibroblast-like or B cell. The second type is rich in Golgi complex, contains little or no RER, and is called the macrophage-like or A cell. The third type has a cellular morphology between cell types A and B. A small amount of a clear, straw-colored viscous fluid, the synovial fluid is found in the articular spaces. It is a lubricant

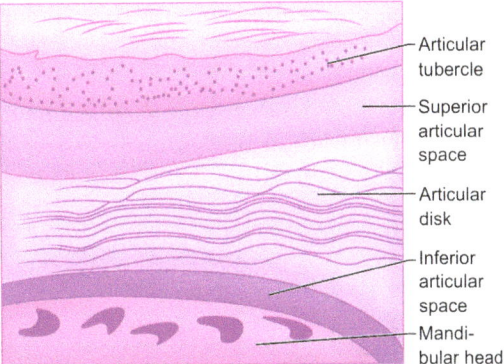

**Fig. 6.6:** Histology of articular disk.

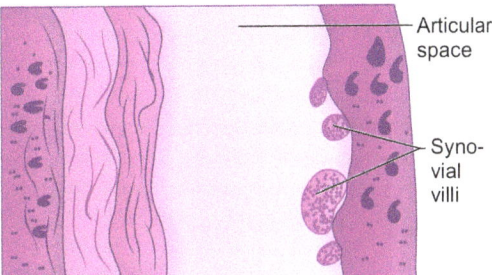

**Fig. 6.7:** Histology of articular capsule.

and also a nutrient fluid for the avascular tissues covering the condyle and the articular tubercle and for the disk. It is elaborated by diffusion from the rich capillary network of the synovial membrane, augmented by mucin possibly secreted by the synovial cells.

## CLINICAL CONSIDERATIONS

1. The thinness of the bone in the articular fossa is responsible for fractures if the mandibular head is driven into the fossa by a heavy blow. In such cases, injuries of the dura mater and the brain have been reported.
2. Abnormal functional activity produces injury to the fibrous covering and the articular bones.
3. In severe trauma, the articular bone is destroyed, and cartilage and new bone develop in the marrow spaces and at the periphery of the condyle. Then the function of the joint is severely impaired.
4. The term "myofacial pain dysfunction syndrome" is used to indicate a dysfunction of the temporomandibular joint.

5. Dislocation of the temporomandibular joint may take place without the impact of an external force. The dislocation of the jaw is usually bilateral and the displacement is anterior. When the mouth is opened unusually wide during yawning, the head of the mandible may slip forward into the infratemporal fossa, causing articular dislocation of the joint.

## MUSCLES OF MASTICATION

### Enumeration

1. Lateral pterygoid
2. Medial pterygoid
3. Masseter
4. Temporalis.

Buccinator is called accessory muscle of mastication as while chewing, it prevents the food to enter the vestibule of the mouth by pressing the cheek on the gum.

### Development

All the muscles of mastication (except buccinator) are developed from the myotome of the first branchial arch whose nerve is the mandibular nerve. So all these muscles are supplied by branches from the mandibular nerve. Buccinator is developed from the myotome of the second branchial arch, so it is supplied by the facial nerve.

### Description of Each Muscle

*Lateral Pterygoid (Fig. 6.8)*

**Origin:** By two heads:
i. *Upper head*: From the infratemporal ridge and infratemporal surface of the greater wing of the sphenoid.
ii. *Lower head*: From the outer surface of the lateral pterygoid plate of the sphenoid.

**Insertion:**
i. Into the pterygoid fossa on the anterior surface of the neck of the mandible.
ii. Into the capsule of the temporomandibular joint.
iii. Into the articular disk of the temporomandibular joint (articular disk is said to be a part of the lateral pterygoid muscle).

**Nerve supply:** Nerve to the lateral pterygoid which is a branch of the anterior division of the mandibular nerve.

*Medial Pterygoid (Fig. 6.8)*

**Origin:**
i. From the medial surface of the lateral pterygoid plate of the sphenoid.
ii. Tubercle (pyramidal process) of the palatine bone, fitting into the pterygoid fissure.
iii. Tuberosity of the maxilla.

**Insertion:** Into the lower and back part of the medial surface of the ramus of the mandible.

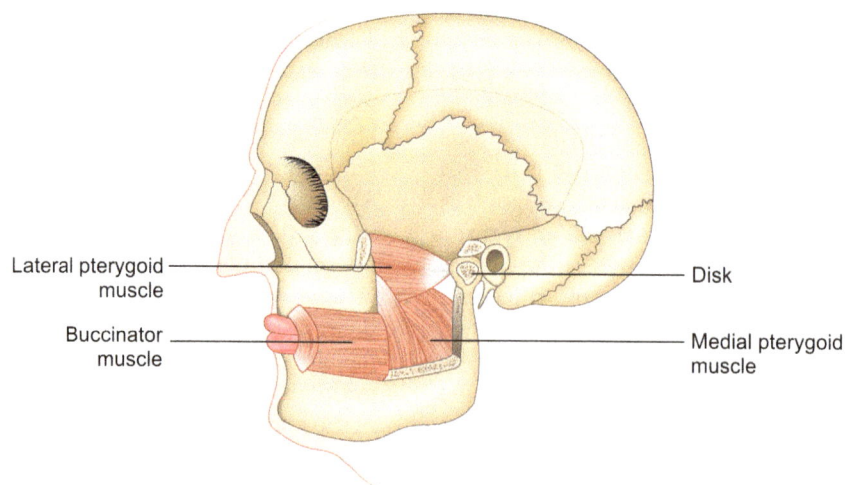

**Fig. 6.8:** Positions of lateral and medial pterygoids and buccinator muscle.

It extends from the mandibular foramen up to the angle of the mandible.

**Nerve supply:** Nerve to the medial pterygoid which is a branch of the trunk of the mandibular nerve.

## Masseter (Fig. 6.9)

**Origin:**
a. *Superficial part*: From the lower border of the anterior two-thirds of the zygomatic arch.
b. *Deep part*: From the posterior one-third of the lower border and whole length of the medial surface of the zygomatic arch.

**Insertion:** To the outer surface of the entire ramus of the mandible.

**Nerve supply:** Masseteric branch of the anterior division of the mandibular nerve.

## Temporalis (Fig. 6.9)

**Origin:**
i. From the whole extent of the bones forming the temporal fossa except the zygomatic bone.
ii. From the temporal fascia.

**Insertion:** Into the tip, anterior border, medial surface of the coronoid process of the mandible. Insertion extends along the anterior border of the ramus of the mandible up to near third molar tooth.

**Nerve supply:** Deep temporal (anterior and posterior) nerves of the anterior division of the mandibular nerve.

## Movements during Mastication

**Opening the mouth:** First there is protrusion of the mandible by two lateral pterygoids. It is followed by depression of the mandible done by the following muscles of both sides acting together:
i. Lower fibers of the lateral pterygoid
ii. Digastric
iii. Mylohyoid
iv. Geniohyoid.

The last three muscles are acting from the hyoid which is kept fixed by the infrahyoid muscles, i.e. sternohyoid, thyrohyoid, and omohyoid.

This movement is exaggerated by the gravity and platysma.

**Closing the mouth:** At first, there is elevation of the mandible done by the following muscles of both sides acting together:
i. Medial pterygoid
ii. Masseter
iii. Anterior fibers of the temporalis.

It is followed by retraction of the mandible done by the posterior fibers of the temporalis of both sides acting together.

**Side-to-side or chewing movement:** Head of the mandible of one side moves forward,

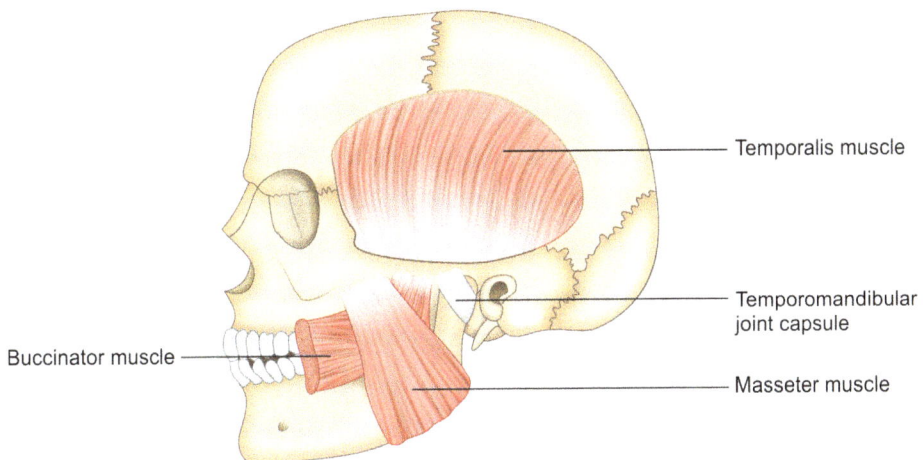

**Fig. 6.9:** Positions of temporalis, masseter, and buccinator muscle.

backward, and rotates alternatively with that of the opposite side. When one side moves forward and rotates, other side moves backward and rotates. It is done by the lateral and medial pterygoids of one side working alternately with those of the opposite side.

## QUESTIONNAIRE

1. What is temporomandibular joint? Discuss in brief about anatomy, histology, and functions of temporomandibular joint.
2. Discuss the movements of temporomandibular joint.
3. Enumerate the muscles of mastication. Discuss the origin, insertion, and nerve supply of all muscles of mastication. Describe the movements during mastication.

## BIBLIOGRAPHY

1. Berkovitz BKB, Holland GR, Moxham BJ. A Colour Atlas and Textbook of Oral Anatomy, Histology and Embryology, 4th edition. Mosby: Elsevier; 2009.
2. Das AK. Dental Anatomy and Oral Histology, 1st edition. West Bengal: Current Books International; 1972.
3. Dutta AK. Essentials of Human Anatomy, Head and Neck, 5th edition. West Bengal: Current Books International; 2010.
4. Dutta AK. Essentials of Human Embryology, 6th edition. West Bengal: Current Books International; 2010.
5. Kumar GS. Orban's Oral Histology and Embryology, 12th edition. Mosby: Elsevier; 2009.
6. Nanci A. Ten Cate's Oral Histology Development, Structure and Function, 7th edition. Mosby: Elsevier; 2008.
7. Nelson SJ, Ash MJ. Wheeler's Dental Anatomy, Physiology and Occlusion, 9th edition. Philadelphia: Elsevier; 2010.
8. Romanes GJ. Cunningham's Manual of Practical Anatomy, 15th edition. London: Oxford University Press; 2002. p. 3.

# CHAPTER 7

# The Maxillary Sinus

The paranasal sinuses are air containing bony spaces around the nasal cavity and lined by the mucous membrane of ciliated columnar epithelium.

## ENUMERATION

- Frontal sinuses
- Ethmoidal sinuses
- Sphenoidal sinuses
- Maxillary sinuses.

## FUNCTIONS

1. These make the cranial bones lighter due to the upward thrust of the air within the sinuses.
2. Regulate the temperature of the inspired air and thus protect the vital structures like brain and eyeball against exposure to cold air.
3. They contribute to resonance of voice.
4. They enhance the craniofacial resistance to mechanical shock.
5. They may produce bactericidal lysozyme to nasal cavity.

## MAXILLARY SINUS

### Definition

It is a pneumatic space within the body of the maxilla and communicates with the environment through the middle nasal meatus and the nasal vestibule. It is the largest of the paranasal sinuses.

### Development

During the seventh week of intrauterine life, there is ventral shifting of the tongue and the palatine processes assume a horizontal position. They fuse with each other and form the permanent palate. Ventrally, the permanent palate meets and fuses with the primitive palate. Ventral three-fourths of the permanent palate is formed by the fusion of palatine processes with each other and with the caudal edge of the nasal septum. This part undergoes membranous ossification and forms the hard palate. The dorsal one-fourth of the permanent palate fails to fuse with the nasal septum and persists as soft palate. The fusion of the palatine processes and primitive palate takes place from before backward and is completed by the eighth week of intrauterine life. The oral cavity is separated from nasal chambers. There is expansion of the lateral wall of the nasal cavity and it exhibits three curved bony plates, the conchae. The mucous lining of the lateral wall of the nose presents a series of tiny pouches which extend outward into the maxilla, ethmoid, and body of the sphenoid bones at the expense of diploic tissue and form rudimentary paranasal sinuses. The maxillary sinus expands vertically into the body of the maxilla and in the perinatal period, the human maxillary sinus measures about 7-16 mm in the anteroposterior direction, 2-13 mm in superoinferior direction, and 1-7 mm in the mediolateral direction. The maxillary sinus appears to expand and modify in the form until the time of eruption of all permanent teeth.

### Dimension

a. Vertical—3.5 cm.
b. Anteroposterior—3.2 cm.
c. Transverse—2.5 cm.

# The Maxillary Sinus

## Boundaries

Each sinus is roughly pyramidal in shape and presents the following boundaries **(Figs. 7.1 and 7.2)**:

**Apex:** By the zygomatic process of maxilla.

**Base:** By the nasal surface of the body of maxilla, in which lies in the recent state the opening of the maxillary sinus close to its roof.

In the disarticulated skull, the base presents a large opening, the maxillary hiatus, which is reduced in size by the following bones:

- Uncinate process of ethmoid bone, from above.
- Ethmoidal process of inferior nasal concha.
- Descending process of lacrimal bone, from the front.
- Perpendicular plate of palatine bone, from behind.

In macerated skull, two openings are present, one above and the other below the uncinate process; in recent state, usually the lower opening is closed by a plug of mucous membrane.

**Roof:** Roof is formed by the orbital surface of the maxilla which is traversed by the infraorbital vessels and nerve in a bony canal.

**Floor:** Floor is supported by the alveolar process of the maxilla and lies about 1.25 cm below the floor of the nasal cavity. Bony projections containing the roots of molar and premolar teeth affect the floor.

**Anterior wall:** Related to the infraorbital plexus of vessels and nerves and the origins of muscles of the upper lip; within the wall anterior-superior alveolar vessels and nerves traverse in a bony canal, the canalis sinuosus.

**Posterior wall:** It is pierced by posterior superior alveolar vessels and nerves, and

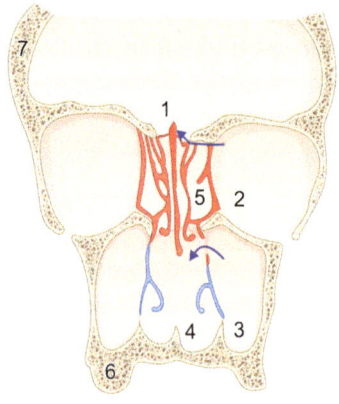

**Fig. 7.1:** Coronal section through skull showing maxillary sinus. 1. Anterior cranial fossa, 2. Orbit, 3. Maxillary sinus, 4. Nasal cavity, 5. Ethmoidal air cell, 6. Alveolar process of maxilla, and 7. Frontal bone.

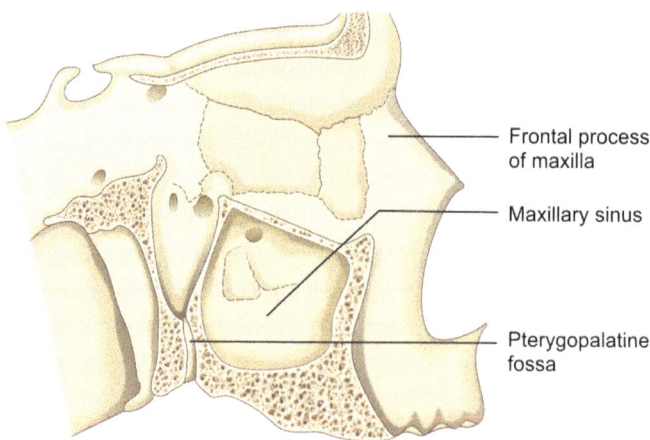

**Fig. 7.2:** Lateral view of sagittal section through the anterior part of skull showing maxillary sinus.

# The Maxillary Sinus

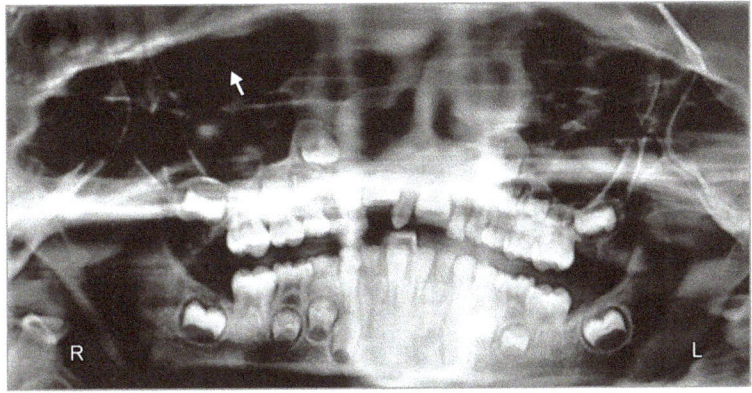

**Fig. 7.3:** OPG showing maxillary sinus.

forms the anterior boundary of infratemporal and pterygopalatine fossae.

## Communication

The maxillary sinus drains into the middle meatus through the floor of hiatus semilunaris and the opening lies just below the bulla ethmoidalis. The opening is located much higher from the floor of the sinus in disadvantageous position for natural drainage.

## Blood Supply

Anterior and middle superior alveolar arteries, branches of the infraorbital arteries. The posterior superior alveolar arteries which are the branches of maxillary artery. The greater palatine artery, a branch of maxillary artery.

## Lymph Drainage

Lymphatic drainage occurs into the submandibular lymph nodes.

## Nerve Supply

The anterior and middle superior alveolar nerves which are branches of infraorbital nerves. Posterior superior alveolar nerve, a branch of maxillary nerve and greater palatine nerve, a branch from the pterygopalatine ganglion.

## Roentgenographic Features

Maxillary sinus is filled with air and radiographically it appears as dark, radiolucent shadow bounded by radiopaque lines representing cortical bones. The radiolucency is not uniform due to superimposition of the zygomatic process and soft tissues of the cheek **(Figs. 7.3 and 7.4)**. The sinus usually extends from premolars to the tuberosity region. The floor of the maxillary sinus is closely related to the root apices of the maxillary teeth.

The most closely related are the roots of the second permanent maxillary molar, especially the apex of its palatal root.

## Microscopic Features

Microscopically, the space of the maxillary sinus is lined by pseudostratified, ciliated,

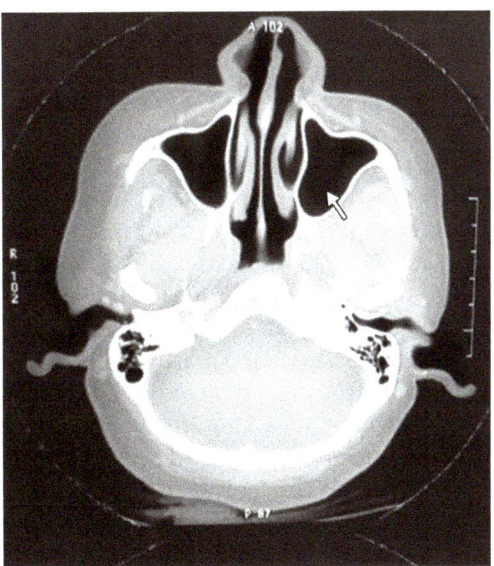

**Fig. 7.4:** CT scan of maxillary sinus.

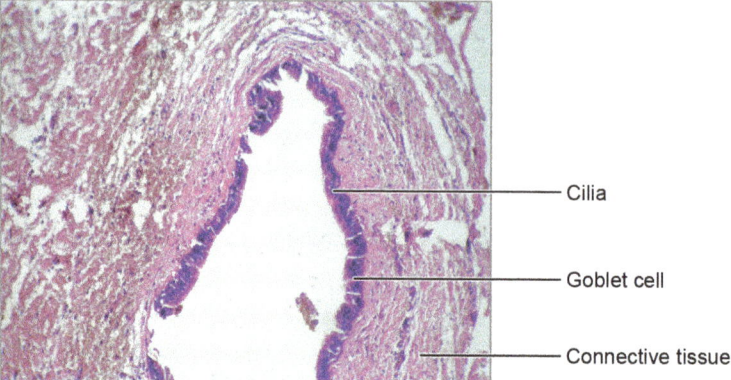

**Fig. 7.5:** Photomicrograph showing lining of maxillary sinus.

columnar epithelium (**Fig. 7.5**), derived from the olfactory epithelium of the middle nasal meatus. There are also numerous mucous-producing goblet cells. The ciliated cell contains nucleus, cytoplasm with numerous mitochondria, and enzyme-containing organelles. The ciliary microtubules are attached to the cells by apical segments. The microtubules provide the motile apparatus and ciliary beating causes movement of mucus from sinus to nasal cavity. The beating pattern and direction are genetically programmed. The epithelial layer is surrounded by subepithelial connective tissue, periosteum, and bone.

## APPLIED ANATOMY

1. Accumulation of infected material in the paranasal sinuses is of frequent occurrence. This is particularly so for maxillary sinus, which being the most dependent part acts as a secondary reservoir for pus from infected frontal or anterior ethmoidal sinuses through hiatus semilunaris. The maxillary sinus surgical drainage is made by breaking the lateral wall of the inferior meatus or through the canine fossa on the anterior surface of the maxilla. Infection of paranasal sinuses is detected by radiological examination, transillumination test, or by proof-puncture.
2. Because of the close relationship of maxillary molar teeth to the maxillary sinus, communication between the sinus and oral cavity (oroantral fistula) following tooth extraction is very common. It is also infected from the carious tooth. Natural drainage from the maxillary sinus is poor, since its opening lies much above the floor. When pus collects in the sinus, it cannot come out through the maxillary hiatus into the nose unless it is filled up to 1.25 cm above the floor as the floor is 1.25 cm below that of the nose.

## QUESTIONNAIRE

1. What are paranasal sinuses? Enumerate paranasal sinuses. Discuss the functions of paranasal sinuses.
2. Discuss structure and microscopic features of maxillary sinus.

## BIBLIOGRAPHY

1. Berkovitz BKB, Holland GR, Moxham BJ. A Colour Atlas and Textbook of Oral Anatomy, Histology and Embryology, 4th edition. Mosby: Elsevier; 2009.
2. Dutta AK. Essentials of Human Anatomy, Head and Neck, 5th edition. West Bengal: Current Books International; 2010.
3. Dutta AK. Essentials of Human Embryology, 6th edition. West Bengal: Current Books International; 2010.
4. Kumar GS. Orban's Oral Histology and Embryology, 12th edition. Mosby: Elsevier; 2009.
5. Romanes GJ. Cunningham's Manual of Practical Anatomy, 15th edition. London: Oxford University Press; 2002. p. 3.

# CHAPTER 8

# Occlusion

The study of occlusion is an important aspect of all specialties of dentistry. It is a complex phenomenon involving the teeth, periodontal ligament, the jaws, the temporomandibular joint, the muscles, and the nervous system.

## DEFINITION

Occlusion is defined as the relationship between the occlusal surfaces of the maxillary and mandibular teeth when they are in contact.

There are three concepts of occlusion in dentistry:
1. *Prosthetic concept*: This is balanced occlusion maintained for full dentures. Functional stability is obtained by bilateral teeth contacts in lateral and protrusive movements.
2. *Orthodontic concept:* This is static occlusion, a norm of occlusion based on cusp–fossa relationship.
3. *Dynamic individual occlusion*: This concept not only considers relation between the teeth, but also other associated structures like the periodontium, the masticatory muscles, the temporomandibular joint, etc.

Occlusion has three components:
1. Interdigitation of teeth of upper and lower jaw.
2. Status of controlling musculature.
3. Morphology and function of temporomandibular joint.

## FEW TERMINOLOGIES

### Balanced Occlusion

It is a type of occlusion where there is simultaneous contact of the upper and lower teeth on the right and left and in the anterior and posterior occlusal areas in centric or any eccentric position. So in this occlusion, balanced and equal contacts are maintained throughout the entire arch during all excursions of the mandible. It is a prosthetic concept of occlusion. It is developed to prevent a tipping or rotating of the denture bases in relation to the supporting structures.

### Centric Relation

It is the relation of the mandible to the maxilla when the mandibular condyles are in the most unstrained, superior, and retruded position in their glenoid fossa with the articular disk properly interposed.

### Centric Occlusion

It refers to the maximum intercuspation of opposing teeth when mandible is in its centric relation.

In centric occlusion and centric relation, mandible is neither protruded nor retruded, neither deviated to right or left. There is full intercuspation and a harmonious balance between the teeth, joint, and neuromuscular system.

### Eccentric Occlusion

It refers to contact of teeth that occurs during movement of mandible. It is of two types:
1. **Functional occlusion** refers to tooth contacts that occur in the segment of the arch, toward which the mandible moves.
2. **Nonfunctional occlusion** refers to tooth contacts that occur in the segment of the arch away from which mandible moves.

### Physiologic Rest Position

It is the postural relation of the mandible to the maxillae when the patient is resting comfortably in upright position and condyles are in a neutral unstrained position in the glenoid fossa. In this position, the teeth of upper and lower jaws are not in contact and the space between the upper and lower teeth is called the freeway space. This measures on average 2–5 mm at incisor area. This position is obtained when all the jaw muscles are at rest. The lips are generally closed. It is constant throughout life and is not dependent on the presence or absence of teeth. All functional movements begin and end with rest position.

### Curve
A nonangular deviation from a straight line.

### Compensating Curve
The anteroposterior and lateral curvature in the alignment of occluding surfaces and incisal edges of artificial teeth which is used to develop balanced occlusion.

### Curve of Spee
It refers to the anteroposterior curvature of the occlusal surfaces beginning at the tip of the lower cuspid and following the cusp tips of the bicuspids and molars continuing as an arc through the condyle **(Fig. 8.1)** as described by Von Spee. The mandibular curve of Spee is concave whereas the maxillary curve is convex. The curves of Spee may help the achievement of occlusal balance during mastication by encouraging simultaneous contact in more than one area of the dental arch.

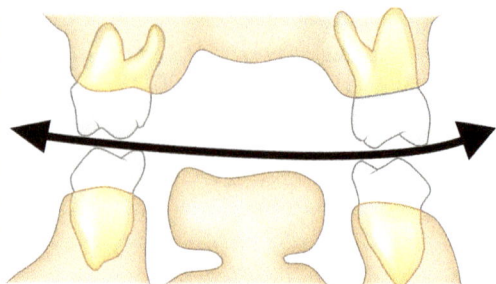

**Fig. 8.2:** Curve of Wilson.

### Curve of Wilson
This is a mediolateral curve on each side of the arch and it contacts the buccal and lingual cusp tips of the maxillary and mandibular posterior teeth **(Fig. 8.2)**. Analysis of the alignment of the long axis of the posterior teeth shows that curves of Wilson are such that the occlusal surfaces of the mandibular molars are directed lingually while the six of the maxillary molars are directed buccally.

### Curve of Monson
The curve of occlusion in which each cusp and incisal edge touches or conforms to a segment of the surface of a sphere 8 inches in diameter with its center in the region of glabella. The curve of Monson is obtained by extending the curve of Spee and curve of Wilson to all cusps and incisal edges.

### Bonwill Triangle
It is an equilateral triangle of 4 inch arm, bounded by lines from contact points of lower central incisors to condyle on either side and from one condyle to the other **(Fig. 8.3)**.

### Plane of Occlusion
It is an imaginary curved surface that touches the incisal edges of incisors and the tips of the occluding surfaces of the posterior teeth.

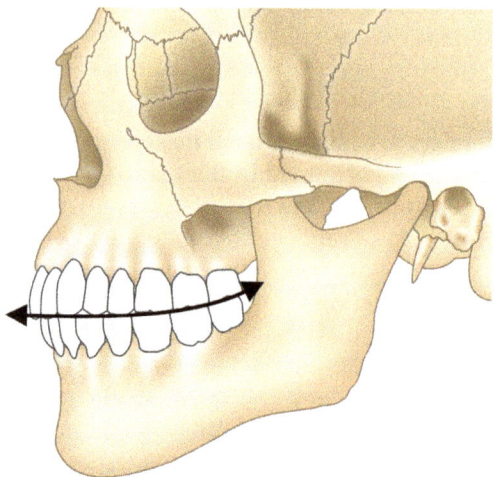

**Fig. 8.1:** Curve of Spee.

# Occlusion

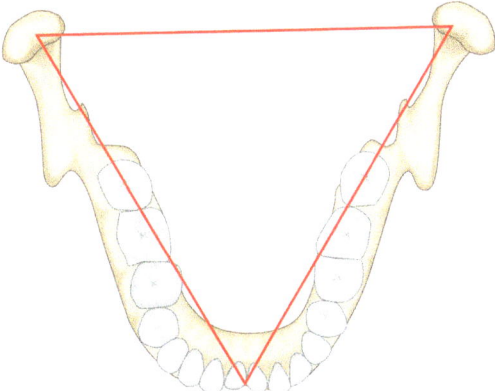

**Fig. 8.3:** Bonwill triangle.

## Incisal Guidance

It refers to the influence of the lingual surfaces of the maxillary incisors on movement of the mandible and is expressed in degrees with the horizontal line.

## Incisal Guide Angle

The angle formed with the horizontal plane by drawing a line in the sagittal plane between the incisal edges of the maxillary and mandibular central incisors when the teeth are in centric occlusion.

## Condylar Guidance

It refers to the path that the horizontal rotation axis of the condyles travels during normal mandibular opening. It is expressed in degrees with the Frankfort plane.

## Guiding Inclines

These are lingual inclines of the buccal cusps of the maxillary posterior teeth, the lingual inclines of the maxillary anteriors, and the buccal inclines of the lingual cusps of the mandibular posterior teeth. The guiding inclines are planes that determine the path of supporting cusps during lateral and protrusive movements.

## DEVELOPMENT OF OCCLUSION

### At Birth

At birth, the oral mucosa over developing alveoli is greatly thickened to form the maxillary and mandibular gum pads.

They show a series of elevations **(Figs. 8.4A and B)** corresponding to underlying deciduous teeth. The elevations associated with the second deciduous molars become prominent at the age of about 6 months.

The groove that marks the distal margin of the canine segment continues into the buccal sulcus and is called lateral sulcus.

The upper arch is horseshoe-shaped and the vault of the palate is very shallow. The alveolar part is separated on its palatal side from the hard palate by a continuous horizontal groove known as the dental or gingival groove. The lower arch is U-shaped and anteriorly the gum pad is slightly everted labially.

The maxillary and mandibular gum pads rarely come into occlusion **(Fig. 8.5)**. The space left between them is occupied by tongue and it projects against the lips anteriorly, the lower lip forming the principal boundary to the front of the oral cavity. The upper lip appears to be very short at this age. The maxillary gum pad overlaps the mandibular gum pad both buccally and labially.

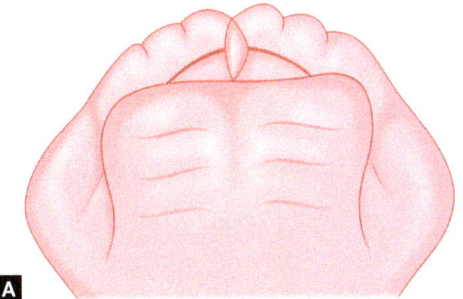
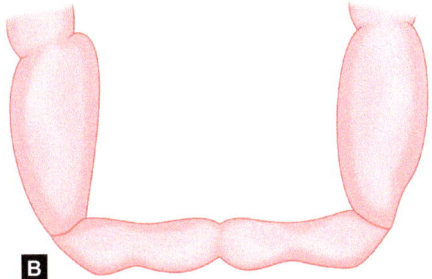

**Figs. 8.4A and B:** Gum pads at birth: (A) Maxillary; (B) Mandibular.

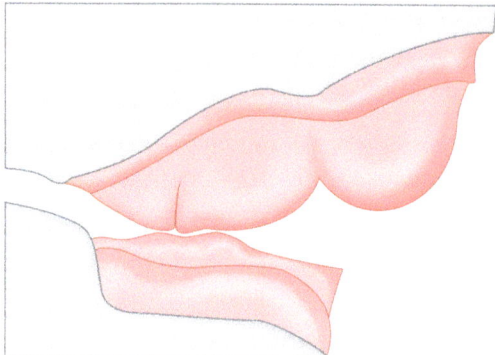

**Fig. 8.5:** Gum pads in occlusion.

The gum pads at birth are not sufficiently wide to accommodate the developing incisors which are crowded and rotated in their crypts, the lateral being rotated distolingually.

During the first year of life, the gum pads grow rapidly, especially in lateral direction. This ultimately permits incisors to erupt in good alignment, helped by pressure from tongue and lips.

## The Deciduous Dentition

The deciduous teeth start to erupt at the age of 6 months and are complete by the age of 3 years. At this time, the occlusion of the deciduous dentition differs from that of the permanent dentition in the following respects **(Figs. 8.6A and B)**:
1. The incisors are more vertically positioned within alveolus and are often spaced.
2. The overbite is usually greater.
3. There may be significant spacings distal to the mandibular canines and mesial to the maxillary canines (the "anthropoid" or primate spacings) **(Fig. 8.7)**.

The distal edges of the maxillary and mandibular deciduous molars are flush **(Fig. 8.8)** and the mesiobuccal cusps of the maxillary first and second deciduous molars occlude in the buccal grooves of the mandibular first and second deciduous molars, respectively.

## Changes in Deciduous Occlusion

Several changes occur in the deciduous occlusion before the appearance of the permanent teeth.
1. The dental arches become wider and longer and the deciduous teeth become more spaced.

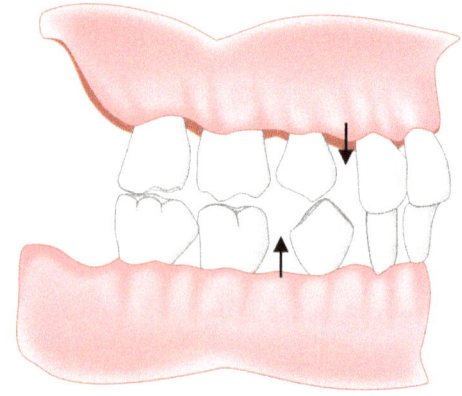

**Fig. 8.7:** Primate spaces.

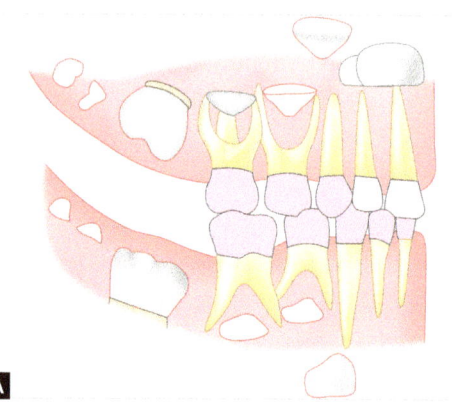

A

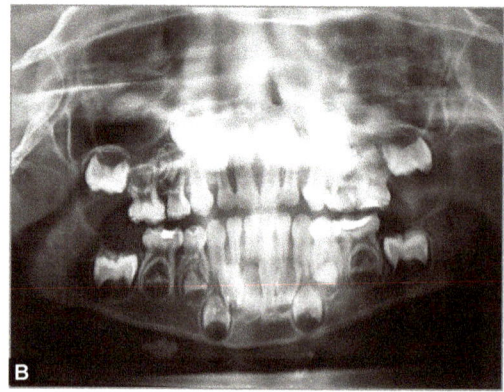

B

**Figs. 8.6A and B:** (A) Dentition at 3 years; (B) OPG showing dentition at 3 years.

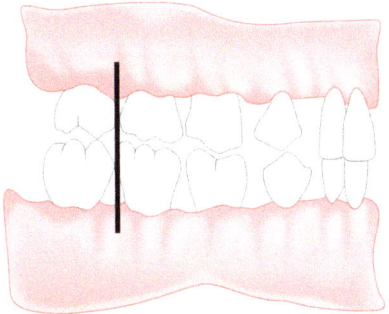

Fig. 8.8: Flush terminal plane.

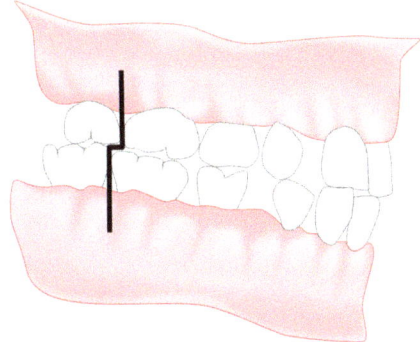

Fig. 8.10: Distal step terminal plane.

2. There is a greater forward growth of the mandible compared to the maxilla. So the lower arch moves forward relative to the upper and that leads to an edge-to-edge incisor relationship.
3. The distal surfaces of the deciduous second molars show a slight mesial step from maxilla to mandible, the mesiobuccal cusp of the maxillary second deciduous molar lying distal to the buccal groove of the mandibular second deciduous molar (**Fig. 8.9**).
Distal step terminal plane (**Fig. 8.10**) is characterized by the distal surface of mandibular second deciduous molar being more distal to that of maxillary one.
4. The deciduous teeth may show signs of considerable wear at the end of their functional lives.

## The Mixed Dentition

After the age of 6 years, the dentition is said to be mixed, comprising both deciduous and permanent teeth.

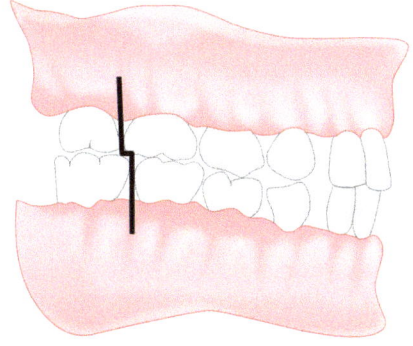

Fig. 8.9: Mesial step terminal plane.

### The Permanent Incisors

The permanent incisors erupt between the ages of 6 years and 9 years (**Figs. 8.11A to C**). The permanent incisors are larger than their deciduous predecessors. So they are accommodated in the dental arch by:
- Utilization of existing spacing between deciduous incisors.
- An increase in intercanine width during the eruption of the incisors.
- The maxillary permanent incisors are more proclined and thus form a larger arch than deciduous incisors.

When the permanent incisors erupt, they fan out (incline distally), so that there may be a significant space or diastema between the central incisors. This appearance has been termed as "ugly duckling" stage (**Figs. 8.12A and B**) and is said to result from pressure on the roots of the permanent incisors from the developing permanent canines. The diastema usually closes following eruption of the permanent canines.

### The Permanent Canines and Premolars

The canines and premolars usually erupt between the ages of 9 years and 12 years (**Fig. 8.13**). They are readily accommodated into the dental arches, as the combined mesiodistal width of the permanent canines and premolars is usually less than that of deciduous canines and molars.

The surplus space, the Leeway space (**Fig. 8.14**), is greater in the lower arch (1.7 mm) and lesser in the upper arch (0.9 mm). The

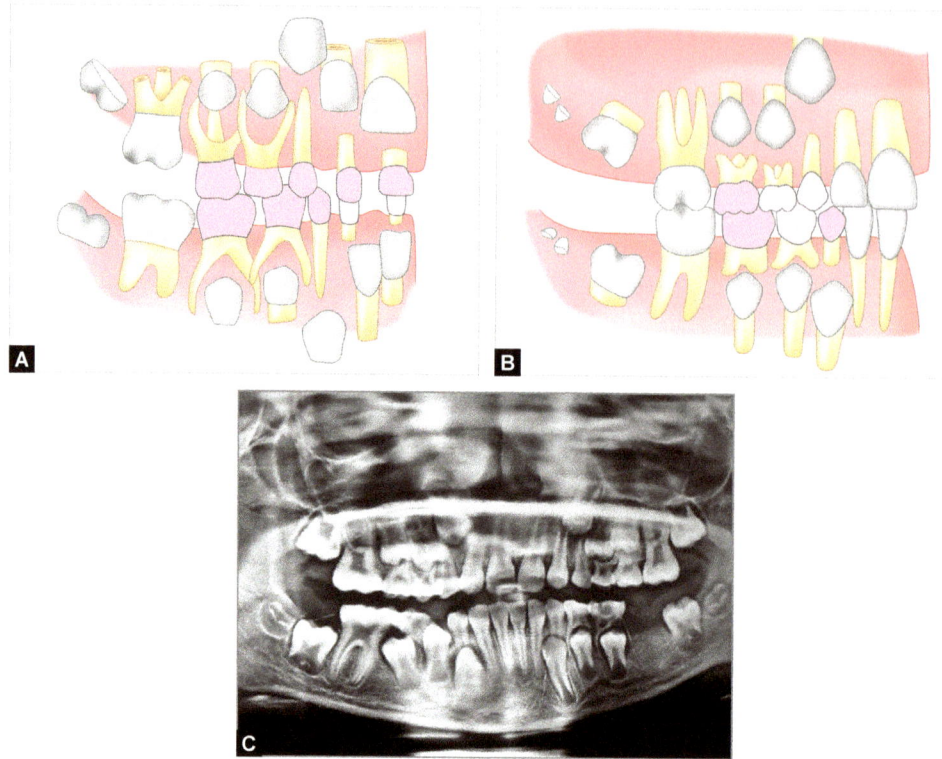

**Figs. 8.11A to C:** (A) Dentition at 6 years; (B) Dentition at 9 years; (C) OPG showing dentition at 9 years.

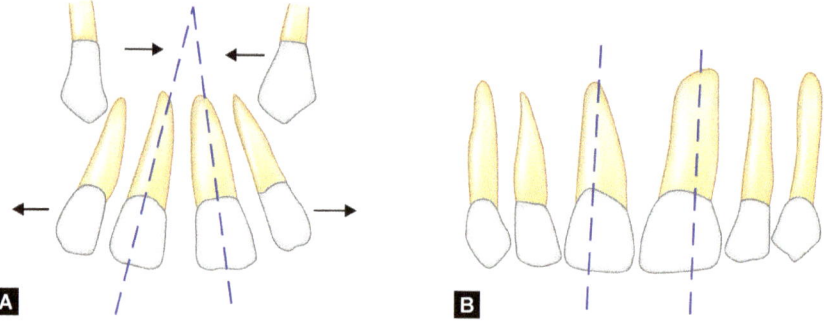

**Figs. 8.12A and B:** Ugly duckling stage: (A) Distal flairing of incisor crowns as canine crowns impinge on roots of lateral incisors; (B) Closure of midline space due to eruption of canine.

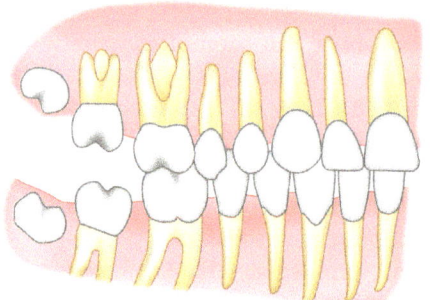

**Fig. 8.13:** Dentition at the age of 12 years.

extra space in the lower arch is taken up by the mesial drift of the first permanent molars.

### The Permanent Molars

The first molars are first permanent tooth to erupt. These are guided into a cusp-to-cusp relationship by the distal surfaces of the second deciduous molars. When the second deciduous molars are shed, the greater Leeway space in the lower arch allows the lower first permanent molars to move forward

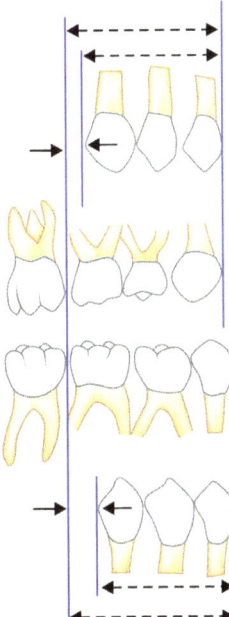

**Fig. 8.14:** Leeway space.

into a correct cuspal relationship with the upper. The second permanent molars should be guided directly into occlusion by the first permanent molars.

## The Permanent Dentition

- The mandibular teeth are set in one inclined plane in advance of the maxillary teeth. This is so because the mandibular central incisor is smaller mesiodistally than the maxillary central incisor.
- The maxillary teeth are half a cusp to the buccal of the mandibular teeth (i.e. they are not cusp-to-cusp).
- The mesiobuccal cusp of the maxillary first permanent molar occludes with the anterior buccal groove of the mandibular first permanent molar. The distobuccal cusp of the maxillary first permanent molar occludes in the embrasure between the mandibular first and second permanent molars.
- The maxillary permanent canine occludes in the embrasure between the mandibular permanent canine and first premolar.
- The maxillary incisors overlap the mandibular incisors in two planes.

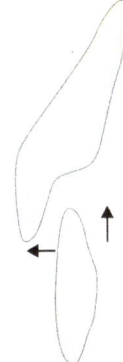

**Fig. 8.15:** Overjet and overbite.

The overlap in the horizontal plane which is known as overjet (**Fig. 8.15**) is approximately 2–3 mm.
- The vertical overlap, peculiar to incisors and canines, is termed overbite (**Fig. 8.15**). The overbite in anatomical centric occlusion is such that the palatal surfaces of the maxillary incisors overlap the incisal third of the labial surfaces of the mandibular incisors.

## Changes in the Permanent Occlusion

- There is a tendency for the mandible to grow slightly further forward than the maxilla after the age of 12 years. Usually, there is no appreciable occlusal change.
- During the later stages of facial growth, there may be an accompanying uprighting of the incisors and they become more crowded.
- Mesial drift may take up any remaining space in the arches and it is responsible for some late crowding.

**Mesial drift:** Wear at the contact points between the teeth, i.e. interproximal wear, is compensated for by a process known as mesial drift. Mesial drift may involve considerable bodily movement of the tooth. Between the ages of 6 years and 18 years, the first permanent molar drifts approximately 4 mm in a mesial direction. Four hypotheses have been postulated to account for this movement:
1. The mesial inclination of teeth produces a resultant force during biting that favors mesial drift.

2. The action of certain jaw muscles, particularly the buccinator, "propels" the teeth forward.
3. Bone deposited preferentially on the distal surface of the sockets pushes the teeth mesially.
4. Contraction of the transseptal fiber system pulls the teeth mesially.

## Cephalometry

It is a standardized radiographic technique of the craniofacial region. It is introduced by Broadbent in the year 1931. It is of considerable importance not only in the study of growth and development but also in clinical evaluation of orthodontic patients.

Cephalometric radiographs are taken under standardized conditions so that measurements can be compared between patients and for the same patient on different occasions. The cephalometric lateral skull radiograph is taken with the head held in a cephalostat, so that the midsagittal plane is at a fixed distance from, and parallel to the film. The target of the X-ray tube is also at a fixed distance from the film, with the central ray directed through the ear rods of the cephalostat, so the enlargement at the midsagittal plane is constant.

The common cephalometric landmarks used in dentistry (**Fig. 8.16**) are as follows:

**Basion (Ba):** The most inferior and posterior point on the basiocciput, lying on the anterior margin of the foramen magnum.

**Sella point (S):** Center of shadow of sella turcica (pituitary fossa).

**Nasion (N):** Junction between frontal and nasal bones in midline on the frontonasal suture.

**Porion (P):** Highest bony point of margin of external acoustic meatus.

**Orbitale (Or):** Lowest point of infraorbital margin.
- Anterior nasal spine (ANS)
- Posterior nasal spine (PNS).

**Subspinale (A):** Position of greatest concavity of maxillary alveolus in the midline.

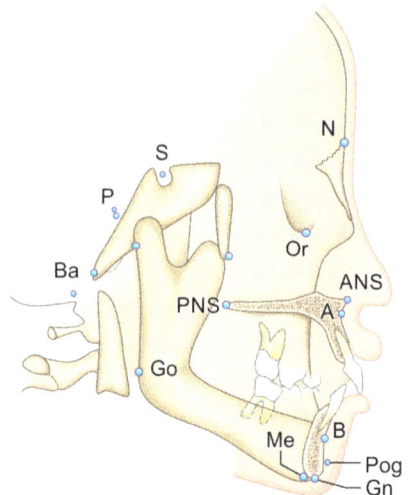

**Fig. 8.16:** Cephalometric landmarks (see text for description).

**Supermentale (B):** Position of greatest concavity of mandibular alveolus in the midline.

**Pogonion (Pog):** Most anterior point on the chin.

**Menton (Me):** Lowest point of the chin.

**Gnathion (Gn):** Point between the most anterior and inferior points of chin established by bisecting the angle formed between the N-pog and mandibular planes.

**Gonion (Go):** Most inferior and posterior point at the angle of the mandible established by bisecting the angle formed between the planes through the lower border of the mandible and posterior border of ramus.

## QUESTIONNAIRE

1. Define occlusion. Discuss development of occlusion at birth, deciduous dentition, and mixed dentition.
2. Write notes on:
    A. Centric occlusion.
    B. Balanced occlusion.
    C. Curve of Spee.
    D. Bonwill triangle.
    E. Leeway space.
    F. Ugly duckling stage.
    G. Cephalometry.

## BIBLIOGRAPHY

1. Berkovitz BKB, Holland GR, Moxham BJ. A Colour Atlas and Textbook of Oral Anatomy, Histology and Embryology, 4th edition. Mosby: Elsevier; 2009.
2. Bhalajhi SI. Orthodontics: The Art and Science, 2th edition. New Delhi: Arya (Medi) Publishing House; 1999.
3. Das AK. Dental Anatomy and Oral Histology, 1st edition. West Bengal: Current Books International; 1972.
4. Houston WJB, Stephens CD, Tulley WJ. A Textbook of Orthodontics, 2nd edition. Bristol: Wright; 1992.
5. Nelson SJ, Ash MJ. Wheeler's Dental Anatomy, Physiology and Occlusion, 9th edition. Philadelphia: Elsevier; 2010.
6. Rani MS. Synopsis of Orthodontics, 1st edition. New Delhi: All India Publishers and Distributors; 1993.

# CHAPTER 9

# Histological Techniques for Study of Oral Tissues

Histology (Greek *Histos*—tissue + *logos*—study) is the study of tissues. It is a science based on the ability to recognize the architectural patterns and cytomorphology of normal tissues. The small size of the cells and matrix components make histology dependent on the use of the microscopes.

## MICROSCOPY

Microscopy is the technical field of using microscopes to view samples and objects that cannot be seen with the unaided eye (objects that are not within the resolution range of the normal eye).

### Light Microscopy

Optical or light microscopy involves passing visible light transmitted through or reflected from the sample through a single or multiple lenses to allow a magnified view of the sample. The resulting image can be detected directly by the eye, imaged on a photographic plate or captured digitally. The single lens with its attachments, or the system of lenses and imaging equipment, along with the appropriate lighting equipment, sample stage, and support, makes up the basic light microscope. Different types of light microscopes are available for the study of tissues.

### Bright-field Microscope

This is a complex, optical instrument which uses visible light. This is the most commonly used microscope. The specimen to be viewed with this microscope needs to be sufficiently thin so that the light can pass through it. The usefulness of this light microscope is its ability to magnify and, more importantly, its ability to resolve structural detail.

With a conventional bright-field microscope, light from an incandescent source is aimed toward a lens beneath the stage called the condenser, through the specimen, through an objective lens, and to the eye through a second magnifying lens, the ocular or eyepiece. A good quality microscope has a built-in illuminator, adjustable condenser with aperture diaphragm (contrast) control, mechanical stage, and binocular eyepiece tube (**Fig. 9.1**). The condenser is used to focus light on the specimen through an opening in the stage. After passing through the specimen, the light is displayed to the eye with an apparent field that is much larger than the area illuminated. The magnification of the image is simply the objective lens magnification times the ocular magnification.

### Dark Ground Illumination

This method allows only that light which is scattered at the periphery of the specimen. It is mainly used for the study of the spirochetes and other microbes, which look like bright objects against a dark background.

### Phase-contrast Microscope

It is used for the examination of unstained specimens especially living cells from body or tissue culture. This technique exploits the fact that light slows slightly when passing through biological specimens. The specimen is illuminated by a hollow cone of light coming through a phase annulus in the condenser. Phase-contrast objectives must be used, which have a corresponding phase plate. Light rays passing through the specimen are

# Histological Techniques for Study of Oral Tissues

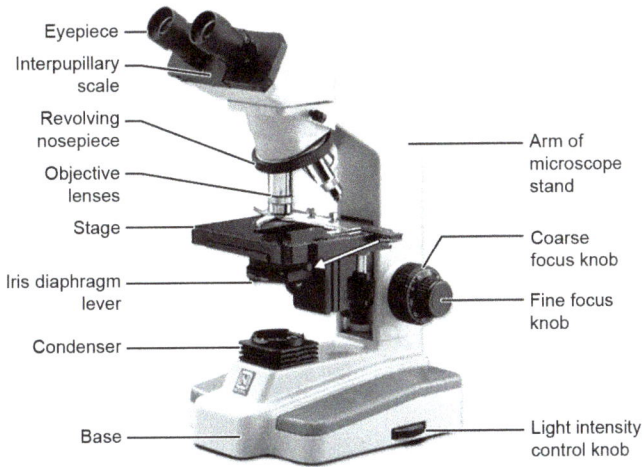

**Fig. 9.1:** Bright-field binocular microscope.

slightly retarded, and further retardation takes place in the phase plate. When these rays combine with rays which have not taken this path, degrees of constructive and destructive interference occur which produce the characteristic light and dark features in image **(Fig. 9.2)**.

## Fluorescence Microscope

The fluorescence microscope detects molecules which are fluorescent, i.e. emit light of wavelengths in the visible range when exposed to an ultraviolet light source. It is used in the detection of the antigens and antibodies in immunocytochemical staining procedure and also in detecting fluorescent growth markers of the mineralized tissues. The key feature of fluorescence microscopy is that it employs reflected rather than transmitted light.

## Confocal Scanning Microscope

This microscope is used to study the structure of the biological material. In the confocal microscope, all out-of-focus structures are suppressed at image formation. This is obtained by an arrangement of diaphragms, which, at optically conjugated points of the path of rays, act as a point source and as a point detector, respectively. The detection pinhole does not permit rays of light from out-of-focus points to pass through it. The wavelength of light, the numerical aperture of the objective, and the diameter of the diaphragm (wider detection pinhole reduces the confocal effect) affect the depth of the focal plane. To obtain a full image, the point of light is moved across the specimen by scanning mirrors. The emitted/reflected light passing through the detector pinhole is transformed into electrical signals by a photomultiplier and displayed on a computer monitor.

## Ultraviolet Microscope

This microscope uses an ultraviolet light source and depends on the absorption of ultraviolet light by the molecules in the specimen. This method is useful for detecting nucleic acid.

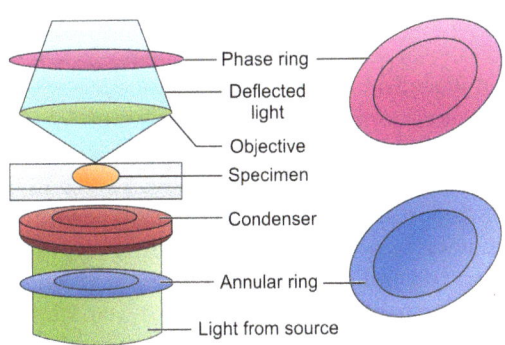

**Fig. 9.2:** Phase-contrast microscope.

## Polarizing Microscope

The polarizing microscope is a simple modification of the light microscope in which polarized light is passed through the specimen and another polarizer is used as a rotator to detect molecular orientation within a tissue sample. Crystalline substances and well-ordered fibrous molecules alter the plane of the entering polarized light and altered plane of light is noted with the detector lens. The rotation of polarized light due to the molecular orientation of tissue components is referred to as birefringence. Enamel, dentin, and cemental tissues show birefringence under polarized light.

The polarized light microscope must be equipped with both—a polarizer, positioned in the light path somewhere before the specimen, and an analyzer (a second polarizer), placed in the optical pathway after the objective rear aperture. Image contrast arises from the interaction of plane-polarized light with a birefringent (or doubly-refracting) specimen to produce two individual wave components that are each polarized in mutually perpendicular planes. The velocities of these components are different and vary with the propagation direction through the specimen. After exiting the specimen, the light components become out of phase, but are recombined with constructive and destructive interference when they pass through the analyzer. Polarized-light microscopy can be used to measure the amount of retardation that occurs in each direction and so it gives information about the molecular structure of the birefringent object.

## Electron Microscopy

An electron microscope is a type of microscope that uses a beam of electrons to illuminate the specimen and produce a magnified image. Electron microscopes (EM) have a greater resolving power than a light-powered optical microscope, because electrons have wavelengths about 100,000 times shorter than visible light (photons), and can achieve better than 50 nm resolution and magnifications of up to about 10,000,000x, whereas ordinary, nonconfocal light microscopes are limited by diffraction to about 200 nm resolution and useful magnifications below 2,000x.

The electron microscope uses electrostatic and electromagnetic "lenses" to control the electron beam and focus it to form an image. These lenses are analogous to, but different from the glass lenses of an optical microscope that form a magnified image by focusing light on or through the specimen. Electron microscopes are used to observe a wide range of biological and inorganic specimens including microorganisms, cells, large molecules, and biopsy samples.

## Transmission Electron Microscope

Transmission electron microscope (TEM) utilizes a beam of electrons instead of light in producing an image. It involves the passage of a high-velocity homogeneous electron beam through a specimen that is thin enough to transmit at least 50% of the incident electrons. The emergent beam of transmitted electrons is then referred by a system of lenses to form a magnified, two-dimensional image of the specimen. The original form of electron microscope, the TEM, uses a high-voltage electron beam to create an image. The electrons are emitted by an electron gun, commonly fitted with a tungsten filament cathode as the electron source. The electron beam is accelerated by an anode typically at +100 keV (40–00 keV) with respect to the cathode, focused by electrostatic and electromagnetic lenses, and transmitted through the specimen that is in part transparent to electrons and in part scatters them out of the beam. When it emerges from the specimen, the electron beam carries information about the structure of the specimen that is magnified by the objective lens system of the microscope. The spatial variation in this information (the "image") may be viewed by projecting the magnified electron image onto a fluorescent viewing screen coated with a phosphor or scintillator material such as zinc sulfide. Alternatively, the image can be photographically recorded by exposing a photographic film or plate directly to the electron beam, or a high-resolution phosphor may be coupled by means of a lens optical system or a fiber optic light guide to the sensor of a CCD (charge-coupled device) camera. The image detected by the CCD may be displayed on a monitor or computer.

## Scanning Electron Microscope (SEM)

Scanning electron microscopy differs from transmission electron microscopy in that the electrons do not pass through the specimen as part of the image-making process. Instead, a beam of electrons is made to scan the surface views. Inside of the organs can be analyzed by freezing the organs and fracturing them to expose their internal surfaces. Unlike the TEM, where electrons of the high-voltage beam carry the image of the specimen, the electron beam of the scanning electron microscope (SEM) does not at any time carry a complete image of the specimen. The SEM produces images by probing the specimen with a focused electron beam that is scanned across a rectangular area of the specimen. When the electron beam interacts with the specimen, it loses energy by a variety of mechanisms. The lost energy is converted into alternative forms such as heat and emission of low-energy secondary electrons and high-energy backscattered electrons, which provide signals carrying information about the properties of the specimen surface, such as its topography and composition.

## FEW ANALYTICAL METHODS

### Autoradiography

It is the study of the biological events in the tissue sections using radioactivity. Various information like divisions of cells, site of protein synthesis, pathway of migration of cell, etc., can be obtained by autoradiography.

### Historadiography

It is actually the production of an X-ray photograph, that is, microradiograph of a specimen on a slide. It is used for quantitative analysis of bone or other mineralized tissues.

## Cell and Tissue Culture

Live cells and tissues can be maintained and studied outside the body. Cell culture has been widely used for the study of the metabolism of normal and cancerous cells, for the development of new drugs, and for the study of chromosomes.

## Histochemistry and Cytochemistry

The terms histochemistry and cytochemistry are used mainly to indicate methods for localizing different substances in tissue section. The procedures are based on specific chemical reactions or on high-affinity interactions between macromolecules. These methods usually produce insoluble colored or electron-dense compounds that enable the localization of specific substances by means of light or electron microscopy.

## ROUTINE LABORATORY TECHNIQUES FOR HISTOLOGIC STUDY

There are different procedures for preparation of tissues for microscopic examination:
1. Paraffin embedding
2. Frozen section
3. Parlodion embedding
4. Ground section

## Paraffin-embedding Procedure

### Indications

1. This is the most commonly used method of preparing tissues for microscopic examination.
2. Both soft tissue and decalcified hard tissues can be prepared by this method.

### Procedure

**Obtaining the specimen:**
- The specimen is surgically removed with minimum trauma.
- Blood clot is removed under running tap water.

## Histological Techniques for Study of Oral Tissues

**Fixation of the specimen:**
- The specimen is fixed in 10% neutral formalin for 24 hours.
- The fixative solution will coagulate the proteins and preserve the tissue.
- It prevents alteration of tissues by subsequent treatment.
- It makes tissue more readily permeable to the subsequent applications of reagent.
- After fixation, the specimen is washed overnight in running tap water.

**Dehydration of the specimen:**
- The specimen is gradually dehydrated in ascending grades of alcohol (40%, 60%, 80%, 95%, and absolute alcohol), 1 hour in each strength.
- The specimen is dehydrated as the subsequent infiltration and embedding are done in molten paraffin which is not miscible with water.

**Clearing:**
- The paraffin is also not miscible with the alcohol. So the alcohol is removed from the specimen by placing it in two changes of xylene, one hour in each.
- Xylene is miscible with both alcohol and paraffin.
- The specimen appears transparent after xylene treatment, hence the name of the step is clearing.

Infiltration of the specimen with paraffin:
- As alcohol in the tissue is totally replaced by xylene, the specimen is ready to be infiltrated in paraffin.
- From xylene, the tissue is placed in three changes of molten paraffin at 60°C in hot air oven, 1 hour in each.

**Embedding the specimen:**
- After infiltration, the tissue is embedded in the center of a block of paraffin.
- Two L-shaped brass pieces (Leuckhard L-pieces) are adjusted to a required size and shape on a metal platform and it is filled with molten paraffin.
- The infiltrated tissue is taken from molten paraffin with a warm forceps and is placed in the center of the box of paraffin with the surface to be cut first toward the bottom of the box.
- The hardened paraffin block is removed, trimmed so that there is about 3 mm of paraffin surrounding the specimen on all four sides, and fixed on a wooden block.

**Cutting sections:**
- The wooden cube to which the paraffin block is attached is clamped on a precision rotary microtome **(Fig. 9.3)**.
- The microtome is adjusted to cut sections of the desired thickness (usually 4–10 mm) and the perfectly sharpened microtome knife is clamped into place for sectioning.
- The sections are placed on warm water bath to spread flat. It is transferred on glass slide, smeared with a mixture of egg albumin in glycerine, and placed on a hot air oven at 42°C for adhering the tissues to the slides.

**Staining the sections:**
- Paraffin is removed from the section by xylene, which is removed by absolute alcohol and the section is brought back to water by treatment with descending grades of alcohol followed by placing it under running tap water.
- The slide is placed in hematoxylin for 5–10 minutes to stain nuclei.
- The section is then placed in distilled water to rinse off excess stain.
- The section is differentiated in ammonium alum.

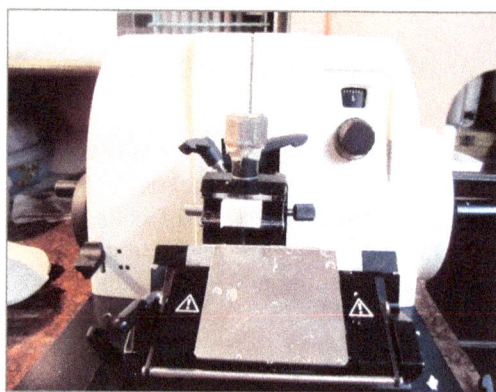

**Fig. 9.3:** Precision rotary microtome.

- Then dipped in eosin solution for 1 minute to stain cytoplasm and intercellular substance.
- The section is washed with distilled water, treated with ascending grades of alcohol, cleared with xylene, mounted with DPX (Dibutylphthalate polystyrene xylene-non-aqueous mounting medium for histology) and cover glass is affixed.
- After the mounting medium hardens, the slides are ready for examination.

## Preparation of Frozen Sections

The fresh, unfixed, or fixed soft tissue may be frozened and sectioned without being embedded.

Such tissue sections are usually referred to as frozen sections.

## Indications

1. It is indicated when immediate histologic examination of a specimen is required.
2. It is also indicated for certain histochemical analysis when the tissue characteristics to be studied would be destroyed by the reagents used in paraffin embedding.
A block of fixed or unfixed soft tissue is frozen with either liquid or solid carbon dioxide.
Sections are taken from frozen tissue in a freezing microtome having 10–15 mm thickness.

## Preparation of Sections of Parlodion-embedded Specimens

## Indications

1. It is indicated for microscopic examination of the delicate pulp tissue and periodontal ligament along with dentin and cementum.
2. It is also indicated for histologic examination of bone with bony matrix.
Tooth and bone specimens are to be decalcified and embedded in parlodion as it is very difficult to get good sections if they are embedded in paraffin.

*Procedure*

1. Obtaining the specimen.
2. Fixation in 10% neutral formalin for a week.
3. Decalcification in any of the following solutions:
    a. 5% nitric acid
    b. 5% formic acid
    c. Mixture of potassium formate and formic acid

    The specimen is suspended in any of the solutions for several days and the solution is changed every day till there is complete decalcification. The specimen may be X-rayed from time to time, a needle may be inserted through the specimen, or the solution may be tested chemically to determine the extent of decalcification.
4. Washing the specimen in running tap water for several hours to remove all of the acid.
5. Dehydration in ascending grades of alcohol. Then specimen is changed to 1:1 proportion of ether and absolute alcohol (as parlodion is dissolved in ether alcohol).
6. Infiltration of the specimen with parlodion.
7. Embedding the specimen in parlodion.
8. *Cutting the sections*: The sections are cut in a precision sliding microtome at a thickness of 15 mm.
9. *Staining the sections*: The sections are first stained with hematoxylin and eosin and then mounted on a slide.

## Preparation of Ground Sections of Teeth or Bone

## Indications

1. Enamel is studied histologically only by ground section as it contains 96% of inorganic material.
2. Inorganic component of dentin, cementum, and bone may be studied by making thin ground sections.

## Equipment

a. A laboratory lathe (**Fig. 9.4**)
b. A coarse and a fine abrasive lathe wheel
c. A stream of water directed onto the rotating wheel

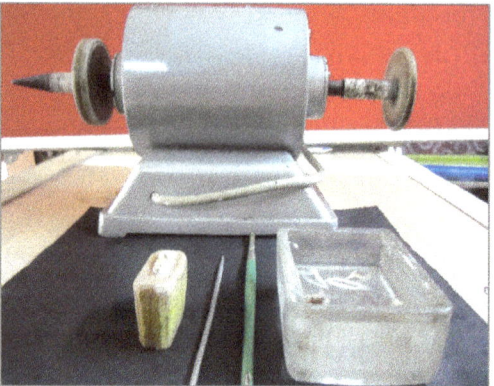

Fig. 9.4: Laboratory lathe.

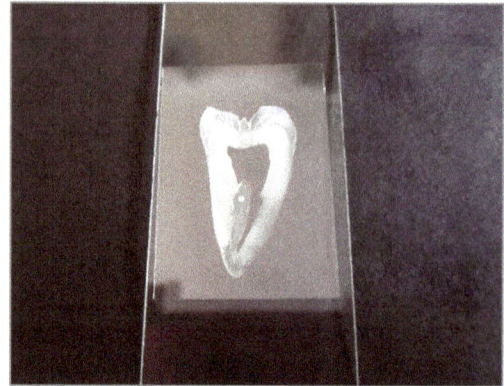

Fig. 9.6: Longitudinal ground section of tooth.

d. A pan beneath to collect the water
e. A wooden block (25 mm³ cube)
f. 13 mm adhesive tape
g. A camel's hair brush
h. Ether
i. Mounting medium
j. Microscope
k. Cover glasses

## Procedure

- The tooth or bone with the desired plane of section is fixed onto a wooden block by means of adhesive tape in longitudinal direction and the wooden block with the tooth is held securely and firmly against the flat surface of rapidly rotating coarse abrasive wheel of a laboratory lathe **(Fig. 9.5)**. Uniform pressure is to be given along the longitudinal axis of tooth to achieve uniform thickness of the section. Water is sprayed constantly onto the wheel to prevent charring. The tooth is ground down nearly to the level of the desired section.
- The coarse wheel is now exchanged for a fine abrasive lathe wheel and the cut surface of the tooth is ground down to a thickness of about 0.5 mm.
- For transverse section, the tooth is held directly against the rotating coarse abrasive wheel under water spray both from coronal and radicular directions. The tooth is ground down uniformly to the level of desired thickness around height of contour of crown. At this point, the cross-section of tooth is pressed onto the wooden block by means of adhesive tape and ground down to a thickness of about 0.5 mm.
- Then specimen is now rubbed on a ground glass with pumice–glycerine paste to remove the scratches on the tooth.
- The section is dipped in ether, dried and mounted with mounting medium on microscope slide **(Fig. 9.6)**, and a cover glass is affixed for microscopic studies under the microscope.

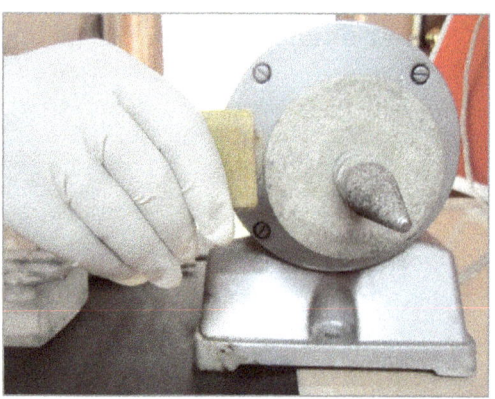

**Fig. 9.5:** Ground sectioning in lathe.

## QUESTIONNAIRE

1. What are the parts and functions of light microscope?
2. What are the different procedures for preparation of tissues for microscopic examination? Discuss the different steps of paraffin-embedding procedure.

3. Write notes on:
   a. Frozen section.
   b. Ground section.
   c. Electron microscopy.

## BIBLIOGRAPHY

1. Bancroft JD, Stevens A. Theory and Practice of Histological Techniques, 2nd edition. China: Churchill Livingstone; 1990.
2. Das AK. Dental Anatomy and Oral Histology, 1st edition. UK; Current Publishers; 1972.
3. Junqueira LC, Jose C. Basic Histology, Text and Atlas, 10th edition. USA: Lange Medical books McGraw-Hill; 1998.
4. Kumar GS. Orban's Oral Histology and Embryology, 12th edition. India: Mosby; 2009.
5. Pease AGE. Histochemistry. Theoretical and Applied, 4th edition. New York: Churchill Livingstone; 1980.

# CHAPTER 10

# Development of Face and Oral Cavity

Prenatal development comprises 10 lunar months, 28 days each. It is divided into three successive phases:
1. Period of ovum—1 week.
2. Embryonic period—second week to eighth week. It is divided into:
   a. Presomite
   b. Somite
   c. Postsomite period.
3. Period of fetus—third month to tenth month.

## ZYGOTE

The mating of male and female gametes in the maternal uterine tube initiates the development of a large, totipotent cell (can give rise to cell of all types), having 100 mm diameter, known as zygote (**Fig. 10.1**).

## MORULA

Zygote undergoes rapid mitotic division to form morula having 16 pluripotent cells (can give rise to specialized form of tissue). It has an inner cell mass which gives rise to embryo proper and is known as embryoblast. The outer layer of cells is trophoblasts which help to provide nutrition to the embryo (**Fig. 10.2**).

## BLASTOCYST

On the fourth day, after conception, the fluid passes from uterine cavity into morula and partially separates the inner cell mass from the trophoblast. The morula now becomes a blastocyst (**Fig. 10.3**) and the cavity is known as blastocele.

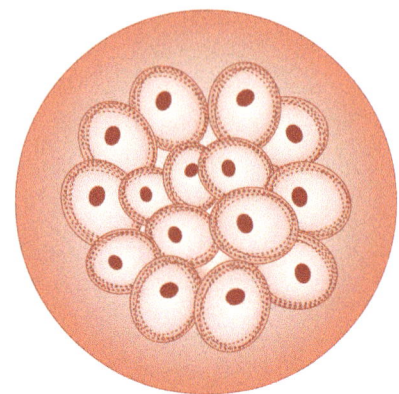

Fig. 10.2: Morula.

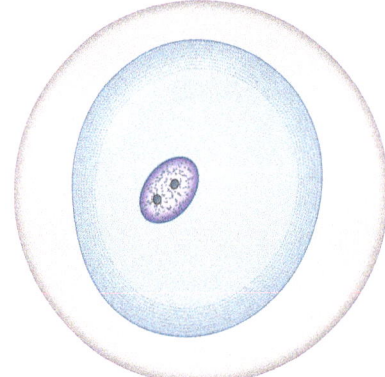

Fig. 10.1: Zygote.

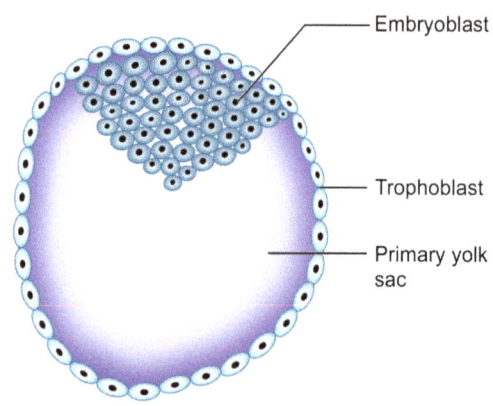

Fig. 10.3: Blastocyst.

# Development of Face and Oral Cavity

## PLACENTA

On the seventh day, the zygote passes through uterine tube and implants into uterine wall. The chorion develops from blastocyst by growth of villi into surrounding maternal uterine wall to tap blood supply. The surface directed villi eventually atrophy while basally directed villi hypertrophy and combine with uterine wall to form placenta (**Fig. 10.4**).

## BILAMINAR GERM DISK

Some cells of the inner cell mass differentiate into flattened cells which constitute endoderm, the first germ layer. The remaining cells of the inner cell mass become columnar and form the ectoderm, the second germ layer. At this stage, the embryo is in the form of a disk having two layers (**Fig. 10.4**).

## AMNIOTIC CAVITY

The space between the ectoderm (below) and the trophoblast (above) is amniotic cavity filled with amniotic fluid.

## YOLK SAC

The space between endoderm (above) and trophoblast (below) is yolk sac. The fluid of amniotic cavity and yolk sac is meant for protection, nutritional exchange, and waste elimination.

## PROCHORDAL PLATE

Around the 14th day of development, at one circular area near the margin of the embryonic disk, the cubical cells of the endoderm become columnar.

This area is called prochordal plate (**Fig. 10.5**). It later forms the endodermal layer of oropharyngeal membrane. It determines the central axis of the embryo and also enables us to distinguish its future head and tail end.

## PRIMITIVE STREAK

Around third week of development, some of the ectodermal cells lying along the central axis, near the tail end of the disk, begin to proliferate and form an elevation that bulges into amniotic cavity. This elevation is called the primitive streak (**Fig. 10.6**).

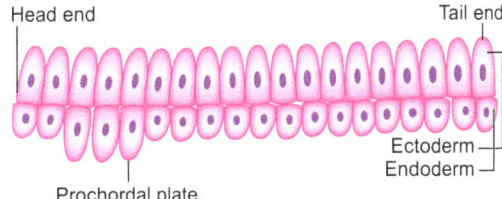

**Fig. 10.5:** Prochordal plate.

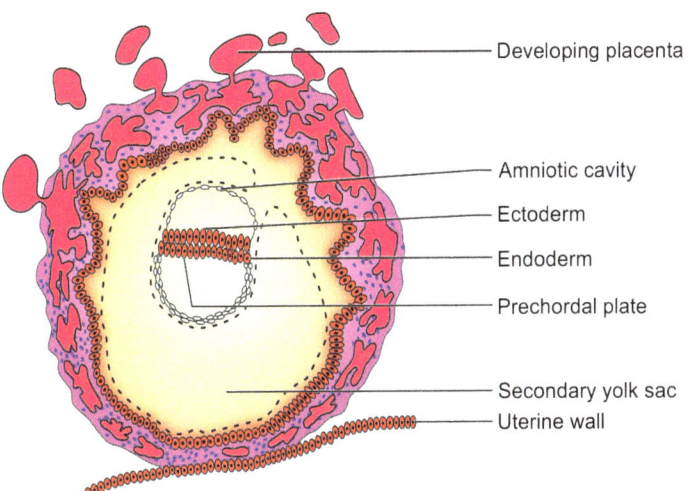

**Fig. 10.4:** Developing placenta and bilaminar germ disk.

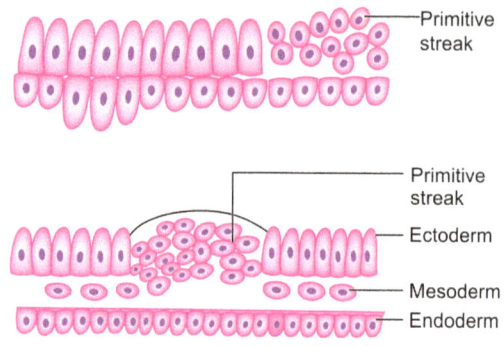

Fig. 10.6: Primitive streak.

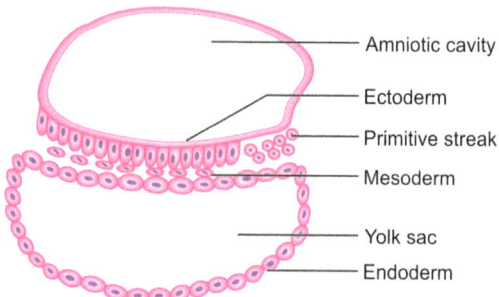

Fig. 10.7: Mesoderm.

## MESODERM

The cells that proliferate in the region of primitive streak pass sideways, pushing themselves between the ectoderm and the endoderm, and form mesoderm, the third germ layer. The mesoderm migrates in all directions between the ectoderm and endoderm excepting near oropharyngeal membrane anteriorly and cloacal membrane posteriorly (**Fig. 10.7**).

## NOTOCHORD

The cells of the primitive streak proliferate and move cranially in the midline between the ectoderm and the endoderm, reaching up to the caudal margin of the prochordal plate. The cells undergo differentiation and form a solid rod called notochord (**Figs. 10.8A and B**) which lies in the midline, in the position to be later occupied by the vertebral column. However, the notochord does not give rise to vertebral column.

The notochord terminates anteriorly at prochordal plate and marks the site of future pituitary gland. Most of the notochord disappears but parts of it persist in the region of each intervertebral disk as the nucleus pulposus.

## DERIVATIVES OF THREE GERM LAYERS

### From Ectoderm

1. Skin and appendages
2. Central and peripheral nervous system
3. Oral mucous membrane
4. Enamel.

### From Mesoderm

1. Cardiovascular system (heart and blood vessel)
2. Locomotor system (bones and muscles)
3. Connective tissue
4. Pulp, dentin, cementum, periodontal ligament, and alveolar bone.

### From Endoderm

1. Lining epithelium of alimentary canal between pharynx and anus
2. Secretory cells of liver and pancreas
3. Lining epithelium of respiratory system.

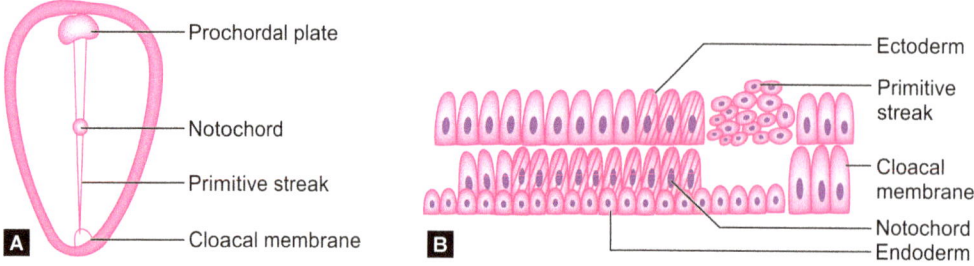

Figs. 10.8A and B: Notochord.

# Development of Face and Oral Cavity

## Neural Crest Cells (Figs. 10.9A to D)

The ectoderm over notochordal process becomes thickened to form the neural plate which is depressed along the midline to form neural groove. The edges of the groove eventually fuse converting the neural groove into the neural tube **(Figs. 10.9A to D)**.

At the junction between the neural tube and the surface (cutaneous) ectoderm on either side, groups of cells appear. They are known as neural crest cells. They are ectodermal in origin but have the properties of mesoderm. So they are known as ectomesenchyme.

They are capable of migrating along the cleavage planes between mesoderm, ectoderm, and endoderm. After reaching their destination, they undergo cytodifferentiation.

Several important structures are derived from neural crest cells. They are:
1. The neurons of the sensory ganglia of the fifth, seventh, eighth, ninth, and tenth cranial nerves.
2. The neurons of the sympathetic ganglia.
3. The Schwann cells.
4. The specific cells of the adrenal medulla and chromaffin tissue.
5. Melanocytes.
6. Calcitonin-secreting cells.
7. Cartilages of the branchial arches.
8. Facial processes.
9. All the tissues of the tooth (except enamel) and its supporting structures.

[*Clinical consideration*: Proper migration of neural crest cells is essential for the development of the face and the teeth. In Treacher Collins syndrome, full facial development does not occur due to failure of migration of neural crest cells to facial region. Depletion of neural crest cells prevents proper dental development.]

## SUBDIVISIONS OF MESODERM (FIGS. 10.10A AND B)

### Paraxial Mesoderm

It is the mesoderm, on either side of the notochord. It becomes segmented to form a number of somites that lie on either side of the developing neural tube **(Figs. 10.11A and B)**; 42-44 paired somites appear in craniocaudal direction of which there are 4 occipital, 8 cervical, 12 thoracic, 5 lumbar, 5 sacral, and 8-10 coccygeal somites. The somite is divisible into three parts:

a. The ventromedial part is called the sclerotome. It gives rise to vertebral column and ribs.
b. The lateral part is called the dermatome. The cells of this part give rise to dermis of the skin and subcutaneous tissue.

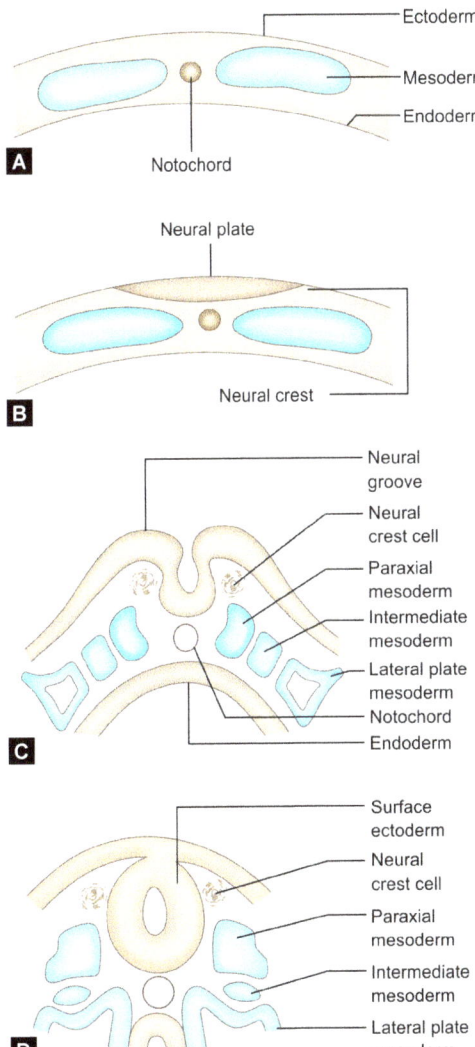

**Figs. 10.9A to D:** (A) Embryonic disk; (B) Formation of neural plate; (C) Formation of neural groove and neural crest cells; (D) The groove is converted to neural tube.

# Development of Face and Oral Cavity

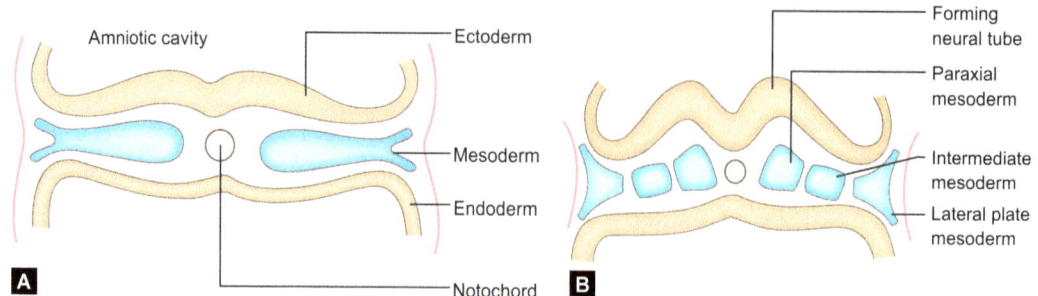

Figs. 10.10A and B: A. Mesoderm between ectoderm and endoderm; B. Differentiation of mesoderm.

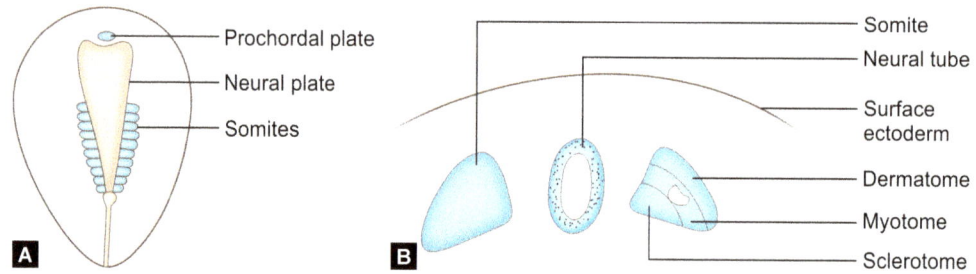

Figs. 10.11A and B: A. Somites on either side of neural tube; B. Subdivisions of somites.

c. The intermediate part is myotome. It gives rise to striated muscle.

In the cervical, thoracic, lumbar, and sacral regions, one spinal nerve innervates each myotome.

In somite period, cardiovascular system, alimentary system, nervous system, primordium of eye, and internal ear develop.

## Lateral Plate Mesoderm

It is laterally placed and gives rise to:
a. Pleural, pericardial, and peritoneal cavities
b. Connective tissue
c. Muscles of viscera
d. Blood
e. Lymph cells
f. Cardiovascular and lymphatic system
g. Spleen
h. Adrenal cortex.

## Intermediate Mesoderm

It gives rise to urogenital system.

## FOLDING OF EMBRYO

At this stage, the embryonic disk undergoes lateral and craniocaudal folds **(Figs. 10.12A and B)**. With the formation of the head and tail folds, parts of the yolk sac become enclosed within embryo and a tube lined by endoderm is formed. This is primitive gut which is in direct communication with yolk sac. The part of the gut cranial to this communication is foregut. The part the gut caudal to this communication is hindgut and the intervening part is called midgut. The whole of the gut is sealed off anteriorly by oropharyngeal membrane and posteriorly by cloacal membrane. Later, it is converted into a canal by breakdown of oropharyngeal and cloacal membrane.

## Derivatives of Foregut Endoderm

1. Laryngotracheal diverticulum (bronchi and lungs)
2. Hepatic and pancreatic diverticulum (liver and pancreas)
3. Pharynx and pouches
4. Esophagus, stomach, and first part of duodenum.

## Derivatives of Midgut Endoderm

1. Rest of duodenum
2. Entire small intestine

# Development of Face and Oral Cavity

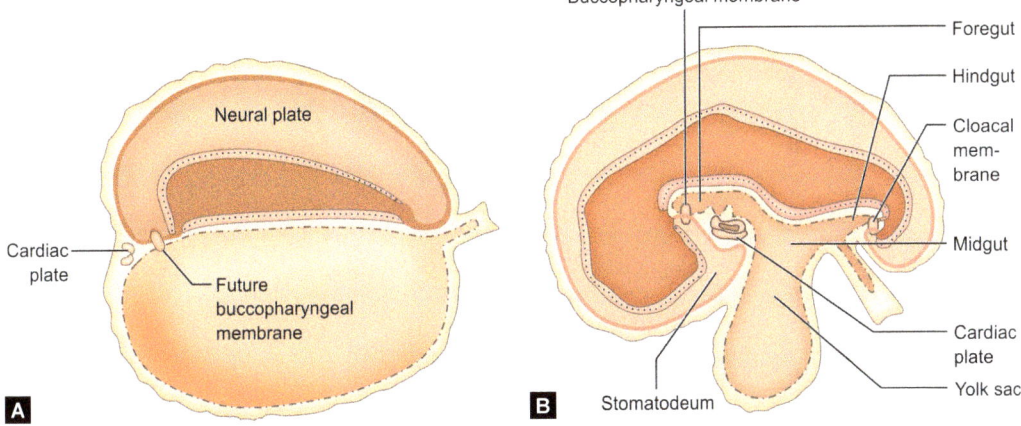

**Figs. 10.12A and B:** A. Craniocaudal folding begins; B. Completion of folding.

3. Ascending colon and transverse colon of large intestine.

## Derivatives of Hindgut Endoderm

Descending colon and rest of alimentary canal.

## EARLY OROFACIAL DEVELOPMENT

Cranial end of embryo develops rapidly compared to caudal end. Stomatodeum, the primitive oral cavity, is a shallow depression, surrounded by neural plate cranially and cardiac plate caudally **(Fig. 10.13)**. The buccopharyngeal membrane separates it from foregut. Stomatodeum forms the topographical center of developing face.

In the early somite period (21–31 days of embryo), five mesodermal elevations, augmented by neural crest cells and lined by ectoderm, appear surrounding the stomatodeum. They are facial processes and constitute the initial features of face. The single, central most, cranially located process is frontonasal process and two bilaterally located processes are maxillary and mandibular processes **(Fig. 10.14)**.

The different facial processes grow differentially and by obliterating the ectodermal grooves between them provide an even contour to the features of face **(Figs. 10.15A to C)**.

The wide frontonasal process intervenes between the laterally placed developing

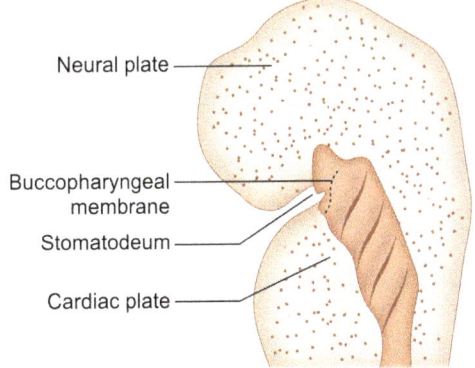

**Fig. 10.13:** Boundaries of stomatodeum between neural plate and cardiac plate.

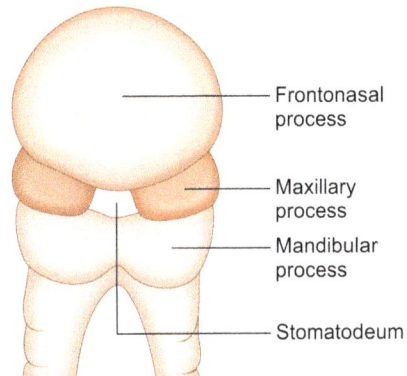

**Fig. 10.14:** Boundaries of stomatodeum between different facial processes.

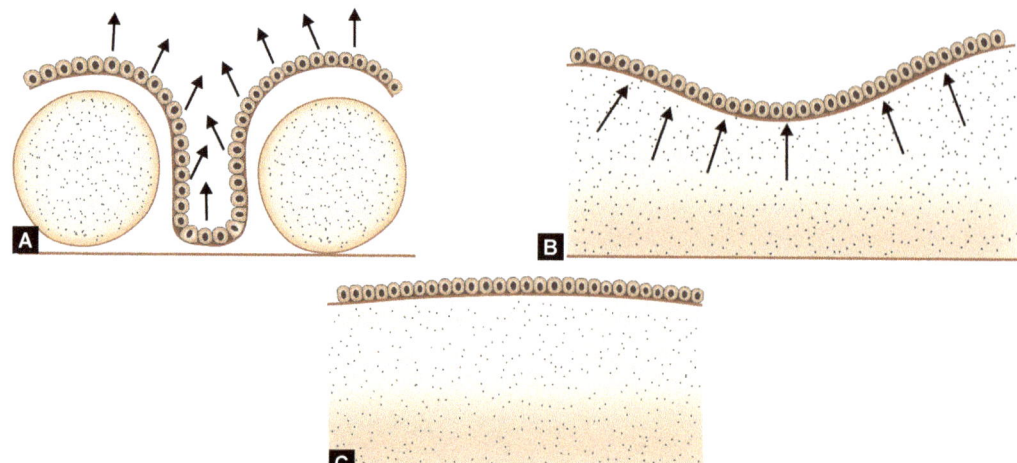

**Figs. 10.15A to C:** Obliteration of ectodermal grooves before fusion of facial processes.

eyes. It contributes to the forehead and nose. The olfactory part of nose develops from nasal (olfactory) placodes, which is formed from specialized epithelial thickening at the inferolateral corners of the frontonasal process.

## Globular Process

During the fifth week of intrauterine life (IU), horseshoe-shaped medial and lateral nasal processes develop surrounding each of the sinking nasal placodes and cause deepening of the nasal pits to form anterior nares. The two medial nasal processes approach each other to form a single globular process **(Fig. 10.16)**. It forms (a) the tip of the nose, (b) the columella, (c) the philtrum, (d) labial tuberculum of upper lip, (e) labial frenum, and (f) primary palate. The elevation of the lateral nasal processes creates the alae of the nose. The maxillary processes of each side form the lateral part of the lip and cheek, and the maxillary processes merge with the frontonasal process by obliteration of intervening ectodermal groove, to provide continuity of upper lip and cheek region.

The two mandibular processes merge in the midline to provide continuity to the lower jaw and lip. The maxillary process and the lateral nasal process are separated by deep furrow. The epithelium in the floor of the furrow forms a solid core which eventually

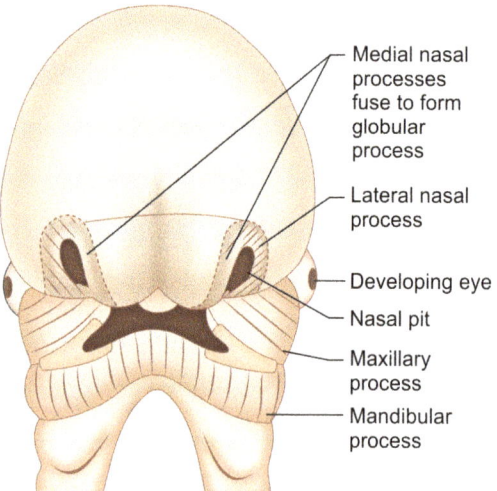

**Fig. 10.16:** Developing face.

canalizes to form nasolacrimal duct. Once the duct is separated, the two processes merge by infilling of the mesenchyme.

## BRANCHIAL ARCHES

During the late somite period (4th week IU), a series of distinct, bilateral mesenchymal swellings, augmented by neural crest tissues, develops on the ventral aspect of the embryo, just caudal to the head fold, in the future mandibulocervical region. These sets of five or six elevations are known as branchial arches. They are separated by four branchial

# Development of Face and Oral Cavity

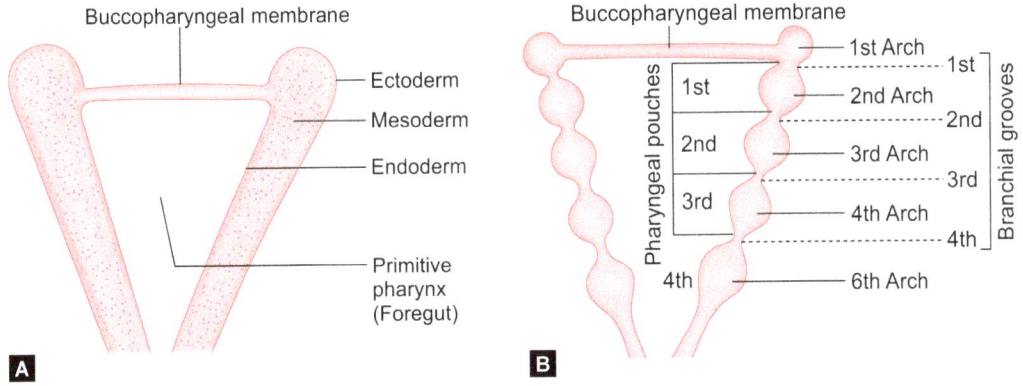

**Figs. 10.17A and B:** A. Formation of branchial arches; B. Branchial grooves and pharyngeal pouches.

grooves on the external aspect of the embryo. Internally, they are separated by the five outpocketings of the elongated pharynx of the foregut, known as pharyngeal pouch **(Figs. 10.17A and B)**. The branchial arches decrease serially in size from the first to the sixth, each pair merging midventrally to form semicircular "collars" around the pharynx. Only five pairs of arches are discernible, however, the fifth being transitory. In each pair of arches, there are:

1. A central cartilage rod that forms the skeleton of the arch and is differentiated from neural crest tissue.
2. A vascular component—originates from lateral plate mesoderm.
3. A nervous element—consisting of sensory special visceral motor fibers of one or more cranial nerves supplying the mucosa and branchial muscle arising from that arch.
4. A muscular component—the branchiomeric muscle component is of lateral plate mesoderm origin **(Table 10.1)**.

## THE BRANCHIAL GROOVES AND PHARYNGEAL POUCHES

After the formation of branchial arches, between primitive stomatodeum and developing heart, they are marked on outside by a series of grooves, lined by surface ectoderm and are known as branchial grooves. On the inner aspect of pharyngeal wall is a corresponding small depression lined by foregut endoderm called pharyngeal pouches that separate each of the branchial arches internally **(Fig. 10.18A)**.

### Fate of Branchial Groove

The first branchial groove persists and deepens to form the external acoustic meatus. The ectomesoendodermal membrane in the depth of the groove, separating it from the first pharyngeal pouch, persists as the tympanic membrane. The second, third, and fourth branchial grooves become obliterated by caudal overgrowth of the second branchial arch, which provides a smooth contour to the neck. Failure to obliterate completely these branchial grooves results in a branchial fistula leading from the pharynx to the outside or a branchial sinus or cyst, forming a closed sac **(Fig. 10.18B)**.

### Fate of Pharyngeal Pouches

The five pairs of pharyngeal pouches on the sides of the pharyngeal foregut form dorsal and ventral pockets, of which endodermal epithelium differentiates into a variety of structures. Elongation of the third, fourth, and fifth pharyngeal pouches during the sixth and seventh weeks IU, increasingly dissociates the pouches from the pharynx and allows their derivatives to form in the lower anterior neck region.

#### First Pharyngeal Pouch

The ventral portion of this pouch is obliterated by the developing tongue. The

## Development of Face and Oral Cavity

**TABLE 10.1:** Derivatives of branchial arches.

| Branchial arch | Skeleton | Muscle | Artery | Nerve |
|---|---|---|---|---|
| 1. Mandibular | Maxillary process, palatal shelf, mandible from Meckel's cartilage, incus, malleus, anterior ligament of malleus, spine of sphenoid bone, and sphenomandibular ligament | Muscles of mastication, (temporalis, masseter, medial and lateral pterygoid), mylohyoid, anterior belly of digastric, tensor veli palatini, and tensor tympani | External carotid and maxillary artery | Mandibular nerve |
| 2. Hyoid | Stapes, styloid process, stylohyoid ligament, lesser horn, and upper part of hyoid body | Stapedius, stylohyoid, posterior belly of digastric, muscles of facial expression, platysma, occipitofrontalis, and auricular muscle | Stapedial and facial artery | Facial nerve |
| 3. Third | Greater horn and lower part of hyoid body | Stylopharyngeus | Internal carotid and common carotid artery | Glossopharyngeal nerve |
| 4. Fourth | Thyroid cartilage | Cricothyroid, constrictors of the pharynx, levator veli palatini, uvular muscles of the soft palate, and palatoglossus muscle | Arch of aorta (left) proximal part of right subclavian artery | Superior laryngeal branch of vagus nerve |
| 5. Sixth | Cricoid and arytenoid cartilage | Intrinsic muscles of larynx | Proximal part of both pulmonary arteries and ductus arteriosus (left) | Recurrent laryngeal nerve of vagus |

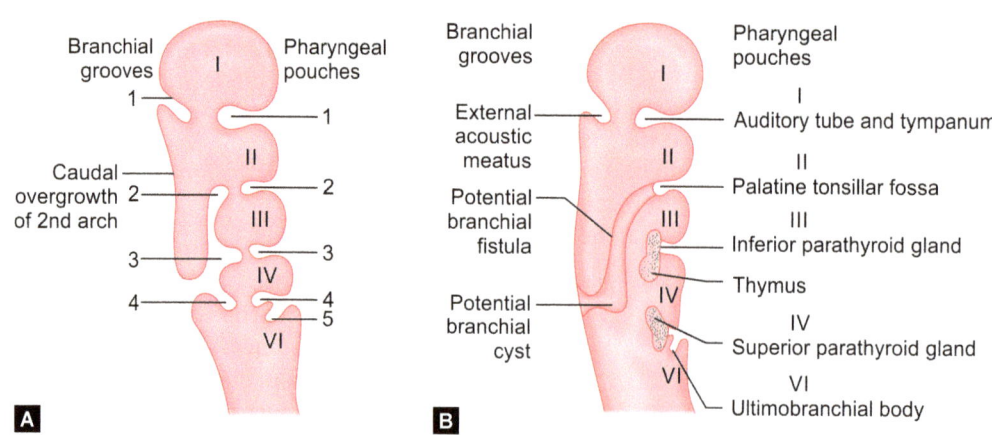

**Figs. 10.18A and B:** A. Fate of branchial groove; B. Pharyngeal pouches.

dorsal diverticulum deepens laterally as the tubotympanic recess to form the auditory tube, widening at its end into the tympanum or middle ear cavity, separated from the first branchial groove by the tympanic membrane.

The tympanum becomes occupied by the dorsal ends of the cartilages of the first and

# Development of Face and Oral Cavity

second branchial arches that later develop into ear ossicles. The tympanum maintains contact with the pharynx via the auditory tube throughout life.

## Second Pharyngeal Pouch

The ventral portion of this pouch is obliterated by the developing tongue. The dorsal portion forms palatine tonsil and tonsillar fossa.

## Third Pharyngeal Pouch

The ventral diverticulum endoderm proliferates and migrates from each side to form single median thymus gland. The dorsal diverticulum endoderm differentiates and migrates caudally to form the inferior parathyroid gland.

## Fourth Pharyngeal Pouch

The fate of endoderm of the ventral diverticulum is uncertain. The lining membrane may possibly contribute to thymus or thyroid tissue. The dorsal diverticulum endoderm differentiates into the superior parathyroid gland, which after losing contact with the pharynx, migrates caudally with thyroid gland.

## Fifth Pharyngeal Pouch

The fifth pouch appears as a diverticulum of the fourth pouch, the endoderm of which forms the ultimobranchial body. The calcitonin-secreting cells of the ultimobranchial body are derived from neural crest tissue and are eventually incorporated into thyroid gland.

## FORMATION OF THE TONGUE

The tongue begins to develop at about fourth week of intrauterine life in the ventral wall of the primitive oropharynx in relation to first four branchial arches. Paired lateral proliferation of mesenchyme appears on the internal aspect of first branchial arch to form lingual swellings **(Fig. 10.19A)**. Between and behind the lingual swellings, there appears a median eminence, the tuberculum impar; its caudal border is marked by a blind pit, the foramen cecum, from which the epithelium proliferates to form a downgrowth, thyroglossal duct, from which the thyroid gland develops. Another midline swelling appears in relation to the medial ends of the second, third, and fourth arches. This swelling is called the hypobranchial eminence **(Fig. 10.19B)** which soon shows a subdivision into a cranial part related to the second and third arches (called the copula) and a caudal part related to the fourth arch **(Fig. 10.20A)**.

The caudal part forms the epiglottis.

The anterior two-thirds of the tongue is formed by fusion of:
a. The tuberculum impar
b. The two lingual swellings.

The anterior two-thirds of the tongue is thus derived from the mandibular arch **(Figs. 10.20B and C)**. According to some, the tuberculum impar does not make a significant contribution to the tongue.

The posterior one-third of the tongue is formed from the cranial part of the hypobranchial eminence (copula) **(Fig.**

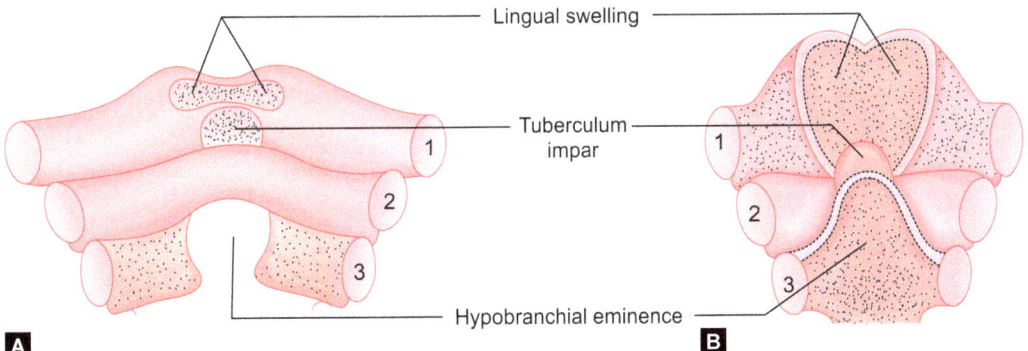

**Figs. 10.19A and B:** Development of tongue.

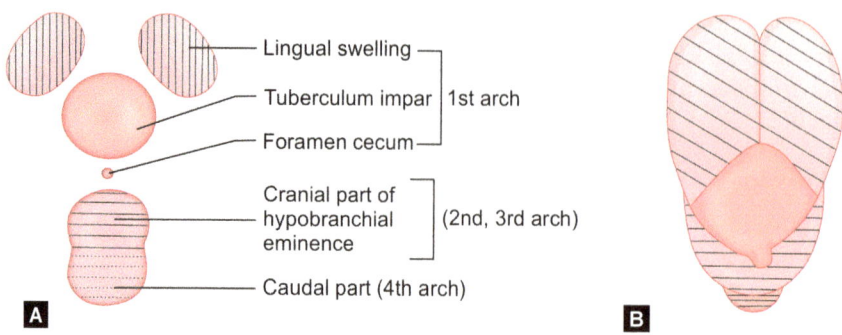

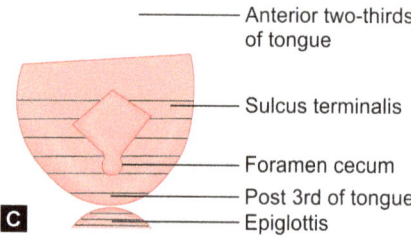

Figs. 10.20A to C: Origin of different parts of tongue.

**10.21A).** In this situation, the second arch mesoderm gets buried below the surface. The third arch mesoderm grows over it to fuse with the mesoderm of the first arch **(Fig. 10.21B).** The posterior one-third of the tongue is thus formed by third arch mesoderm. The posterior most part of the tongue is derived from the fourth arch **(Fig. 10.22).** A V-shaped sulcus terminalis, whose apex is the foramen cecum, demarcates the junction between anterior two-thirds and posterior one-third of tongue. According to the embryological origin, the anterior two-thirds of the tongue is supplied by the lingual branch of the mandibular nerve, which is the posttrematic nerve of the first arch and by the chorda tympani which is pretrematic nerve of this arch. The posterior one-third of the tongue is supplied by the glossopharyngeal nerve, which is the nerve of the third arch. The most posterior part of the tongue is supplied by the superior laryngeal nerve, which is the nerve of the fourth arch. The musculature of the tongue is derived from the occipital myotomes and is supplied by the hypoglossal nerve, which is the nerve of these myotomes.

The epithelium of the tongue is at first made up of a single layer of cells. Later, it becomes stratified and papillae become evident.

The line of the sulcus terminalis is marked by 8–12 circumvallate papillae that develop at 2–5 months of IU. The mucosa of the dorsal surface of the body of the tongue develops filiform and fungiform papillae at 11 weeks

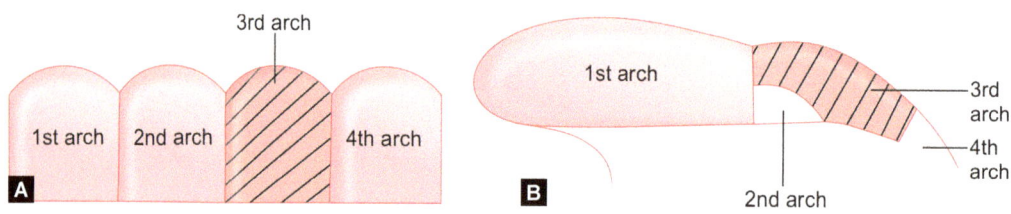

Figs. 10.21A and B: Second arch is buried by the overgrowth of the third arch.

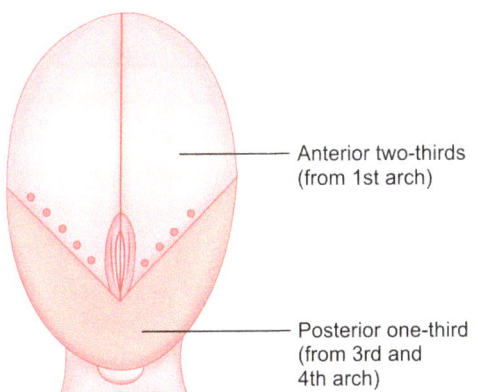

**Fig. 10.22:** Final disposition of the tongue and the relative contributions from branchial arches.

IU. At birth, the root mucosa becomes pitted by deep crypts that develop into lingual tonsil, the completion of which is marked by lymphocytic infiltration. Taste buds arise by inductive interaction between epithelial cells and nerve cells from the chorda tympani, glossopharyngeal, and vagus nerves.

## DEVELOPMENT OF PALATE

The palate is developed from three components:
1. The primitive palate, formed from globular process.
2. The two palatal processes from maxillary process.

Initially, there is a common oronasal cavity bounded anteriorly by the primary palate and occupied mainly by the developing tongue. Around 7-8 weeks of development, the maxillary processes which form the lateral wall of primitive oronasal cavity develop processes on each side at the lateral portion of oral roof. They grow downward vertically on either side of tongue. The processes are called palatine processes (palatine shelves). After the seventh week of development **(Figs. 10.23A and B)**, the tongue is withdrawn from between the shelves, which now elevate and fuse with each other above the tongue and with the primary palate **(Fig. 10.24)**. The fusion begins anteriorly and proceeds backward. The closure of the secondary palate involves:

a. An intrinsic force in the palatal shelves.
b. The high concentration of glycosaminoglycans, which attract water and make shelves turgid.
c. Presence of contractile fibroblasts in the palatine shelves.
d. Displacement of the tongue from between the palatine shelves by the growth pattern of the head.

About 24-36 hours before fusion of palatine processes, there is cessation of DNA synthesis within epithelium.

Surface epithelial cells are sloughed off as they undergo physiologic cell death (*apoptotic cell death).

The basal cells have a carbohydrate-rich surface coat that permits adhesion between processes. The single layer of basal cells ultimately breaks into discrete islands of epithelial cells and there is ectomesenchymal continuity between the fused processes.

At a later stage, the mesoderm in the palate undergoes intramembranous ossification to form the hard palate. However, ossification does not extend into the most posterior portion, which remains as the soft palate.

## DEVELOPMENT OF THE JAWS

At about sixth week of intrauterine life, the first indication of bone formation for the jaws is seen. Both the mandible and maxilla form

---

*Apoptosis (derived from the Greek and meaning "dropping off" or "falling off") is the process by which cell numbers are reduced physiologically. The cell condenses, apparently due to the loss of water, to form a pyknotic nuclear mass surrounded by a variable amount of cytoplasm in which the organelles are still easily recognizable. This is called an "apoptotic body" and it undergoes nuclear fragmentation and the separation of protuberances that appear on the cell surface. These apoptotic bodies are then phagocytosed by macrophages and also often by neighboring epithelial cells, in which they are incorporated in lysosomes where they are digested, finally to form small, optically dense, residual bodies. Apoptotic bodies derived from the epithelial cells lining free mucosal surfaces are also shed directly to the exterior.

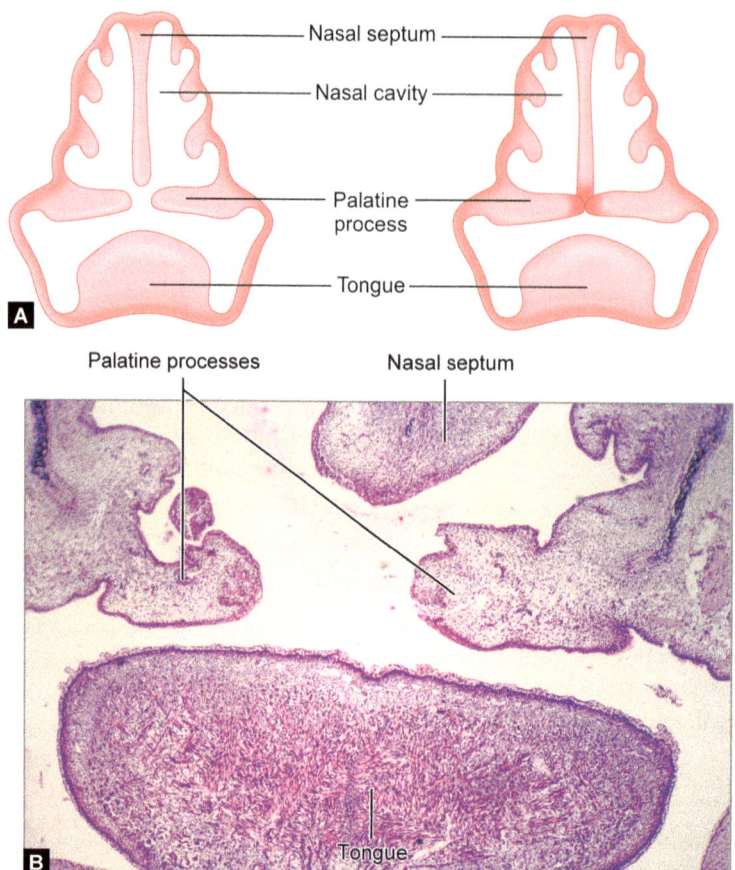

**Figs. 10.23A and B:** Fusion of palatine processes.

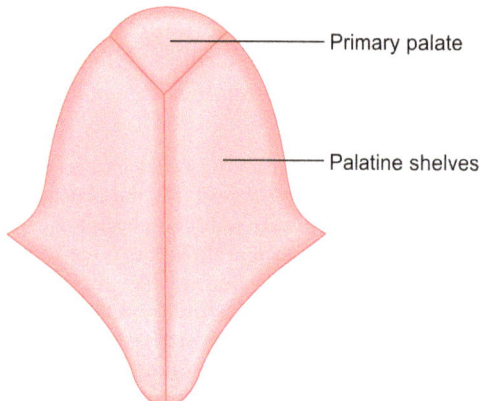

**Fig. 10.24:** Fusion of palatine shelves and primary palate.

from the tissues of the first branchial arch, the mandible forming within the mandibular process and maxilla within the maxillary process.

## Development of the Mandible

The mandible is partly intramembranous and partly intracartilaginous in origin. Greater part of body, ramus, and condyloid and coronoid processes are intramembranous in origin. Only the tip of the condyloid and coronoid processes and symphyseal region is of endochondral origin. Meckel's cartilage, the cartilage of the first arch, has a close positional relationship to the developing mandible but makes no contribution to it. It only acts as a scaffold and a guideline.

The cartilage attains its full form by 6 weeks and grows forward and downward toward midline. It is surrounded by a thick fibrocellular tissue. The mandibular nerve and mandibular artery are in close contact with Meckel's cartilage. The mandibular nerve divides into the lingual and inferior dental branches near about the junction of dorsal and middle-third of the cartilage. The lingual nerve runs medially and the inferior dental nerve runs laterally and divides into mental and incisive branches. The mental branch runs away from the cartilage and the incisive branch runs along with the cartilage (**Fig. 10.25**). At the seventh week, first intramembranous ossification is observed in the dense fibrocellular tissue outside and lateral to Meckel's cartilage, at the fork formed by the incisive nerve and mental nerve (in the region of future mental foramen).

From this center of ossification, bone formation spreads rapidly anteriorly to the midline and posteriorly toward the point where the mandibular nerve divides into its lingual and inferior alveolar branches. This spread of new bone consists of lateral and medial plates that unite beneath the incisive nerve. This trough of bone extends to the midline, where it comes into close approximation with a similar trough formed in the adjoining mandibular process. The two separate centers of ossification remain separated at the mandibular symphysis until shortly after birth. This trough is soon converted into a canal as bone forms over the nerve joining the lateral and medial plates.

Similarly, a backward extension of ossification along the lateral aspect of Meckel's cartilage forms a trough, later converted into a canal that contains the inferior alveolar nerve.

From the bony canal which extends from division of the mandibular nerve to the midline, medial, and lateral alveolar plates of bone develop in relation to the forming tooth germs, which occupy a secondary trough of bone. This trough of bone is partitioned and thus each developing tooth occupies individual compartment which finally is totally enclosed by growth of bone over the tooth germ. In this way, the body of the mandible is essentially formed.

The ramus of the mandible develops by rapid spread of ossification posteriorly into the mesenchyme of the first arch, turning away from Meckel's cartilage (**Fig. 10.26**). This point of divergence is marked by the lingula in the adult mandible, the point at which the inferior alveolar nerve enters the body of the mandible.

By the 10th week, the rudimentary mandible is formed entirely by membranous ossification. The further growth of the mandible until birth is strongly influenced by the appearance of three secondary cartilages and the development of muscular attachment. The secondary cartilages are

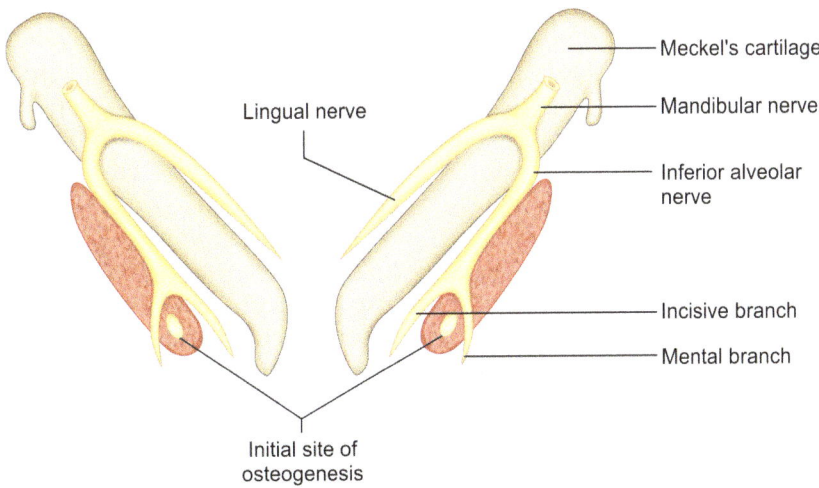

**Fig. 10.25:** Site of initial osteogenesis related to mandible formation.

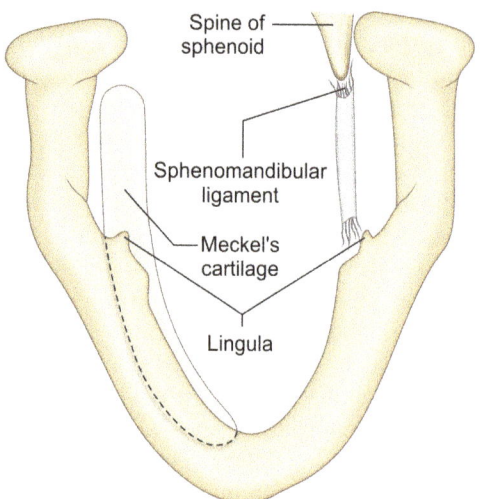

Fig. 10.26: Spread of mandibular ossification away from Meckel's cartilage at the lingula.

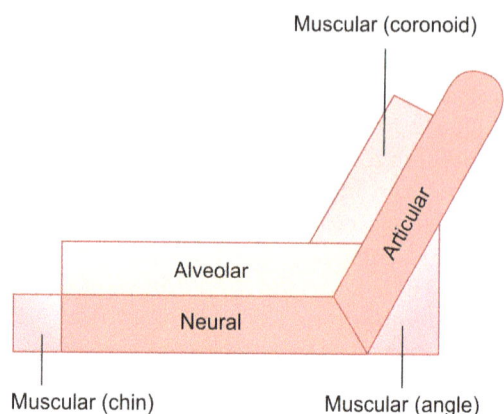

Fig. 10.27: Different developmental blocks for the mandible.

condylar cartilage, coronoid cartilage, and symphyseal cartilage.

The condylar cartilage appears during the 12th week of development and rapidly forms a cone or carrot-shaped mass that occupies most of the developing ramus. The mass of cartilage is quickly converted to bone by endochondral ossification, so that at 20 weeks only a thin layer of cartilage remains at condylar head. This remnant of cartilage persists until the end of the second decade of life. The coronoid cartilage appears at about 4 months of development and disappears long before birth.

The symphyseal cartilages, two in number, appear in the connective tissue between the two ends of Meckel's cartilage, but are entirely independent of it.

They are obliterated within the first year after birth.

Small islands of cartilage may also appear as variable and transient structures in the developing alveolar processes.

Secondary cartilages have larger cells and less intercellular matrix compared to primary cartilage.

Thus, the mandible is a membrane bone, developed in relation to the nerve of the first arch and almost entirely independent of Meckel's cartilage. It has neural, muscular, and alveolar elements **(Fig. 10.27)** and its growth is assisted by development of secondary cartilage.

**Meckel's cartilage:** It is the cartilage of first arch, attains its full form by 6 weeks, and then grows forward and downward toward midline. Two solid hyaline cartilaginous rods of each side do not meet at midline but are separated by a thin band of mesenchyme. Mandibular nerve and artery have close relationship to Meckel's cartilage.

**Functions:**
1. It has a close positional relationship to the developing mandible but makes no contribution to it. It acts as scaffold and a guideline for formation of mandible.
2. The dorsal end of cartilage gives rise to two middle ear bones, incus and malleus by intracartilaginous ossification.
3. Formation of sphenomandibular ligament.

**Fate:** From the sphenoid bone to the division of mandibular nerve into its alveolar and lingual branches, the cartilage is totally lost, but its fibrocellular capsule persists as sphenomandibular ligament. From the lingula forward to the division of the alveolar nerve into its incisive and mental branches, Meckel's cartilage is totally resorbed. Near the midline, one or two nodules of cartilage are seen in late fetal life and at birth. These cartilages may ossify to form small contribution to mandible at symphysis.

## DEVELOPMENT OF MAXILLA

The maxilla is formed by maxilla proper and premaxilla. The maxilla proper is developed as an extension of mandibular arch. It forms by intramembranous ossification. Ossification starts at about 6 weeks of intrauterine life. The ossification center appears near the part which forms enamel organ of the canine tooth germ and also lateral and below the fork formed by infraorbital nerve and anterior superior alveolar nerve. From this center, bone formation spreads posteriorly below the orbit toward the developing zygoma and anteriorly toward premaxilla. It unites with premaxilla at an early stage. Ossification also spreads superiorly to form the frontal process. As a result of this pattern of bone deposition, a bony trough forms for the infraorbital nerve. From this trough, a downward extension of bone forms lateral to alveolar plate for the maxillary tooth germ. Ossification also spreads into palatine process to form the hard palate. The medial alveolar plate develops from the junction of the palatal process and the main body of the forming maxilla. This plate, together with its lateral counterpart, forms a trough of bone around the maxillary tooth germs, which eventually become enclosed in bony crypts. A secondary cartilage also contributes to the development of maxilla. A zygomatic cartilage appears in the developing zygomatic process and adds to the development of maxilla. The maxillary sinus appears at the 16th week fetal life as a projection from nasal cavity. It comes in contact with maxilla after cartilage of nasal capsule atrophies. It increases gradually and separates the orbital surface from dental surface. The final height is reached after eruption of all permanent teeth.

## DEVELOPMENT OF THE TEMPOROMANDIBULAR JOINT

The temporomandibular joint (TMJ) is an articulation between two bones initially formed from membranous centers of ossification. At the seventh week, the Meckel's cartilage extends from chin to base of the skull. This joint is replaced by the temporomandibular joint near the end of fetal life. Articular disk seems to be a muscle derivative of first branchial arch. There is first a mesenchymal condensation on the upper end of mandibular ramus. Anteriorly, this mesenchyme extends from superior border of lateral pterygoid muscle to medial side of masseter muscle. The lateral pterygoid muscle contributes to the formation of medial part of articular disk.

Mesenchymal condensation forms the fibrous covering on the joint surfaces. At the 12th week, mandibular condylar cartilage appears. At the 13th week, the condyle with articular disk comes in contact with temporal bone and inferior joint cavities develop, followed by superior cavity. The disk is first vascular. Later on, as the disk is compressed, central and anterior parts become avascular. The disk loses its connection with malleus and attaches itself to the squamotympanic fissure. The synovial lining of the joint cavities appears later.

## DEVELOPMENT OF THE SKULL

The skull can be divided into three components **(Fig. 10.28)**:
1. The cranial vault
2. The cranial base
3. The face.

Biologically, the skull consists basically of two bones, mandible and cranium. For

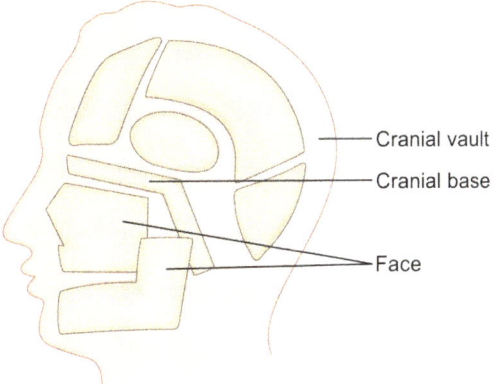

**Fig. 10.28:** Subdivisions of skull.

the purpose of understanding the growth of head, face, and jaw may be described under following headings:
1. Growth of cranium:
   a. Growth of cranial vault
   b. Growth of cranial base.
2. Growth of face:
   a. Growth of upper face
   b. Growth of lower face.
3. Growth of air sinuses.

## Growth of Cranial Vault

The cranial vault is made up of the following membrane bones: The frontal, parietals, and squamous part of the temporalis and part of occipital and sphenoid. These bones grow as different parts of a single bone and then fuse to form the cranial vault.

The cranium grows because the brain grows **(Fig. 10.29)**. The brain grows quicker than the face. The brain triples in volume in first 2 years of life and then slows down considerably. By 5 years, 90% of brain growth has taken place. The growth of cranial vault is accomplished primarily:
1. By proliferation and ossification of connective tissue at sutural lines.
2. By appositional growth of individual bones.
3. By selective resorption in early postnatal life at the inner surface in the areas close to sutural borders.
4. Apposition of bone on the inner surface in the central areas.

This selective resorption helps in flattening of the skull as it grows.

Apposition is seen on both inner and outer plates of bones. This thickening of bone is not uniform throughout because the outer plate of bone of the cranial superstructure is under the influence of masticatory and other mechanical forces. Thickening is specially seen on supraorbital region, mastoid region, and tympanic region. Increase in length of the cranial vault is due to active growth at the frontoparietal suture and parietooccipital suture. Increase in width is due to growth at interparietal, parietosphenoidal, and parietotemporal sutures. The height of the brain case grows due to the growth at parietooccipital, parietosphenoidal, and parietotemporal sutures.

## Growth of Cranial Base

In contrast to the cranial vault, the base grows primarily by growth of cartilage. The areas participating in the growth are sphenoethmoidal, spheno-occipital, and intraoccipital synchondrosis. The growth activity at intersphenoidal synchondrosis disappears after birth. The activity of interoccipital synchondrosis is up to 5 years, of sphenoethmoidal synchondrosis is from 5 years to 25 years and of sphenooccipital synchondrosis is up to 20 years.

## Growth of Face

Facial bones grow at a faster rate than bones of the vault after first year and continue to grow for a long time.

### The Upper Face

The upper face consists of a nasomaxillary complex. It is attached to the base of the skull. The growth of the cranial base is due to endochondral ossification and the growth of the maxillary complex is mostly a sutural growth like that in the cranial vault.

The maxilla is joined to the cranium via four pairs of sutures **(Fig. 10.30)**:
1. Frontomaxillary suture

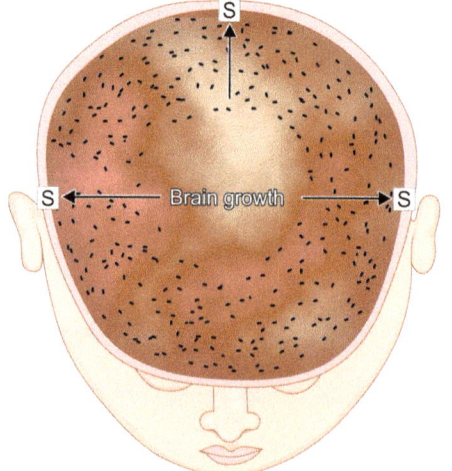

**Fig. 10.29:** Growth of the brain stimulates the sutural growth of the skull cap.

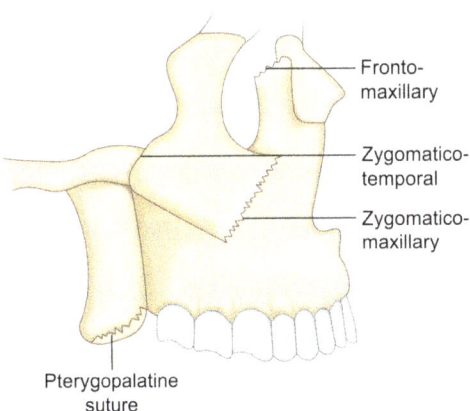

**Fig. 10.30:** Growth mechanism at upper face.

2. Zygomaticomaxillary suture
3. Zygomaticotemporal suture
4. Pterygopalatine suture.

The downward and forward growth of maxilla is due to:
1. Growth of connective tissue in the suture
2. Endochondral growth of cranial base and nasal septal cartilage.

Increase in height of maxillary complex is due to continued apposition of alveolar bone during eruption of teeth. Growth in width is due to growth along median palatal suture. Other sutures that contribute to the width are in relation to ethmoid, zygomatic, lacrimal, and nasal bones.

### The Lower Face

The lower face consists of mandible which is formed at fetal period. At birth, the condyles are short; right and left halves are separated in the midline by a thin line of fibrocartilage. By the end of the first year, the symphyseal cartilage is replaced by bone. There is proliferation of the condylar cartilage and its replacement by bone in the deepest layer. Condylar growth pushes mandible downward and forward.

There is apposition along the posterior border of ramus with resorption along the anterior border. This increases the length of the body of mandible. There is apposition on the alveolar border and consequently there is increase in height. The width increases by apposition on outer surface and posterior border.

The additive growth on the posterior border increases the distance between the terminal points of angles of the mandible.

Additive growth at the coronoid process, sigmoid notch, and condyle also increases superior inter-ramus dimension. Along with the developing dentition, alveolar border increases the height of the body of mandible. Growth of alveolus also increases the width of the body of the mandible.

### Growth of Air Sinuses

Air sinuses develop as: (1) Evaginations of the nasal cavity or (2) expansion of the cavity of middle ear into the adjacent bones. Air sinuses reduce the weight of the bones without reducing the functional efficiency considerably. The growth of the sinuses is secondary to the growth of bone. The frontal sinus starts forming in the second year of life. The two frontal sinuses grow at a different rate and are separated by a thin septum. The air sinuses increase in volume at old age.

The sphenoid sinus develops in the second year of life as the body of the sphenoid bone hollows out. It gradually increases in size.

The maxillary sinuses develop as an evagination from middle nasal meatus just before birth. Its growth is dependent upon eruption of teeth. It expands throughout life. The mastoid air sinuses develop along mastoid process. In the second year of life, the formation of mastoid sinus commences.

## DEVELOPMENT OF SALIVARY GLAND

There are three pairs of major and innumerable minor salivary glands in the oral cavity. They arise as buds from oral epithelium and grow into the underlying connective tissue. The parotid and submandibular buds appear during the sixth week and that of sublingual gland appear during the seventh week. Minor salivary glands appear later. The epithelial buds ramify as solid cords with small terminal enlargements, the acini. Later, the solid cords are canalized to give rise to duct system. The cells of acini are specialized for secretion. The majority of glands are ectodermal in origin, though some glands about the base of the tongue are entodermal. The connective tissue component and nervous system play an important role in the growth of salivary gland.

## CLINICAL CONSIDERATIONS

Nonunion of the part or whole of one process with another frequently results in malformation of face, lip, palate, and jaws. Nonunion of processes may be due to deficiency of mesenchyme in the facial region, failure of facial mesenchyme to proliferate, and failure of the neural crest cells to migrate.

**Cleft lip:** It may be unilateral or bilateral. It is the result of nonunion of globular process and maxillary processes.

**Cleft palate:** It may be unilateral, bilateral, incomplete, or complete involving both soft and hard palates.

Cleft palate is due to nonunion of two palatine processes. Anteriorly nonunion of premaxilla (globular process) and maxilla (palatine process) results in a complete bilateral Y-shaped cleft palate.

**Oblique facial cleft:** It is due to nonunion of maxillary and lateral nasal process.

**Lateral facial cleft and macrostomia:** They are due to failure of maxillary and mandibular processes to fuse.

**Microstomia:** It is overclosure of mouth opening due to excessive merging of the maxillary and mandibular processes.

**Labial pits:** Small pits may persist on either side of midline lower lip. They are caused by failure of embryonic labial pits to disappear.

**Bifid tongue:** It is due to lack of fusion between two lateral lingual prominences.

**Lingual thyroid:** Thyroid tissue may be present in the base of tongue. Part of thyroglossal duct may persist and form cysts at the base of tongue.

**Branchial cleft cyst or fistulas:** They may arise from the rests of epithelium in the visceral arch area and are laterally disposed on the neck.

**Thyroglossal duct cyst:** It may occur at any place along the course of the duct, usually at or near the midline.

**Fissural Cyst**

*Median palatine cyst*: Arises from epithelial inclusions at the line of fusion of palatal processes. In relation to other facial processes, fusion occurs by obliteration of ectodermal grooves and not by apoptotic cell death of intervening epithelium. So the cysts in other line of fusion are not fissural cyst.

**Cleft mandible:** It is a rare condition found due to nonunion of two mandibular processes.

## QUESTIONNAIRE

1. What are the neural crest cells? Discuss the formation and derivatives of neural crest cells.
2. What are the derivatives of different germ layers?
3. What is globular process? Describe development of face.
4. What are branchial arches and pharyngeal pouches? Enumerate derivatives of branchial arches and pharyngeal pouches.
5. Describe the development of tongue with neat diagram. Discuss innervation of tongue.
6. Discuss the development of palate.
7. Describe the development of mandible. What is Meckel's cartilage? What are functions and fate of Meckel's cartilage?
8. Write notes on:
    a. Notochord.
    b. Globular process.
    c. Tuberculum impar.
    d. Prochordal plate.

## BIBLIOGRAPHY

1. Antonio N. Ten Cate's Oral Histology Development, Structure, and Function, 7th edition. Mosby: Elsevier; 2008.

2. Berkovitz BKB, Holland GR, Moxham BJ. A Colour Atlas and Textbook of Oral Anatomy Histology and Embryology, 4th edition. Mosby: Elsevier; 2009.
3. Das AK. Dental Anatomy and Oral Histology, 1st edition. West Bengal: Current Books International; 1972.
4. Kumar GS. Orban's Oral Histology and Embryology, 12th edition. Mosby: Elsevier; 2009.
5. Singh Pal GP. Human Embryology, 7th edition. Uttar Pradesh: Macmillan India Limited; 2001.
6. Sperber GH. Craniofacial Embryology, 4th edition. Bristol, UK: Butterworth-Heinemann Ltd; 1989.

# CHAPTER 11

# Development of Tooth

The primitive oral cavity or stomodeum is lined by epithelium (two or three cell layer thick).

Beneath the epithelium, there is an embryonic connective tissue, enriched with neural crest cells and is termed ectomesenchyme. In hematoxylin and eosin stained section, the epithelial cells appear vacuolated (once filled with glycogen which is washed out of cells during tissue preparation). The ectomesenchyme consists of a few spindle-shaped cells separated by gelatinous ground substance.

At about fourth week of development, buccopharyngeal membrane ruptures and primitive oral cavity establishes a connection with foregut. The neural crest cells are thought to induce the overlying ectoderm to start tooth development.

## PRIMARY EPITHELIAL BAND

At about 6th week of development, certain areas of basal cells of oral ectoderm proliferate at more rapid rate than do the cells of the adjacent areas. There is condensation of mesenchymal tissue and of capillary network beneath the proliferating epithelium. The thickened oral epithelium invaginates into mesenchyme to form the primary epithelial band **(Fig. 11.1)**.

By the 7th week, the primary epithelial band divides into two processes by invagination of underlying ectomesenchyme. The processes are buccally located vestibular lamina and lingually located dental lamina **(Fig. 11.2)**.

The vestibular lamina contributes to the development of the vestibule, delineating the lips and cheeks from the tooth bearing region.

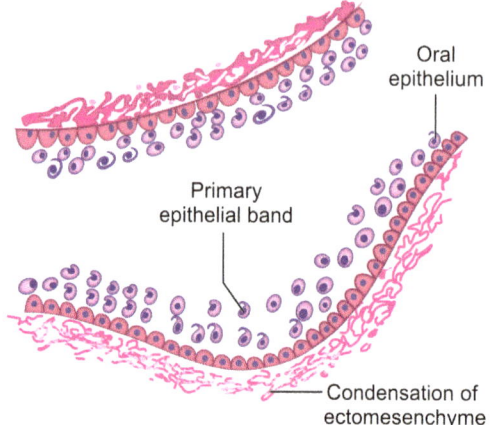

**Fig. 11.1:** Primary epithelial band.

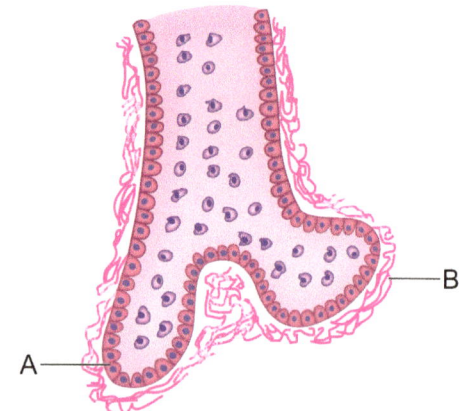

**Fig. 11.2:** Primary epithelial band divides into: A. Buccally located vestibular lamina and B. Lingually located dental lamina.

The dental lamina contributes to the development of the teeth. The cells of the vestibular lamina proliferate. Subsequently, there is degeneration of the central epithelial cells, which results in the formation of a sulcus, the vestibule between the alveolar portion of the jaws and lips and cheeks.

## Dental Lamina

The dental lamina is the primordium for the ectodermal portion of the teeth. By the 8th week to 10th week of utero, a series of swellings or epithelial ingrowths into underlying ectomesenchyme occur at certain points along dental lamina (10 areas on each arch, corresponding to future deciduous central incisor to the second deciduous molar) **(Fig. 11.3)**.

Later, during the development of the jaws, the permanent molars (4th month of utero for first permanent molar, first year of life for second permanent molar, and 4-5 years of life for third permanent molar) arise directly from a distal extension of the dental lamina. The distal proliferation of the dental lamina is responsible for the location of the germs of the permanent molars in the ramus of the mandible and tuberosity of maxilla.

The successors of the deciduous teeth develop from lingual extension of the free end of dental lamina opposite to the enamel organ of each deciduous tooth **(Fig. 11.4)**. The lingual extension of the dental lamina is named as successional lamina and develops from the 5th month in utero (permanent central incisor, lateral incisor, canine, first premolar) to the 10th month of age (second premolar).

*Timing for initiation of tooth development*

| | |
|---|---|
| 8th–10th week of utero | Deciduous central incisor to deciduous second molar |
| 5th month of utero | Permanent central incisor to first premolar |
| 10th month of utero | Second premolar |
| 4th month of utero | First permanent molar |
| 1st year of life | Second permanent molar |
| 4–5 years of life | Third molar |

## Fate of Dental Lamina

It is evident that the total activity of dental lamina extends over a period of at least 5 years. It is not equally active in all the region at the same time. The dental lamina may still be active in the third molar region after it has disappeared elsewhere. As the teeth continue to develop in early bell stage, the dental lamina joining the tooth germ to oral epithelium breaks into discrete islands of epithelial cells by mesenchymal invasion, separating the developing tooth germ from oral epithelium. The clusters of epithelial cells normally degenerate and are resorbed. If they escape degeneration, they may form small

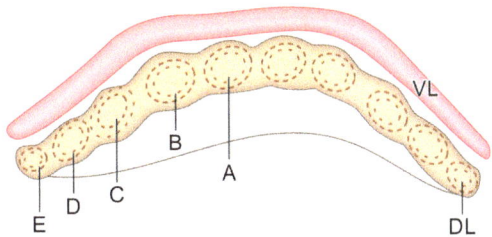

**Fig. 11.3:** Diagram to represent swelling in 10 areas in each arch corresponding to future deciduous tooth. A—Tooth bud of deciduous central incisor; B—Tooth bud of deciduous lateral incisor; C—Tooth bud of deciduous canine; D—Tooth bud of deciduous first molar; E—Tooth bud of deciduous second molar; VL—Vestibular lamina; DL—Dental lamina.

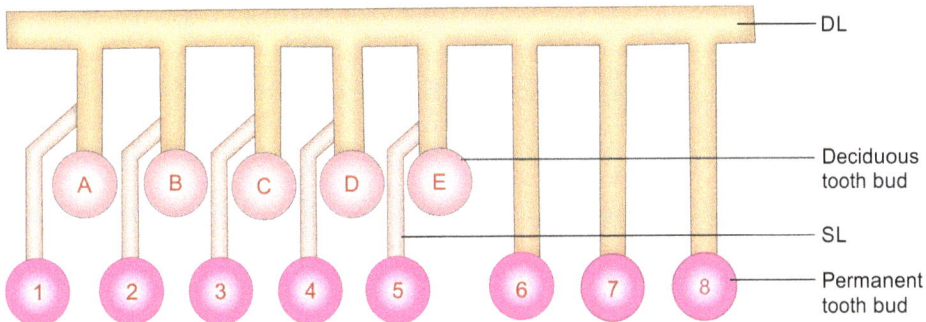

**Fig. 11.4:** The relationship between the deciduous and the permanent tooth bud. **Deciduous tooth bud**—A B C D E. **Permanent tooth bud**—1 2 3 4 5 6 7 8. Deciduous tooth bud and permanent molar tooth bud arise from DL. Other permanent teeth arise from SL.
(DL: dental lamina; SL: successional lamina)

cyst (eruption cyst) over developing tooth and delay eruption or the remnants of dental lamina persist as epithelial pearl within the jaws as well as in gingiva. The epithelial pearls are known as cell rests of Serre.

## DIFFERENT STAGES OF TOOTH DEVELOPMENT

Within the dental lamina, continued and localized proliferative activity leads to the formation of a series of epithelial ingrowths into the ectomesenchyme at the sites corresponding to the positions of 10 maxillary and 10 mandibular deciduous teeth. At this time, the mitotic index and the growth of the epithelial cells are significantly lower than corresponding index in the underlying ectomesenchyme, which suggests that part of the "ingrowth" is achieved by ectomesenchymal upgrowth. The epithelial downgrowth is known as enamel organ. All the enamel organs do not develop at the same time and the first tooth to appear is those of the anterior mandibular region.

As cell proliferation continues, the enamel organ increases in size and due to differential growth, it changes its shape. Although tooth development is a continuous process, it is divided into several morphologic stages. They are named after the shape of the enamel organ and are called:
1. The bud stage (stage of initiation)
2. The cap stage (stage of proliferation)
3. The early bell stage (stage of morphodifferentiation and stage of histodifferentiation)
4. The late bell stage (stage of apposition).

## Bud Stage (Stage of Initiation)

The bud stage is represented by the first epithelial incursion into the ectomesenchyme of the jaw. The ectodermal component in the bud stage appears as a simple, spherical to ovoid epithelial condensation (resembling a bud) which is poorly morphodifferentiated and histodifferentiated (show little change in shape and function). It consists of peripherally located low columnar cells and centrally located polygonal cells. The cells of the tooth bud have a higher RNA content, a lower glycogen content, and an increased oxidative enzyme activity. The cells are separated from underlying ectomesenchyme by a basement membrane. There is condensation of ectomesenchymal cells adjacent to the bud **(Figs. 11.5A to C)**.

## Cap Stage (Stage of Proliferation)

By the 11th week of utero, epithelial bud continues to proliferate into the ectomesenchyme. It does not expand uniformly and unequal growth in different parts of the tooth bud leads to cap stage, which is characterized by a shallow invagination on the deep surface of the bud.

The epithelial ingrowth which superficially resembles a cap is called enamel organ or

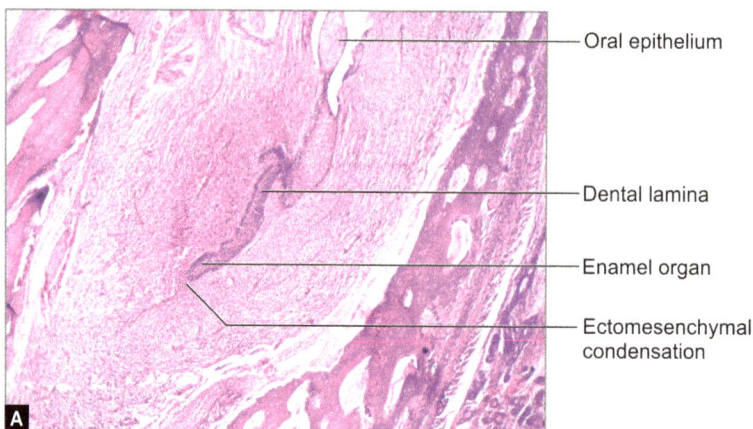

**Fig. 11.5A:** *Contd...*

# Development of Tooth

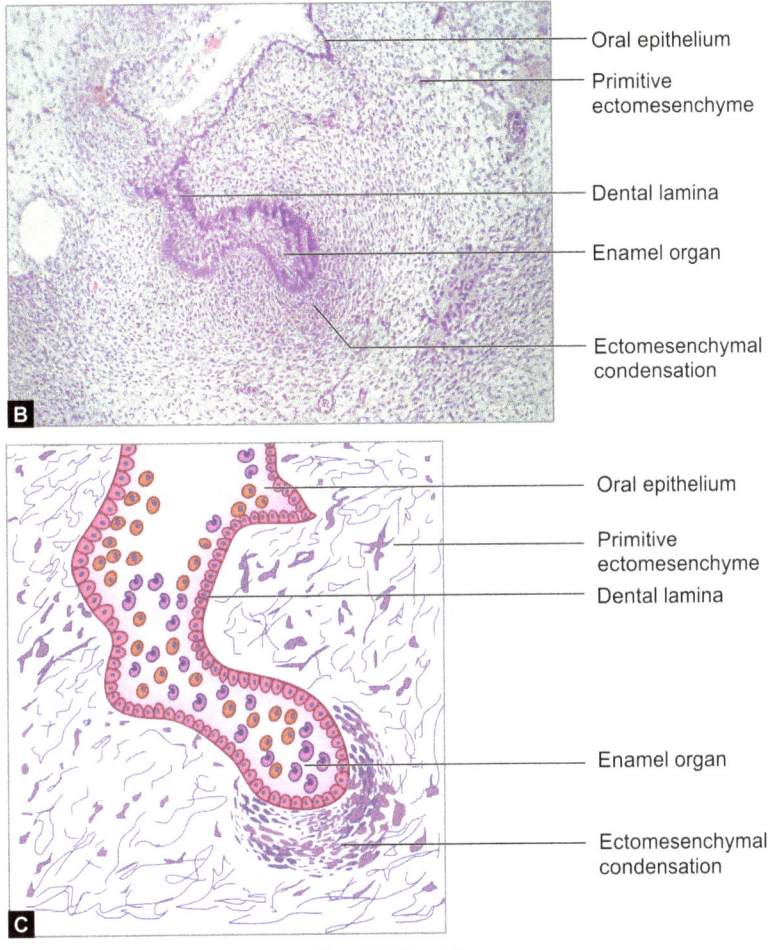

**Figs. 11.5B and C**

**Figs. 11.5A to C:** Bud stage of tooth development.

dental organ. Among other functions, it eventually forms enamel of the tooth. Adjacent to the concave portion of the enamel organ, there is condensation of ectomesenchyme. This condensation of cells results from failure to produce extracellular substance and thus not separated from each other. The condensed ectomesenchymal cells are called dental papilla which forms dentin and pulp. The condensed ectomesenchyme limiting the dental papilla and encapsulating the enamel organ is known as dental follicle or dental sac. It gives rise to cementum, periodontal ligament, and alveolar bone **(Figs. 11.6A and B)**.

The enamel organ or dental organ at this stage consists of distinct cell layers:

## Outer Enamel (Dental) Epithelium

These are cuboidal cells covering the convexity of the cap. They are separated from dental follicle by delicate basement membrane and hemidesmosomes anchor the cells to the basal lamina. The cells of the outer enamel epithelium contain large centrally placed nucleus. Organelles associated with protein synthesis (e.g. endoplasmic reticulum, Golgi material, and mitochondria) are present in small amount.

## Functions

They are involved (a) in the maintenance of the shape of the enamel organ and (b) in the exchange of substances between enamel organ and surrounding tissues.

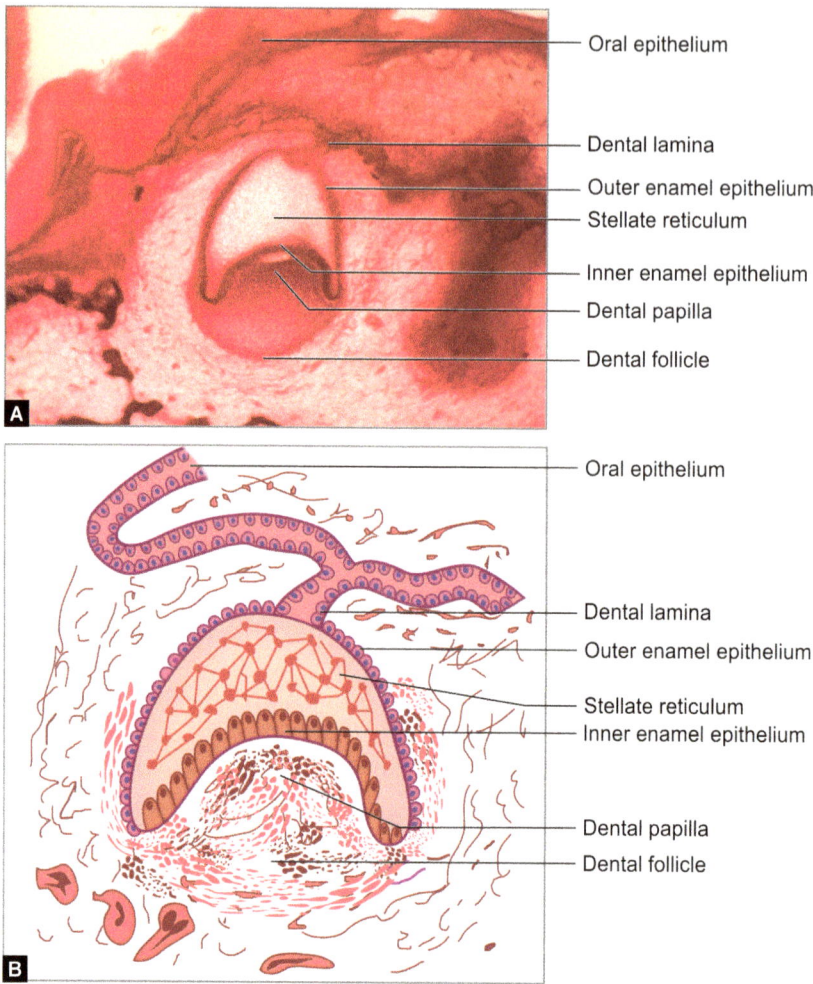

**Figs. 11.6A and B:** Cap stage of tooth development.

### Inner Enamel (Dental) Epithelium

The cells at the concavity of cap of enamel organ are tall, columnar, and are known as inner enamel epithelium. They show an increase in RNA content, hydrolytic, and oxidative enzyme activity. They are separated from dental papilla by basement membrane.

### Function

In later stages, they are transformed into enamel-forming cells, the ameloblast.

### Stellate Reticulum

They are polygonal cells, located in the center of the enamel organ. They synthesize and secrete glycosaminoglycans into extracellular compartment between the cells. Glycosaminoglycans are hydrophilic, so they pull water into enamel organ. The increasing amount of fluid increases the volume of the extracellular compartment of enamel organ and the cells are forced apart. Because the cells retain connections with each other through their desmosomal contacts, they become star-shaped. So the central part of enamel organ is known as stellate reticulum. The cell bodies contain large nucleus with many branching processes. In addition to glycosaminoglycans, the cells also contain alkaline phosphatase and small amounts of RNA and glycogen.

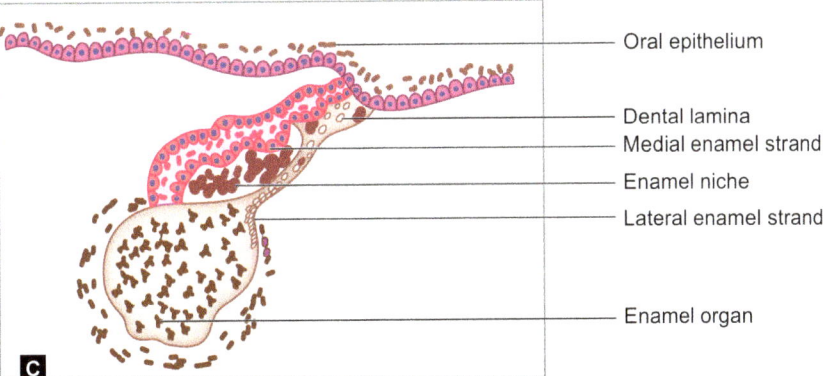

Fig. 11.6C: Enamel niche.

*Functions*
a. It gives a cushion-like consistency that may support and protect the delicate enamel-forming cells.
b. It gives nutrition to the enamel-forming cells.

During early stages of tooth development, the following transitory structures may be seen:
- **Enamel niche (Fig. 11.6C):** It is a funnel-shaped depression enclosing ectomesenchyme and is created as the dental lamina is a sheet rather than a single strand. A section through this arrangement creates the impression that the tooth germ has a double attachment to the oral epithelium by two separate strands. The significance of this structure is unknown.
- **Enamel knot:** It is a localized mass of cells produced by a rapid multiplication of cells in the center of the inner enamel epithelium. It forms a bulge into the dental papilla, at the center of the enamel organ.

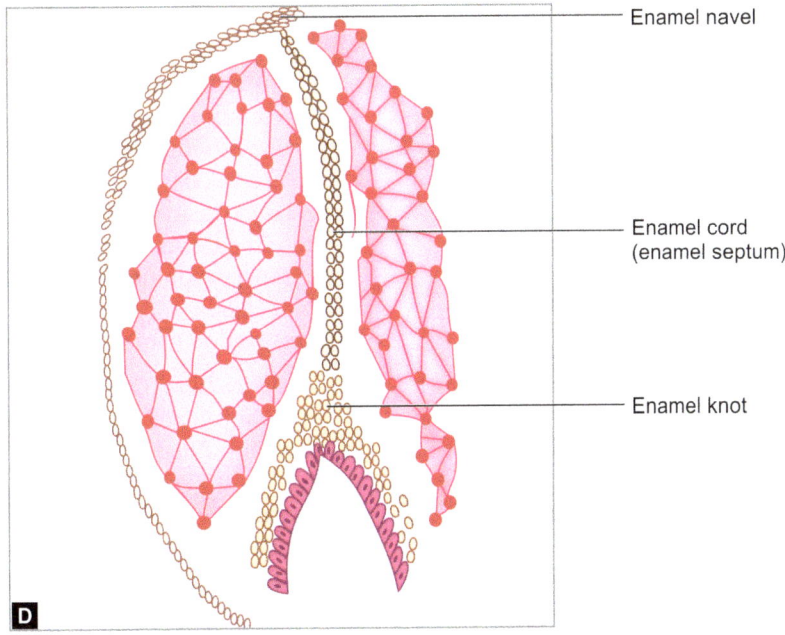

Fig. 11.6D: Part of enamel organ in early bell stage.

It was once thought that the enamel knot played a role in the formation of crown pattern by outlining the central fissure. But its role is unknown as it disappears very soon. It contributes cells to the enamel cord. The current view states that the enamel knot represents the organizational center for cuspal morphogenesis.

- **Enamel cord:** It is a strand of cells extending from enamel knot to stellate reticulum. It overlies the incisal margin of a tooth or to the apex of the first cusp to develop. The cells of the enamel cord are distinguished from their surrounding stellate reticulum cells by their elongated nuclei. It is a focus for the origin of stellate reticulum cells.
- **Enamel septum:** When the enamel cord completely divides the stellate reticulum into two parts, reaching the outer enamel epithelium, it is termed enamel septum.
- **Enamel navel:** Where the enamel cord meets the outer enamel epithelium, a small invagination is termed enamel navel **(Fig. 11.6D)**.

## Early Bell Stage (Stage of Morphodifferentiation and Histodifferentiation)

By the 14th week of development, the tooth germ continues to grow to the next stage of tooth development, the bell stage **(Figs. 11.7A and B)**. It is so called because the enamel organ resembles the shape of a bell as the undersurface of the epithelial cap deepens.

### Enamel Organ in Early Bell Stage

***Inner enamel epithelium:*** The cells of this layer are columnar at early bell stage. They have a centrally placed nucleus and cytoplasm contains free ribosomes, scattered rough endoplasmic reticulum, evenly dispersed mitochondria, some tonofilaments, and a Golgi complex. The cells are connected by desmosomal connections.

They are rich in RNA and glycogen but do not contain alkaline phosphatase. The cells lie between two opposing pressures of stellate reticulum and growing dental papilla and are in a state of equilibrium. The inner enamel epithelium is separated from peripheral cells of dental papilla by a basement membrane and a cell-free zone 1–2 µm wide.

***Morphodifferentiation:*** The configuration of the inner enamel epithelium broadly maps out the occlusal pattern of the tooth. This folding is related to differential mitosis along the inner enamel epithelium. The future cusps and incisal margin are sites of precocious cell maturation associated with cessation of mitosis, while areas corresponding to the fissures and margins of the tooth remain mitotically active **(Fig. 11.8)**. The differential cell division of inner enamel epithelium clearly demarcates the crown pattern of the tooth germ and it is known as morphodifferentiation.

***Stratum intermedium:*** These cells first appear at the early bell stage and consist of two or three layers of flattened cells lying over the inner enamel epithelium.

The cells of the stratum intermedium resemble the cells of the stellate reticulum, although the intercellular spaces are smaller and the cells contain more alkaline phosphatase.

***Functions:*** The stratum intermedium is concerned with:
a. The synthesis of protein.
   (Inner enamel epithelium cannot form enamel without stratum intermedium as they lack alkaline phosphatase. Both the layers are considered as a single functional unit for the formation of enamel).
b. The transport of materials to and from the ameloblasts.
c. Concentration of materials.

***Stellate reticulum:*** This tissue is most fully developed at the bell stage. The intercellular spaces become filled with fluid due to osmotic effects arising from high concentration of glycosaminoglycans. The cells are star-shaped with bodies containing conspicuous nuclei and many branching processes. The cells contain glycosaminoglycans, alkaline phosphatase, and a small amount of RNA and glycogen. The cells possess endoplasmic

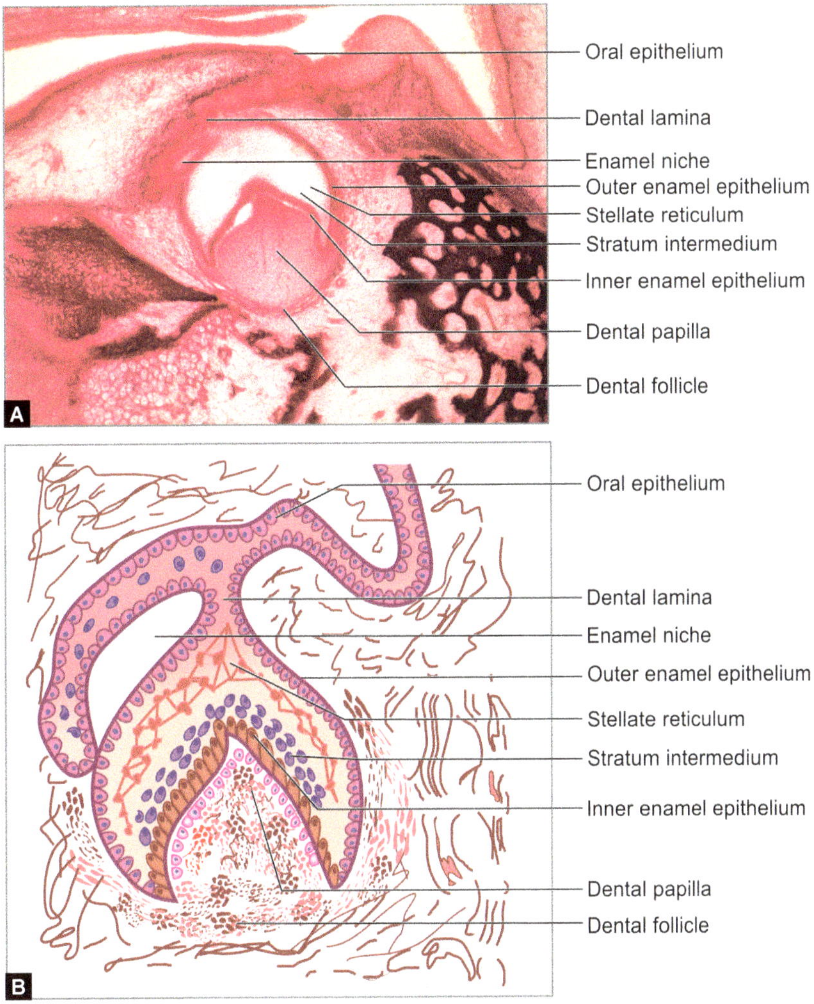

**Figs. 11.7A and B:** Early bell stage of tooth development.

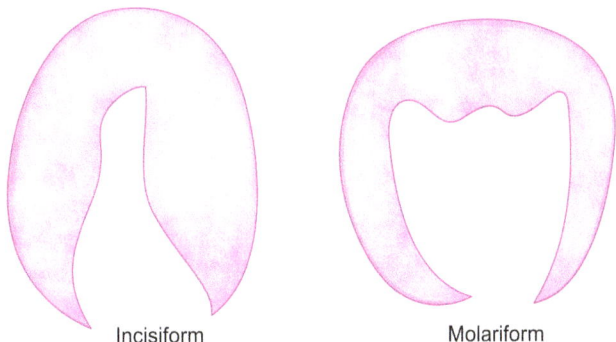

**Fig. 11.8:** Differential cell division of internal enamel epithelium determines the crown pattern.

reticulum, mitochondria, Golgi complex, and microvilli on the cell surface. It indicates that the cells contribute to the secretion of the extracellular material.

## Functions:
a. Protection of underlying tissues.
b. The hydrostatic pressure generated within stellate reticulum is in equilibrium with that of the dental papilla, allowing the proliferative pattern of the intervening inner enamel epithelium to determine crown morphogenesis.
c. The stellate reticulum produces macrophage colony-stimulating factor (MCSF), transforming growth factor (TGF)-$\beta_1$, and parathyroid hormone-related protein (PTHrP) which are released into the dental follicle and activate the osteoclasts to resorb the adjacent alveolar bone for enlargement and eruption of tooth.

*Outer enamel epithelium:* The cells of the outer enamel epithelium flatten to a low cuboidal form. The inner enamel epithelium meets the outer enamel epithelium at the rim of the enamel organ.

This junctional zone is known as cervical loop **(Fig. 11.9)**.

- **Dental papilla:** The dental papilla consists of closely packed mesenchymal cells with only a few delicate extracellular fibrils. Histochemically, the dental papilla becomes rich in glycosaminoglycans.
- **Dental follicle:** Interposed between the enamel organ and the wall of the developing bony crypt is the mesenchymal tissue of the dental follicle **(Fig. 11.10)**.

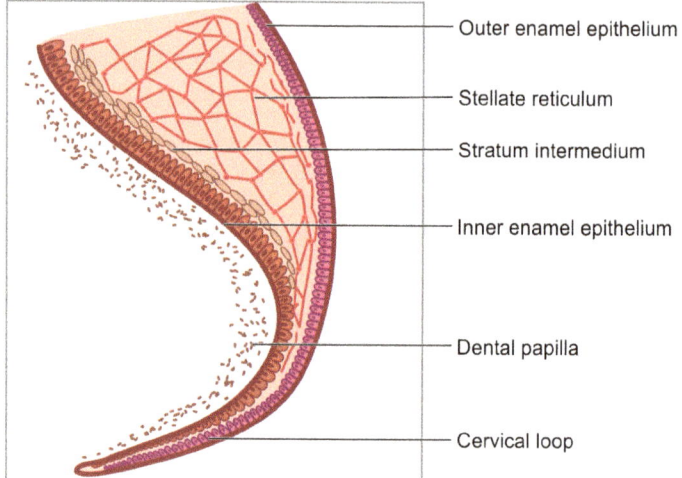

**Fig. 11.9:** Cervical loop.

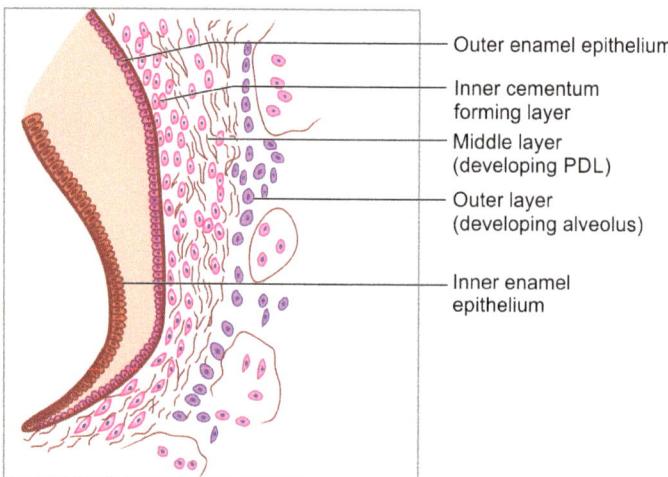

**Fig. 11.10:** Dental follicle.

It has three layers. The inner investing layer is a vascular, fibrocellular condensation, three to four cells thick, immediately surrounding the tooth germ. The nuclei of the cells tend to be elongated circumferentially. This layer is responsible for formation of cementum. The outer layer of the dental follicle is represented by a vascular mesenchymal layer which lines the developing alveolus.

Between the two layers is loose connective tissue with no marked concentration of blood vessels. This layer forms the periodontal ligament.

# HISTODIFFERENTIATION OF TOOTH GERM PRIOR TO ENAMEL AND DENTIN FORMATION

Prior to amelogenesis (enamel formation), the cells of the inner enamel epithelium differentiate into tall columnar cells called ameloblasts. These cells are 4–5 mm in diameter and about 40 mm high. Before enamel formation begins, the stellate reticulum collapses, reducing the distance between the ameloblasts and the nutrient capillaries near outer enamel epithelium. This change begins at the height of the cusp or incisal edge and progresses cervically.

Prior to enamel and dentin formation, the outer enamel epithelium is laid in folds.

Between the folds, the adjacent mesenchyme of the dental follicle forms papillae that contain capillary loops and thus provide a rich nutritional supply for the intense metabolic activity of the avascular enamel organ. Once enamel and dentin deposition start, nutritional supply from dental papilla cannot reach the enamel-forming cells. So the change in stellate reticulum and outer enamel epithelium facilitates the reversal of nutrition from dental follicle.

The cells of the inner enamel epithelium exert an organizing influence on the underlying mesenchymal cells in the dental papilla, which later differentiate into odontoblast, the dentin-forming cells. The basement membrane that separates the enamel organ and the dental papilla just prior to dentin formation is called the membrana preformativa.

## Advanced Bell Stage (Late Bell Stage or Stage of Apposition)

This stage is associated with the formation of the dental hard tissues, commencing at about 18th week of utero. Under the inductive influence of developing ameloblasts (preameloblasts), the adjacent mesenchymal cells of the dental papilla become columnar and differentiate into odontoblasts **(Figs. 11.11A to C and 11.12)**.

The odontoblasts then lay down a layer of dentin along membrana preformativa.

The dentin induces the ameloblasts to secrete enamel. The boundary between the enamel and dentin forms dentinoenamel junction.

The formation of hard tissues gradually progresses from future incisal edge or tip of the cusp to cervix and from dentinoenamel junction to outer periphery in case of enamel and in reverse direction in case of dentin **(Fig. 11.13)**.

The cervical portion of enamel organ gives rise to epithelial root sheath of Hertwig, which acts as a scaffold for root formation.

## Formation of Root

The development of the roots begins after enamel and dentin formation has reached the future cementoenamel junction. At early bell stage, inner and outer enamel epithelia meet at the rim of the enamel organ to form cervical loop. The epithelial cells of inner and outer enamel epithelia of cervical loop proliferate to form a double-layered sheath around the dental papilla between the papilla and the dental follicle.

The sheath is known as Hertwig's epithelial root sheath. It molds the shape of the roots and initiates radicular dentin formation. The outer and inner enamel epithelia bend at the future cementoenamel junction into a horizontal plane, narrowing the wide cervical opening of tooth germ. This rim of the root sheath, the epithelial diaphragm encloses the primary apical foramen **(Fig. 11.13)**.

## Development of Tooth

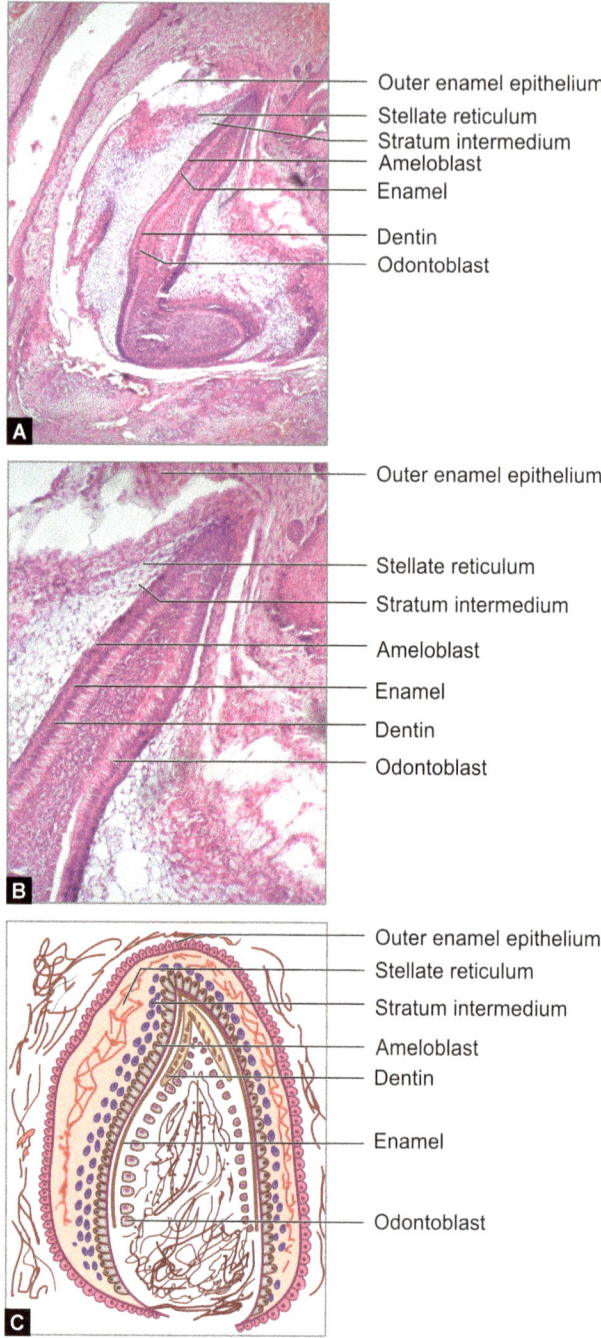

**Figs. 11.11A to C:** Late bell stage.

As the inner epithelial cells of root sheath progressively enclose more and more of the expanding dental papilla, they initiate the differentiation of odontoblasts from the cells at the periphery of the dental papilla. The cells eventually form dentin of the root. Once the first layer of radicular dentin is laid down, the epithelial root sheath loses its structural continuity. It fragments to form a fenestrated network around the tooth. Through the break

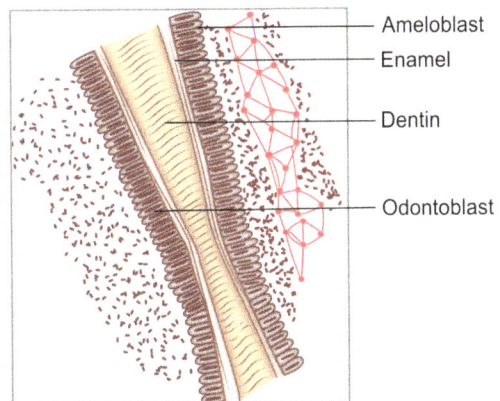

**Fig. 11.12:** Part of developing tooth at late bell stage.

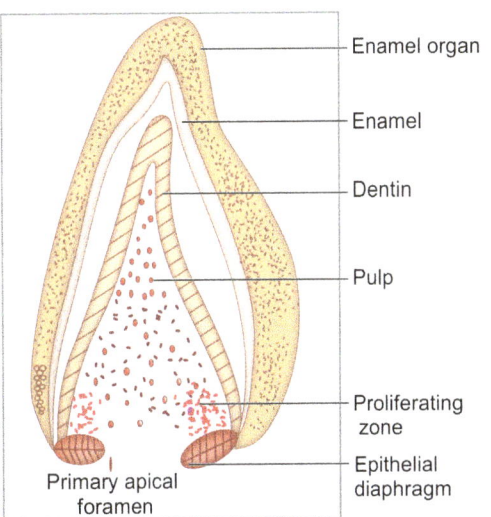

**Fig. 11.13:** Formation of hard tissue progresses from incisal edge to cervix. Formation of epithelial diaphragm and primary apical foramen.

in the root sheath, the newly formed dentin comes in direct contact with the connective tissue of the dental follicle **(Figs. 11.14A and B)**.

Under the influence of dentin, cells of the dental follicle are differentiated into cementoblasts which are responsible for formation of cementum. This initiates the formation of root of single-rooted tooth.

In case of multirooted tooth, the differential growth of the epithelial diaphragm causes the division of the root trunk into two or three roots.

During the general growth of the enamel organ, the expansion of its cervical opening occurs in such a way that long tongue-like extensions of the horizontal diaphragm develop **(Figs. 11.15A to C)**.

Two such extensions are found in the germs of tooth having two roots and three in the germs of teeth having three roots. Before division of the root trunk occurs, the free ends of these horizontal epithelial flaps grow toward each other and fuse. The single cervical opening of the coronal enamel organ is then divided into two or three openings. On

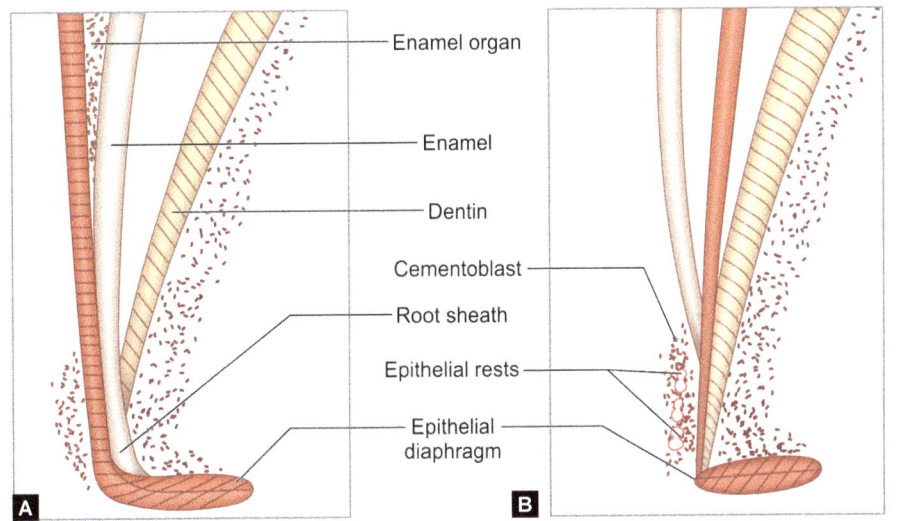

**Figs. 11.14A and B:** (A) Elongation of Hertwig's epithelial root sheath coronal to diaphragm; (B) Root sheath is broken into epithelial rest, differentiation of cementoblast.

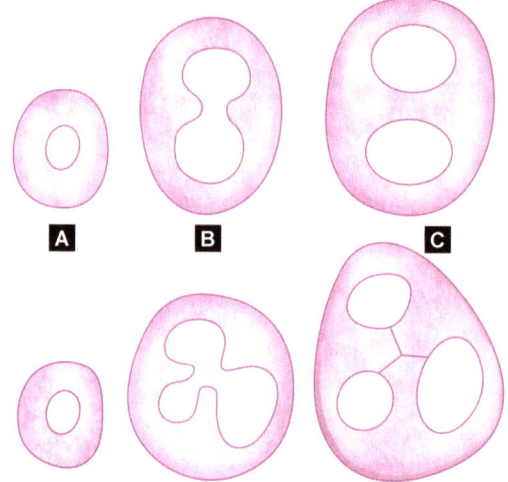

**Figs. 11.15A to C:** Surface view of epithelial diaphragm. (A) Simple diaphragm; (B) Tongue-like extensions of epithelial diaphragm proliferate; (C) The flaps unite and divide single cervical opening into two or three openings.

the pulpal surface of the dividing epithelial bridges, dentin formation starts and on periphery of each opening, root development follows in the same way as single-rooted tooth.

### Growth of Root

The plane of the diaphragm remains relatively fixed during the development and growth of the root. With the onset of root formation, as gradually dentin and cementum are deposited, the crown of the tooth is growing away from the bony base of the crypt and the root sheath is not actually growing into jaw **(Fig. 11.16)**. So with the elongation of the root, crown moves in the upward direction and the plane which was once the cervical region gradually forms wide apical foramen. Later, it is further narrowed by apposition of dentin and cementum to the apex of the root.

### Fate of The Hertwig's Epithelial Root Sheath

The Hertwig's epithelial root sheath loses its structural continuity after the first layer of radicular dentin is laid down. Its remnants persist as an epithelial network of strands or tubules near the external surface of root. These epithelial remnants are found in the periodontal ligament of erupted teeth and are called cell rests of Malassez.

Although apparently functionless, they are the source of the epithelial lining of dental cysts that develop in reaction to inflammation of the periodontal ligament.

### Clinical Consideration

1. Tooth may develop in abnormal location like in ovary as in dermoid tumors or cysts or in the hypophysis. This happens as dental papilla mesenchyme can induce tooth epithelium to form enamel.
2. *Anodontia*: Absence of single or multiple teeth due to the lack of initiation of tooth-forming epithelium is anodontia and most frequently occurs in relation to permanent maxillary lateral incisor, third molar, and mandibular second premolar.
3. *Supernumerary tooth*: Abnormal initiation may result in development of single or multiple supernumerary teeth.
4. Disturbances in morphodifferentiation may affect the form and size of the tooth, e.g. congenital syphilis may lead to mulberry molar and peg-shaped lateral incisor.

### Hard Tissue Formation

The development of hard tissues consists of two phases **(Table 11.1)**:

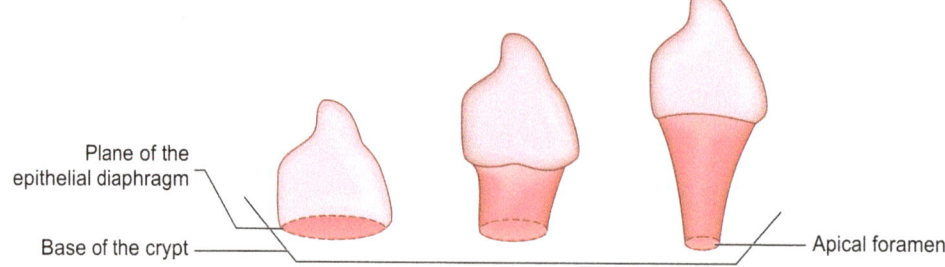

**Fig. 11.16:** Crown moves in upward direction with elongation of root.

1. Initially, there is extracellular secretion of an organic matrix.
2. In the next phase, there is deposition of mineral (primarily in the form of calcium hydroxyapatite crystals) within organic matrix surrounding a nucleus.

## Amelogenesis (Development of Enamel)

Amelogenesis or formation of enamel is a complex process and under genetic control. The deposition of enamel begins at the late bell stage, immediately after dentinogenesis has commenced.

> Ameloblasts are differentiated from the inner enamel epithelium. Under the inductive influence of ameloblasts, the adjacent ectomesenchymal cells of dental papilla are differentiated to odontoblasts which lay down a layer of dentin along membrana preformativa. The dentin then induces the ameloblasts to initiate their secretory activities.

In a single developing tooth, amelogenesis will be present at different stages. When enamel is being formed, the ameloblasts at different locations in the inner enamel epithelium will beat different stages of enamel-forming process but, by the time enamel formation is complete, each ameloblast will have completed a similar life cycle. Different tooth types form enamel at different times, at different rates, and with different final morphological outcomes.

## Life Cycle of the Ameloblasts

An understanding of amelogenesis is best approached by outlining the life cycle of the ameloblasts. It is divided into six stages which are described below.

1. ***Morphogenic stage***

   The differential cell division of the inner enamel epithelium and their interaction with adjacent ectomesenchyme determine the crown pattern of the tooth germ.

   The inner enamel epithelial cells are short columnar with large oval nuclei that almost fill the cell body **(Fig. 11.17A)**. The Golgi apparatus and the centrioles are located in the proximal end (toward stratum intermedium) of the cells. The mitochondria and other cytoplasmic components are evenly dispersed throughout the cytoplasm. During ameloblast differentiation, mitochondria migrate to basal region of the cells and terminal bars appear. They are the point of close contact between the cells. They comprise thickening of the opposing cell membranes associated with condensation of underlying cytoplasm.

2. ***Organizing stage (presecretory stage)***

   The inner enamel epithelium interacts with the adjacent connective tissue which differentiates into odontoblast. This differentiation is controlled by the cells of the inner enamel epithelium that release transforming growth factor (TGF)-β. The inner enamel epithelium becomes longer and the nucleus-free-zones at the distal end of the cells become as long as the proximal part containing the nuclei **(Fig. 11.17B)**. There is migration of centrioles and Golgi apparatus from

**TABLE 11.1:** Differences in the processes of mineralization between enamel and other hard tissues (dentin, cementum, and bone).

| Enamel | Dentin, cementum, and bone |
|---|---|
| 1. Only dental hard tissue which is ectodermally derived | 1. Derived from ectomesenchymal tissue |
| 2. Organic matrix is composed of protein and not collagenous in nature | 2. Organic matrix is collagenous in nature |
| 3. Initial mineralization of enamel matrix takes place almost simultaneously with organic matrix deposition. Thus, unmineralized layer of organic matrix is not found | 3. There is a lag period between matrix formation and mineralization, resulting in the presence of a layer of unmineralized organic matrix, a few micrometers thick |
| 4. The organic matrix of enamel is removed during the final mineralization phase (maturation), leaving less than 1% by weight of organic matrix in fully formed enamel | 4. The organic matrix of dentin, cementum, and bone forms a substantial part of mineralized tissue |

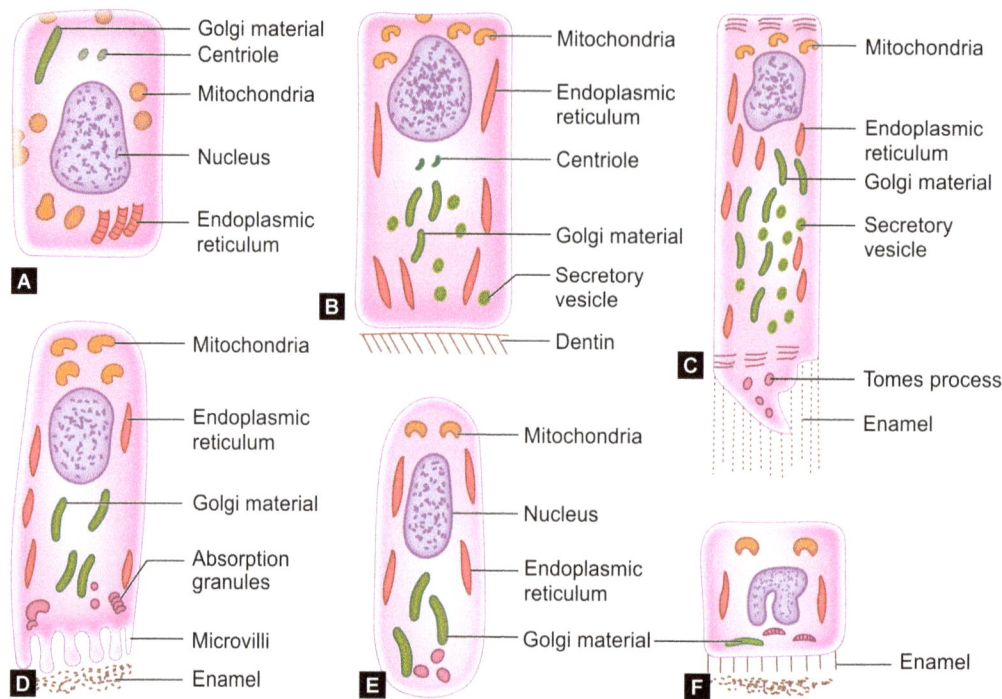

**Figs. 11.17A to F:** (A) Morphogenic stage; (B) Organizing stage; (C) Formative stage; (D) Maturative stage; (E) Protective stage; (F) Desmolytic stage.

the proximal end of the cells into their distal end. Fine acidophilic granules (EM study reveals them as mitochondria) are concentrated in basal or proximal part of cell.

Once the odontoblasts have differentiated, the basal lamina separating them from preameloblasts disappears and future ameloblasts and odontoblasts are in intimate contact, allowing inductive signaling to occur between them.

Before formation of enamel and dentin, there is reversal of nutritional source for ameloblasts as they can no more receive nutrient material from blood vessels of dental papilla. The capillaries of the dental sac proliferate into the corrugated folds of outer enamel epithelium. The stellate reticulum collapses, reducing the distance between the ameloblasts and nutrient capillaries. The change in stellate reticulum and outer enamel epithelium facilitates the reversal of nutrition from dental follicle. In the initial stages of enamel formation until the collapse of the enamel organ, ameloblasts utilize the stored glycogen, accumulated before beginning their secretory activity.

During the terminal phase of the organizing stage, the odontoblasts lay down the first layer of dentin. This provides the signal for the ameloblasts to begin secretion. The odontoblasts produce noncollagenous proteins like dentin sialophosphoprotein (DSPP). A small amount of DSPP is also formed by preameloblasts. This initial matrix defines dentinoenamel junction.

3. **Formative stage (secretory stage)**
In the formative stage, the ameloblasts are 2–4 mm in diameter and about 60 mm in height, with their nuclei at the basal end (away from forming enamel). The ameloblasts enter their formative stage after the first layer of dentin has been formed. The earliest apparent change is the development of blunt cell processes on the ameloblast surfaces, which penetrate the basal lamina and enter the predentin **(Fig. 11.17C)**.

4. *Maturative stage*

   Enamel maturation (full mineralization) occurs after most of the thickness of the enamel matrix has been formed in the occlusal or incisal area.

   In the cervical parts of the crown, enamel matrix formation is still progressing. At this stage, the cells of the stratum intermedium lose their cuboidal shape and regular arrangement and assume a spindle shape. Ameloblasts play a part in the maturation of enamel. They are slightly reduced in length and are closely attached to the enamel matrix. They display microvilli at their distal extremities, and cytoplasmic vacuoles containing material resembling enamel matrix are present (**Fig. 11.17D**). These structures indicate an absorptive function of these cells.

5. *Protective stage*

   After complete calcification of enamel, the ameloblast cell layer cannot be differentiated from stratum intermedium and outer enamel epithelium. The three cell layers form a stratified epithelial covering of the enamel, the reduced enamel epithelium (**Fig. 11.17E**). The function of the reduced enamel epithelium is to protect the mature enamel by separating it from surrounding connective tissue until the tooth erupts. If the connective tissue comes in contact with the enamel, it may be either resorbed or covered by a layer of cementum. During this phase of the life cycle of ameloblasts, the epithelial enamel organ may retract from the cervical edge of the enamel. The adjacent mesenchymal cells may then deposit afibrillar cementum on the enamel surface.

6. *Desmolytic stage*

   The reduced enamel epithelium proliferates, inducing atrophy of the connective tissue separating it from oral epithelium. The epithelial cells elaborate enzymes which destroy the connective tissue fibers by desmolysis. After the desmolysis of connective tissue, the reduced enamel epithelium fuses with oral epithelium and it facilitates eruption of tooth (**Figs. 11.17A to F**). Premature degeneration of reduced enamel epithelium may prevent the eruption of a tooth.

### Prerequisite for Amelogenesis

a. Differentiation of inner enamel epithelium to ameloblasts.
b. Deposition of dentin as a phase of reciprocal induction.
c. High alkaline phosphatase activity of stratum intermedium.
d. Reversal of nutritional source.

On the basis of ultrastructure and composition, two processes are involved in the development of enamel: a) organic matrix formation and b) mineralization.

### Formation of Enamel Matrix

After the formation of first layer of dentin, the earliest apparent change is the development of blunt cell processes on the ameloblast surfaces, which penetrate the basal lamina and enter the predentin. After a small amount of dentin has been laid down, the ameloblasts lose the projections that had penetrated the basal lamina separating them from predentin and the islands of enamel matrix are deposited along the predentin. Following the deposition of the initial, thin, aprismatic enamel, the ameloblasts begin to move away from the dentin surface. As a result of that, each cell forms a cone-shaped process, called *Tomes' process* (**Fig. 11.18**), at the distal, secretory end of the ameloblasts. The shape of Tomes

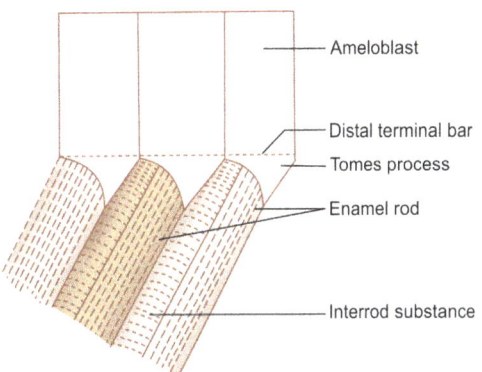

**Fig. 11.18:** Relationship between Tomes' processes and enamel prism formation.

processes is responsible for the prismatic structure of enamel. The processes jut into the newly formed enamel giving the junction between the enamel and ameloblast a "picket fence" or "saw-toothed" appearance. The interdigitation is due to the fact that the long axes of the ameloblasts are not parallel to the long axes of the rods.

The junctional complexes which encircle the ameloblast at their distal and proximal ends have fine radiating actin filaments extending into cytoplasm, forming webs. The junctional complexes which format the distal end are called distal terminal bars **(Fig. 11.18)**. These terminal bars separate the Tomes processes from the cell proper. Ameloblasts are joined to each other by terminal bar apparatus.

The junctional complexes consist of desmosomes and tight junctions. The tonofilaments associated with the desmosomes pass, for a short distance, into the cell and form an incomplete septum between the Tomes process and the rest of the ameloblast. The junction of the distal terminal bars is zonular (encircling the cell) and effectively separates the developing enamel from enamel organ such that all secretion and modification of the matrix occur, via the Tomes processes.

Junctions at the basal end of the ameloblasts, adjacent to the stratum intermedium, are macular and provide mechanical union.

The basic enamel matrix proteins are assembled in the endoplasmic reticulum and carried by transitional vesicles to the Golgi apparatus where glycosylation and sulfation take place before packaging into electron-dense secretory granules 0.25 μm in diameter. The secretory granules are transported along microtubules toward the Tomes process. There is marked aggregation of vesicles with organic matrix at the distal end of the ameloblast. The contents of the vesicles are discharged into the extracellular space, both at the distal end of the cell and between the cell membranes of adjacent ameloblasts. The ameloblasts are pushed away from dentin surface along with progression of enamel matrix formation.

The organic matrix consists of enamel proteins, an array of enzymes including serine proteases, metalloproteinases, and phosphatases and traces of other proteins analogous to various glycosylated, sulfated, and phosphorylated noncollagenous proteins found in the calcifying connective tissues. Developing enamel contains two main groups of proteins: the amelogenins comprise 90–95% and nonamelogenins (enamelin, ameloblastin, tuftelin, and amelotin) comprise the remaining 5–10%.

**Amelogenin:** It is a hydrophobic, proline-rich, heterogenous group of gene-specific, low molecular weight protein. It has high level of histidine, glutamine, and leucine. It has specific functions as in regulating crystal growth and has been shown to form minute nanospheres between which enamel crystals form. So it maintains the spaces between the crystals. In fully formed enamel, amelogenin remains in between the crystals and also surrounding them. It is broken down by proteolytic cleavage with increasing depth of enamel and is absent from inner layer of enamel. Most of the secreted amelogenin is removed during maturation. They form thixotropic gels in that they can be easily squeezed out by the pressure from growing crystals.

**Enamelins:** These are glycine-rich parent molecules and largest enamel proteins, found in the outermost layer of newly secreted enamel. They are primarily located in the prism core and help in nucleation and growth of crystals.

**Ameloblastin (amelin):** The protein is located initially in the region of the prism core near secretory ameloblasts, while smaller breakdown products are found at the prism boundary. They are responsible for generation of prism structure and may play a role in cell adhesion. Ameloblastin is also produced by the epithelial root sheath during root formation.

**Tuftelin:** It is localized to dentinoenamel junction and functions as a signaling molecule during epithelial/mesenchymal interactions.

**Sulfated enamel proteins:** These represent acidic enamel proteins that are present in small amounts and appear to be degraded within about 1–2 hours after their secretion.

**Serum-derived products:** These proteins are not secreted by ameloblasts but are derived from serum. Because of their affinity for hydroxyapatite, these are absorbed into developing enamel. The major serum protein identified in developing enamel is albumin, which has the property of inhibiting mineral growth.

**Amelotin:** This is a recently discovered protein produced by ameloblasts at the maturation stage. It may have a role in cell adhesion.

## Mineralization and Maturation of the Enamel Matrix

In the first stage, the initial hydroxyapatite crystallites of the enamel appear within organic matrix almost immediately, before the matrix is 50 nm thick. An immediate partial mineralization occurs in the enamel matrix. The initial influx may amount to 25–30% of the eventual total mineral content.

> A distinct zone of unmineralized matrix analogous to predentin or osteoid is never seen in enamel.

As enamel protein is deposited directly on mineralized dentin, the first enamel crystallites are nucleated by apatite crystallites located within dentin. Enamel protein tuftelin also acts as a nucleator for the first enamel crystal. The first formed crystallites are thin needle-like, 10–15 nm wide and 1–2 nm thick. As enamel deposition proceeds, a thin continuous layer of enamel is formed along the dentin. This junction is termed as the dentinoenamel membrane. Its presence accounts for the fact that the distal ends of the enamel rods are not in direct contact with the dentin.

There are a number of possible sources for calcium that mineralizes the enamel matrix. Calcium reaches the matrix principally, via the enamel organ (rather than the dental papilla). Possibly, it travels by an extracellular route, or there may be an active transport mechanism utilizing carriers in the cell membranes of the ameloblasts, or the calcium may flow passively from high concentrations in the blood plasma to low concentration in the enamel matrix.

The enamel crystallites are aligned perpendicular to the distal surface of the ameloblasts. The crystallites appear as flattened hexagons when viewed in cross-section. The crystallites that elongate around the tip of the Tomes process form the region of the prism core. Crystallites extending from where the ameloblasts are joined to each other form the region at the prism boundary. Enamel is identical at the prism core and prism boundary except for the orientation of the crystallites. The prism core crystallites are parallel to the long axis of the prism and the prism boundary deviates from this by up to 40–65° **(Fig. 11.18)**. Four ameloblasts contribute to the formation of a single prism and each ameloblast is involved in the development of four prisms **(Fig. 11.19)**.

Enamel crystallites grow rapidly in length within the organic matrix. Enamel prisms elongate incrementally. Each daily increment

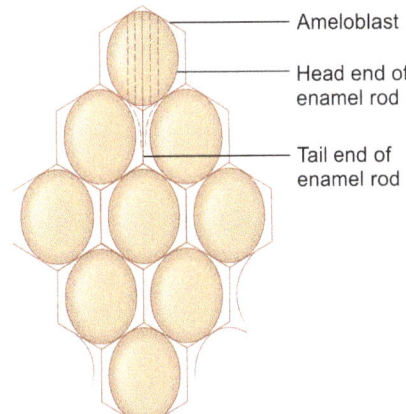

**Fig. 11.19:** Diagrammatic representation of relationships between enamel rods and ameloblasts. The hexagonal lines represent the cross-sections of ameloblasts. Curved, black lines indicate enamel rods, revealing keyhole-shaped rods. Dotted lines represent orientation of crystals, which are parallel to long axes of rods in the "head" and perpendicular to long axes in "tails." The drawing shows that each rod is formed by four ameloblasts and each ameloblast contributes to four different rods.

leads to a cross-striation. Approximately at every 7 days, prominent cross-striations produce the appearance of enamel striae.

The secretory phase ends once the entire thickness of enamel has been laid down. The second stage or maturation is characterized by the gradual completion of mineralization. The process of maturation starts from the height of the crown and progresses cervically. However, at each level, maturation seems to begin at dentinal end of the rods. Each rod matures from the depth to the surface, and the sequence of maturing rods is from cusps or incisal edge toward the cervical line **(Figs. 11.20A to D)**.

As much maturation proceeds, the ribbon-shaped crystals increase in thickness and width. Concomitantly, the organic matrix gradually becomes thinned to make room for growing crystals. The loss of organic matrix is caused by withdrawal of a substantial amount of protein as well as water. Mostly the amelogenins and its degraded products are squeezed out from between the growing crystals leaving behind at inorganic matrix surrounding the crystallites in fully mature enamel matrix.

## Ameloblasts Covering Maturing Enamel

The ameloblasts over maturing enamel are short and have villous surface near the enamel. The ends of the cells are packed with mitochondria and are responsible for transporting organic components from the matrix. The Tomes' processes retract and the distal end becomes flat. A thin layer of aprismatic enamel is formed at the surface.

## Clinical Consideration

1. **Enamel hypoplasia:** It is the defect in matrix formation of enamel and manifested by pitting, furrowing, or even total absence of enamel.
2. **Enamel hypocalcification:** It is characterized by the formation of normal amount of enamel matrix which is not fully matured. It appears dull, opaque white, and it is easily discolored, abraded by mastication, or peeled off in layers. The defective enamel formation is known as amelogenesis imperfecta.

## Dentinogenesis (Development of Dentin)

Dentin formation begins when the tooth germ has reached the bell stage of development and the enamel organ is fully formed with inner enamel epithelium differentiated to secrete enamel matrix. Dentin formation follows a specific anatomical pattern. It begins where cusps will later be formed and continues uniformly down the slopes of the cusp

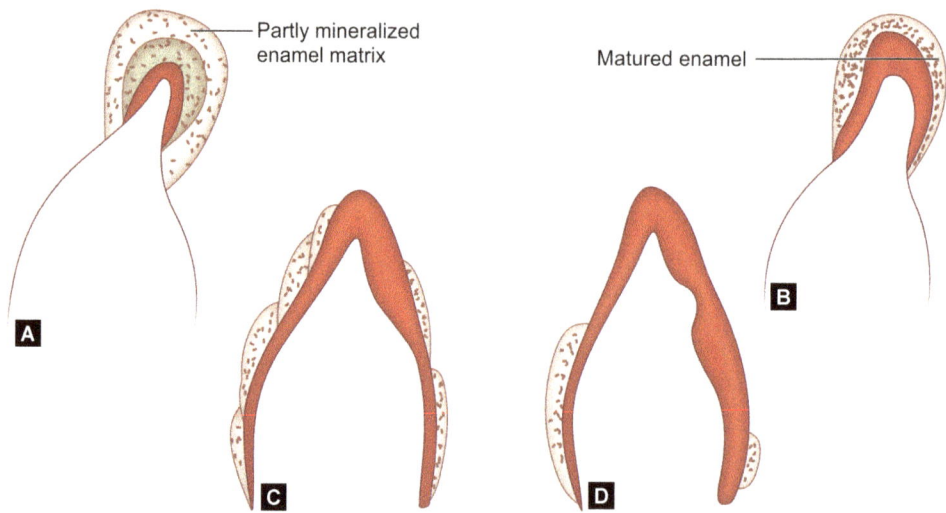

**Figs. 11.20A to D:** Pattern of mineralization and maturation of enamel.

and walls of the crown to the cervical loop, forming coronal dentin. The root dentin forms as the root sheath extends and odontoblasts differentiate on its pulpal surface. Dentinogenesis continues and thickness of dentin increases until at a predetermined point, when it slows down and secondary dentin starts depositing slowly.

*Dentinogenesis* is a continuous process and subdivided into five stages:
1. Differentiation of odontoblasts
2. Deposition of organic matrix
3. Mineralization of organic matrix
4. Peritubular and secondary dentin formation
5. Tertiary dentin formation.

## Differentiation of Odontoblasts

The dentin-forming cells, the odontoblasts are highly specialized connective tissue cells that differentiate from the peripheral cell layer of dental papilla under the influence of ameloblast **(Fig. 11.21)**. The odontoblasts are columnar in shape with 40 mm in length and 7 mm in width.

The nucleus is basally placed **(Fig. 11.22)**. There is a large supranuclear Golgi material and a profuse rough endoplasmic reticulum **(Fig. 11.23A)**. A series of processes develop at the distal end of the cell **(Fig. 11.23B)**. One process becomes more pronounced and it is through this that the matrix is secreted **(Fig. 11.23C)**.

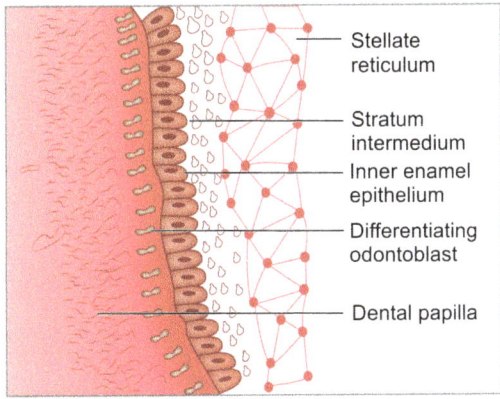

**Fig. 11.21:** Differentiation of odontoblast.

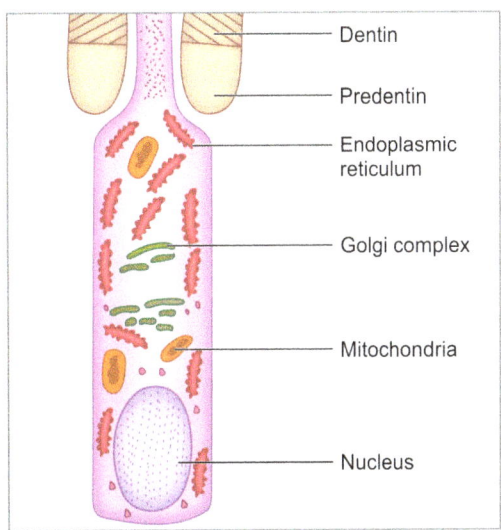

**Fig. 11.22:** Odontoblast.

## Deposition of Organic Matrix

Initially, collagen fibers are formed by subodontoblastic cells in the ground substance of pulp. Later odontoblasts secrete both collagen (Type I, V and VI) and intercollagen substance, proteoglycans, glycoproteins, phosphoproteins, lipid, and growth factors.

Bundles of Type I collagen (composed of large diameter fibrils—0.1-0.2 mm in diameter) formed by the activity of the cells of subodontoblastic layer, pass spirally (corkscrew appearance) between odontoblasts to fan out against the surface of basal lamina supporting the inner enamel epithelium **(Fig. 11.24)**. The fibers are argyrophilic (stain black with silver) and are known as von Korff fibers. The fibers are deposited in structure less ground substance (acid mucopolysaccharide, carbohydrate, and protein). The von Korff fibers are intermingled with fine network of collagenous fibrils (formed by odontoblasts and have a diameter of 0.05 mm).

Electron microscopic existence of von Korff fibers is doubtful. It reveals that the silver staining is of ground substance among the cells and not collagen.

The matrix thus formed consists of Type I collagen fibrils, dentin phosphoprotein (DPP), and dentin sialoprotein (DSP). DPP has a significant role in dentin mineralization and

## Development of Tooth

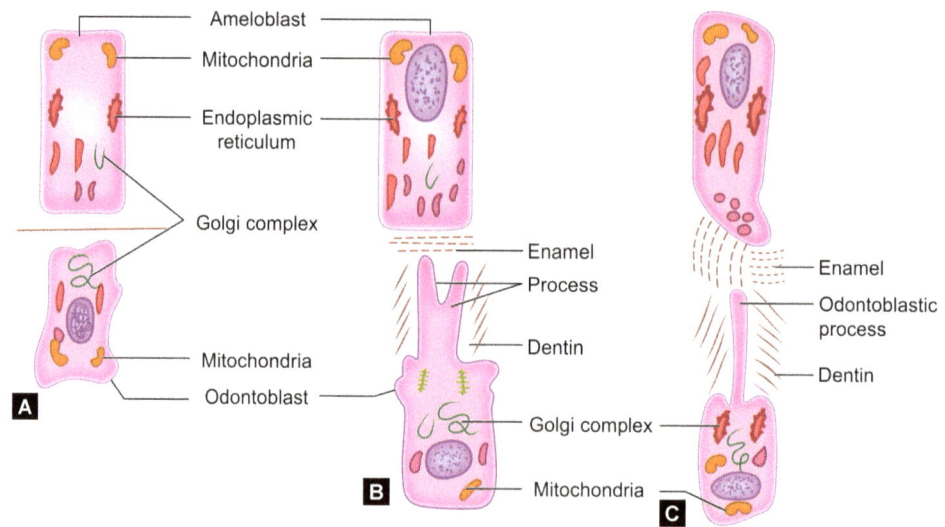

**Figs. 11.23A to C:** Life cycle of odontoblast.

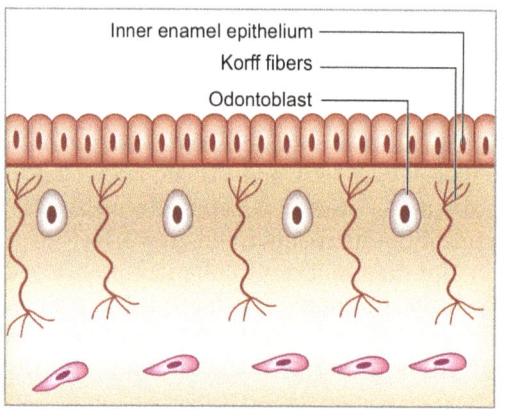

**Fig. 11.24:** Von Korff fibers.

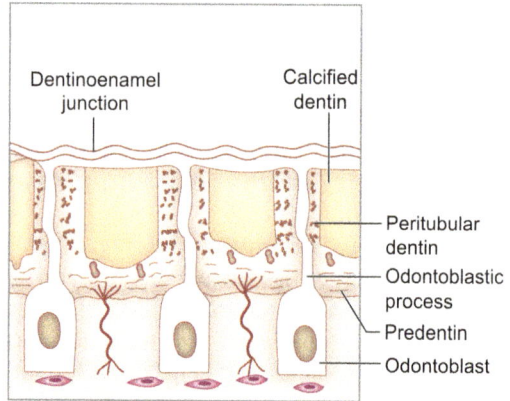

**Fig. 11.25:** Development of dentin.

it is involved in signaling during epithelial-mesenchymal interactions. The large collagen fibrils, together with the ground substance, constitute the organic matrix of first formed or mantle dentin. In mantle dentin, some of the matrix components may be contributed by dental pulp cells beneath the odontoblasts. Once the mantle layer has been deposited, the bulk of the primary circumpulpal dentin is laid down in a regular incremental pattern. After deposition of matrix, the odontoblasts begin to move toward the pulp leaving behind an elongated process, the principal extension of the cell, the odontoblast process **(Fig. 11.25).**

Initial daily increments of matrix deposition are approximately 4 mm. This continues up to the stage of crown formation, eruption of teeth, and movement of the teeth into occlusion. After this stage, dentin production slows down to about 1 mm per day. After root formation dentin deposition may decrease further 2–6 mm wide, unmineralized matrix of dentin is always present along the pulp border as the deposition of mineral lags behind the formation of organic matrix.

### Mineralization of Organic Matrix

The earliest crystal deposition is in the form of very fine plates of hydroxyapatite on the surfaces of the collagen fibrils and in the ground substance with long axis of the crystals parallel to the fibril axis.

Mineralization also occurs by globular calcification. It involves the deposition of crystals in several discrete areas of matrix. With continued crystal growth, globular masses are formed, continue to enlarge, and eventually fuse to form single calcified mass. Throughout dentinogenesis, mineralization is achieved by continuous deposition of mineral, initially in the matrix vesicle and then at the mineralization front. Calcium channels of the L type are present in the basal plasma membrane of the odontoblast. The presence of alkaline phosphatase activity and Ca-ATPase activity at the distal end of the cell indicates a mechanism for the release of mineral from the cell.

## Peritubular and Secondary Dentin Formation

Peritubular dentin consists of small crystals in an amorphous (nonfibrillar) matrix consisting of glycoproteins, proteoglycans, lipids, osteonectin, osteocalcin, and bone sialoprotein. Secondary dentin is formed from original odontoblast and it is a preprogrammed age change rather than a response to external activity. As the pulp volume decreases with continuing dentin deposition, odontoblasts die and that may lead to the change in direction of the tubules, establishing a contour line.

## Tertiary Dentin Formation

Tertiary dentin is the tissue that is laid down in response to a stimulus of any kind. It is a response rather than an age change. Tertiary dentin takes one of two forms depending on the severity of the stimulus. If the stimulus is mild and the original odontoblasts remain alive, they will lay down a tubular form of tertiary dentin, reactionary dentin. If the stimulus is more severe and sufficient to kill the original odontoblasts, new odontoblasts will differentiate from pulpal stem cells and lay down another form of tertiary dentin, reparative dentin, which is atubular and bone-like.

## Clinical Consideration

1. *Dentinogenesis imperfecta*: The condition of defective dentin formation is known as dentinogenesis imperfecta.
2. Exposed dentin should be sealed with nonirritating, insulating substance as thermal, bacterial, chemical, or mechanical trauma may lead to damage of pulp.
3. Tubule system of dentin causes rapid spread of dental caries.

## Cementogenesis (Development of Cementum)

Cementum formation in the developing tooth is preceded by the deposition of dentin along the inner aspect of Hertwig's epithelial root sheath. Once dentin formation is underway, breaks occur in the epithelial root sheath allowing the newly formed dentin to come in contact with the connective tissue of dental follicle and the cells of the follicle are induced to differentiate into cement blast, the cementum-forming cells.

### Primary (Acellular) Cementum

**Matrix formation:** Much of the collagen in primary cementum is derived from Sharpey's fibers of the periodontal ligament and cementoblasts secrete little collagen. The cementoblasts secrete ground substance as it contains intracytoplasmic organelles necessary for protein synthesis and secretion.

**Mineralization:** The presence of the hydroxyapatite crystals in the neighboring dentin initiates mineralization in cementum. The adjacent periodontal ligament fibroblasts, which are rich in alkaline phosphatase, may play a role in mineralization.

Mineralization proceeds in a linear fashion. There is always a thin, unmineralized layer of precementum present on the developing surface of the cementum **(Fig. 11.26)**.

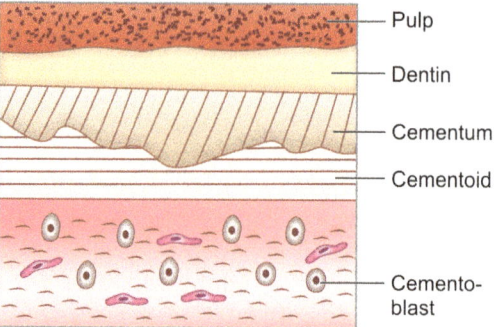

Fig. 11.26: Formation of acellular cementum.

## Secondary (Cellular) Cementum

Following the formation of primary cementum in the cervical portion of the root, secondary cementum appears in the apical region of the root (at about the time of eruption, when approximately two-thirds of the root has formed). Following the loss of continuity of the epithelial root sheath, large basophilic cells are seen to differentiate from the adjacent cells of dental follicle against the surface of root dentin. These cementoblasts secrete the collagen fibers and ground substance and form the intrinsic fibers of cellular cementum. These fibers are oriented parallel to the root surface and do not extend into the periodontal ligament. Associated with the increased rate of formation, a thin unmineralized precementum layer (about 5 µm thick) will be present on the surface of cellular cementum. Cementoblasts at the surface become incorporated into the forming matrix and are converted into cementocytes (Fig. 11.27).

Matrix contains both extrinsic fibers from periodontal ligament arranged perpendicular to root surface and that secreted by cementoblasts.

## QUESTIONNAIRE

1. What is dental lamina? Discuss the function and fate of dental lamina.
2. Enumerate the stages of development of tooth. Describe the early bell stage and advanced bell stage of development of tooth.
3. Describe the formation and growth of root of tooth. Discuss fate of Hertwig's epithelial root sheath.
4. What is amelogenesis? Describe the life cycle of ameloblast. Discuss amelogenesis with diagram.
5. Discuss dentinogenesis.
6. Discuss cementogenesis.
7. Write notes on:
    a. Bud stage of development of tooth.
    b. Cap stage of development of tooth.
    c. Amelogenin.
    d. Hertwig's epithelial root sheath.
    e. Tomes' process.

## BIBLIOGRAPHY

1. Antonio N. Ten Cate's Oral Histology Development, Structure, and Function, 7th edition. Mosby: Elsevier; 2008.
2. Berkovitz BKB, Holland GR, Moxham BJ. A Colour Atlas and Textbook of Oral Anatomy Histology and Embryology, 4th edition. Mosby: Elsevier; 2009.
3. Das AK. Dental Anatomy and Oral Histology, 1st edition. West Bengal: Current Books International; 1972.
4. Kumar GS. Orban's Oral Histology and Embryology, 12th edition. Mosby: Elsevier; 2009.

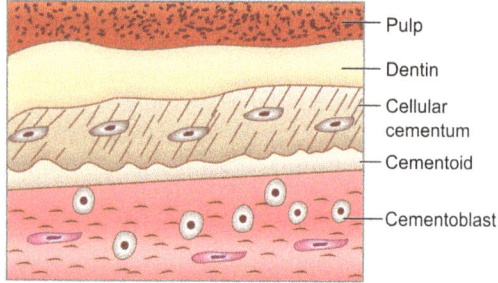

Fig. 11.27: Formation of cellular cementum.

# CHAPTER 12

# Eruption and Shedding of Tooth

## ERUPTION

Eruption (LATIN—*ERUMPERE*, TO BREAK OUT) is defined as axial or occlusal movement of the tooth from its developmental position within the jaw to its functional position in the occlusal plane.

For the teeth to become functional, considerable movement is required to bring them into the occlusal plane. The physiologic movements made by teeth are complex and may be described as:

**Preeruptive tooth movement:** It is made by the deciduous and permanent tooth germs within tissues of the jaw before they begin to erupt. Preeruptive stage extends from initiation of tooth germ to beginning of root formation.

**Eruptive tooth movement:** It is made by a tooth to move from its position within the bone of the jaw to its functional position in occlusion. The eruptive stage starts from the beginning of root formation and extends till the tooth reaches the occlusal plane.

**Posteruptive tooth movement:** It is maintaining the position of the erupted tooth in occlusion while the jaws continue to grow and compensate for occlusal and proximal tooth wear. Posteruptive stage starts from the tooth reaching the occlusal plane and extends till the tooth is lost.

Superimposed on these movements is the replacement of entire deciduous dentition by the permanent. The movement of tooth in relation to bone is called active eruption. The exposure of the erupting tooth by recession of gingiva and peeling of the epithelial attachment is called passive eruption.

### Preeruptive Tooth Movement

Throughout the preeruptive phase of tooth development, there is concentric growth of the tooth within its follicle without any active bodily movement in a direction indicating eruption toward the oral cavity. When the deciduous tooth germs first differentiate, they are extremely small, and there is a good deal of space for them in the developing jaw. Because they grow rapidly, they become crowded. This crowding is gradually alleviated by a lengthening of the infant jaws, which provides room for the second deciduous molars to drift backward and the anterior teeth to drift forward. At the same time, the tooth germs also move outward as the jaws increase in width, and upward (downward in the upper jaw) as the jaws increase in height. Permanent teeth with deciduous predecessors also undergo complex movements before they reach the position from which they will erupt. The permanent incisors and canines first develop lingual to the deciduous tooth germs at the level of their occlusal surfaces and in the same bony crypt (**Fig. 12.1**). As their deciduous predecessors erupt, they move to a more apical position and occupy their own bony crypts (**Fig. 12.2**). Permanent premolars begin their development lingual to their predecessors at the level of their occlusal surfaces and in the same bony crypt. They also shift so that they are eventually situated in their own crypts beneath the divergent roots of the deciduous molars (**Fig. 12.3**).

The permanent molars, which have no deciduous predecessors, also move considerably from the site of their initial differentiation. For example, the upper

# Eruption and Shedding of Tooth

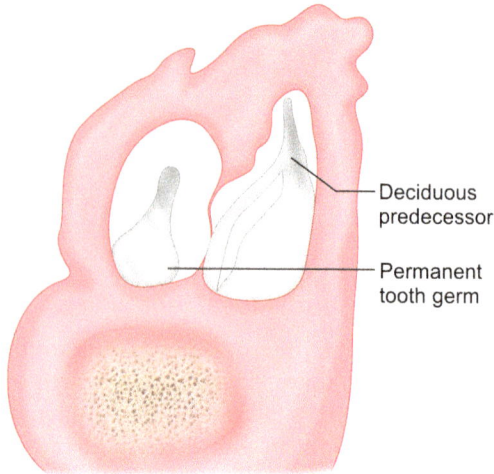

Fig. 12.1: Relationship between developing permanent incisor with deciduous predecessor.

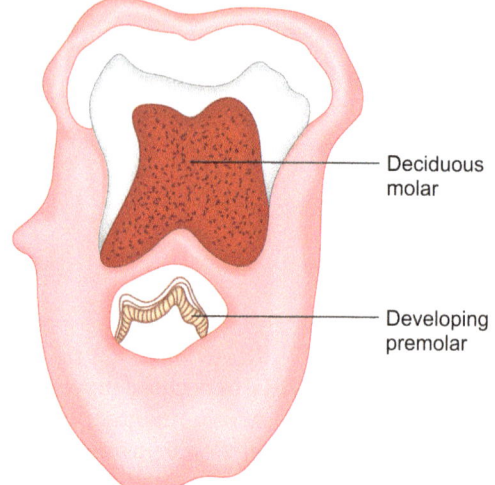

Fig. 12.3: Developing premolar beneath the divergent roots of deciduous molars.

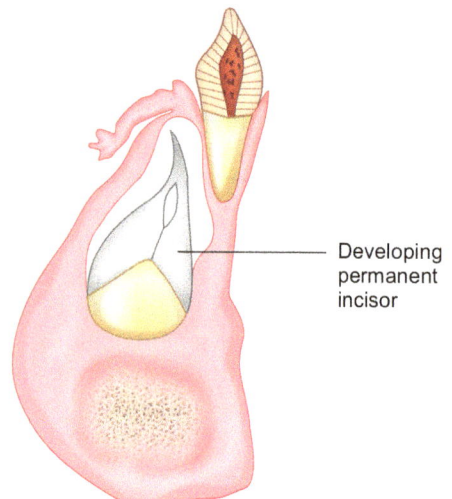

Fig. 12.2: Apical movement of developing permanent incisor.

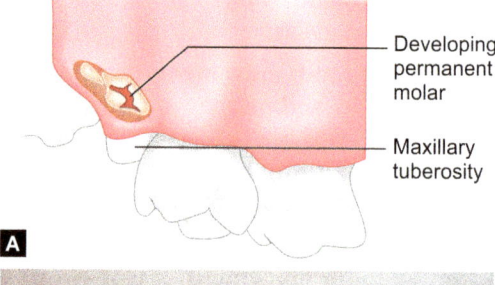

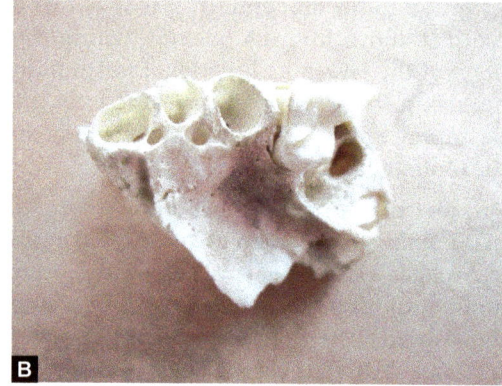

Figs. 12.4A and B: Developing permanent molar in maxillary tuberosity.

permanent molars, which develop in the tuberosity of the maxilla (**Figs. 12.4A and B**), at first have their occlusal surfaces facing distally and swing around only when the maxilla has grown sufficiently to provide the necessary space.

Similarly, mandibular molars develop with their occlusal surfaces inclined mesially and only become upright as room becomes available. All these movements are linked to jaw growth and may be considered as movements positioning the tooth and its crypt within the jaws preparatory to tooth eruption.

## Eruptive Tooth Movement

During the phase of eruptive tooth movement, the tooth moves from its position within the bone of the jaw to its functional position in occlusion and the principal direction of movement is occlusal or axial (movement along the long axis of tooth). However, it is important to recognize that jaw growth is normally occurring while most teeth are erupting, so that movement in planes other than axial is superimposed on eruptive movement.

Movements in other planes account for tilting and drifting.

## Posteruptive Tooth Movement

Posteruptive tooth movements are those that:
1. Maintain the position of the erupted tooth while the jaw continues to grow.
2. Compensate for occlusal and proximal wear. The former movement, like eruptive movement, occurs principally in an axial direction to keep pace with the increase in height of the jaws. It involves both the tooth and its socket and ceases when jaw growth is completed. The movements compensating for occlusal and proximal wear continue throughout life and consist of axial and mesial migration, respectively.

# HISTOLOGY OF TOOTH MOVEMENT

## Preeruptive Phase

During the preeruptive phase, positioning of the developing tooth within the growing jaws is achieved in two ways:
1. There is a total bodily movement of the germ.
2. There is its eccentric growth which means that one part of the developing tooth germ remains stationary while the remainder continues to grow, leading to a shift in its center. This type of growth explains how the deciduous incisors maintain their superficial position as the jaws grow in height. Histologically, preeruptive tooth movement is reflected by bone remodeling at the periphery of the dental follicle, bringing about bone remodeling of the crypt wall. Thus, during bodily movement of the tooth, osteoclastic bone resorption occurs on the surface of the crypt wall in advance of the moving tooth while bone deposition occurs on the crypt wall behind it. During eccentric movement, bone resorption is seen on the surface of the crypt that faces the growing tooth germ.

## Eruptive Phase

During the eruptive phase of physiologic tooth movement, significant developmental changes occur, including the formation of the roots, periodontal ligament, and dentogingival junction of the tooth.

Root formation is initiated by proliferation of Hertwig's epithelial root sheath. The forming root first grows toward the floor of the bony crypt and as a result, there is resorption of bone in this location to provide room for the advancing root tip. However, with the onset of eruptive tooth movement, space is created for the forming root and resorption no longer occurs on the floor of the crypt. Indeed, in some instances, the distance moved by the tooth outstrips the rate of root formation and bone deposition occurs on the crypt floor **(Fig. 12.5)**.

As the roots of the tooth form, important changes associated with the development of the supporting apparatus of the tooth occur in the dental follicle. There is bone deposition on the crypt wall, cement deposition on the

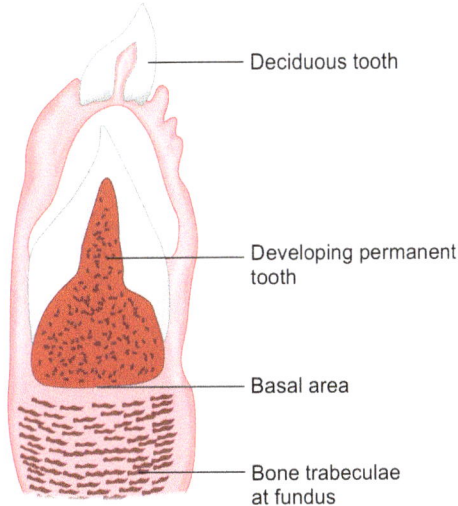

**Fig. 12.5:** Bone deposition on crypt floor.

newly formed root surface, and organization of a periodontal ligament from the dental follicle. These changes lag behind root formation. There are a number of important histologic features in the periodontal ligament that are important in explaining eruptive tooth movement:

1. Occurrence of cell-to-cell contacts of the adherence type between periodontal ligament fibroblasts.
2. Presence of contractile elements in ligament fibroblasts.
3. Occurrence of a structure called the fibronexus. This describes a morphologic relationship between intracellular microfilaments in the fibroblast, a corresponding increased density of fibroblast cell membrane, extracellular filaments, and fibronectin. Fibronectin is a sticky glycoprotein that sticks to a number of extracellular components, including collagen.
4. Active ingestion and degradation of old collagen fibrils by many of the fibroblasts of the ligament and the concurrent formation of new collagen fibrils. Thus, the continual degradation and synthesis of collagen by fibroblasts permit remodeling of the principal fiber bundles of the periodontal ligament.

Significant changes occur within the tissues that cover the erupting tooth. There is a loss of the intervening connective tissue between the reduced enamel epithelium covering the crown of the tooth and the overlying oral epithelium by the enzymes secreted by epithelial cells. The breakdown products of connective tissues are removed by reduced enamel epithelium. Then two epithelia proliferate and form a solid plug of cells in advance of the erupting tooth. The central cells of this epithelial mass degenerate and form an epithelium-lined canal through which the tooth erupts without any hemorrhage. This epithelial cell mass is also involved in the formation of the dentogingival junction **(Fig. 12.6)**. Once the tooth has broken through the oral mucosa, it continues to erupt at the same rate until it reaches the occlusal plane and meets its antagonist. As further occlusal movement is restricted, additional root growth is accommodated by the removal of bone on the socket floor.

Successional teeth possess an additional anatomic feature, the gubernacular canal and its contents, the gubernacular cord, which may have an influence on eruptive tooth movement. The cord is composed of central strand of epithelium (derived from dental lamina) surrounded by connective tissue.

When the successional tooth germ first develops within the same crypt as its deciduous predecessor, bone surrounds both tooth germs but does not completely close over them. As the deciduous tooth erupts, the permanent tooth germ becomes

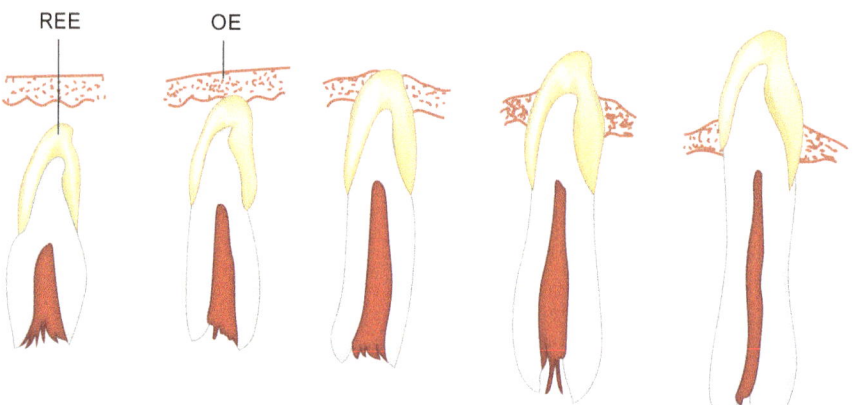

**Fig. 12.6:** Diagrammatic representation of development of the dentogingival junction during eruption of tooth.
(REE, Reduced enamel epithelium; OE, Oral epithelium).

situated apically and entirely enclosed by bone and except for a small canal that is filled with connective tissue and often contains epithelial remnants of the dental lamina. This connective tissue mass is termed the "gubernacular cord" **(Fig. 12.7)** and it may have a function in guiding the permanent tooth as it erupts. But surgical removal of cord does not prevent eruption of permanent tooth.

> Eruption rates of teeth are greatest at the time of crown emergence. The rate differs according to the tooth type. The permanent maxillary central incisors are reported to erupt at about 1 mm/month; the rates for mandibular second premolars have been determined to be about 4.5 mm in 14 weeks. For permanent third molars, where space is available, eruption rates of 1 mm in 3 months have been recorded. The rate of eruption represents a balance between forces tending to move the tooth into the mouth (eruptive force) and forces tending to prevent this movement (resistive force). Resistance may be produced by overlying soft tissues and alveolar bone, the viscosity of the surrounding periodontal ligament/dental follicle, and occlusal forces.
>
> The molecular events associated with the initiation of eruption are not well understood. The epidermal growth factor (EGF), transforming growth factor α, and macrophage colony-stimulating factor (MCSF) can induce tooth eruption. Signaling from stellate reticulum of the enamel organ also appears to have a role in regulating eruption. This signaling seems to occur, via parathyroid-hormone-related protein and interleukin 1α.

## Posteruptive Phase

In the posteruptive phase, the tooth makes movements primarily to accommodate the growth of the jaws. The principal movement is in an axial direction. It occurs most actively between the ages of 14 years and 18 years and is associated with condylar growth, which separates the jaws and teeth. Although bone deposition occurs at the alveolar crest and on the socket floor, this is not responsible for tooth movement. The same forces responsible for eruptive tooth movement achieve axial posteruptive movement with bone deposition occurring later.

There are also movements made to compensate for occlusal and proximal wear of the tooth. It is generally assumed that the continuous deposition of cementum around the apices of the roots of teeth is sufficient to compensate for occlusal wear.

It is more likely that the forces causing tooth eruption are still available to bring about sufficient axial movement of the tooth to compensate for occlusal wear. The cementum deposition that occurs is probably an infilling phenomenon.

Wear also takes place at the contact points between teeth and to maintain tooth contact mesial or proximal drift takes place. Histologically, this drift is seen as a selective deposition and resorption of bone on the socket walls by osteoblasts and osteoclasts, respectively.

## MECHANISM OF ERUPTION OF TOOTH

The mechanism that causes eruption of tooth is a combination of factors. They are (1) bone remodeling, (2) root growth, (3) vascular pressure, and (4) ligament traction.

### Bone Remodeling

Bone remodeling of the crypt wall is important to achieve tooth eruption and in experiments where tooth germ is removed but the follicle is left in position, the eruptive pathway still forms in bone. Such experiments properly indicate dental follicle (not bone), as the major determinant in tooth eruption.

### Root Growth

This theory states that pulp grows and pushes against the cushion hammock ligament which

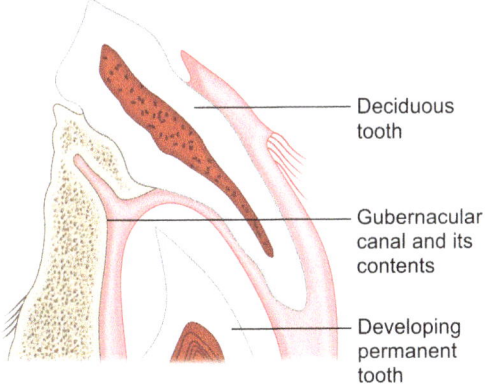

**Fig. 12.7:** Gubernacular cord.

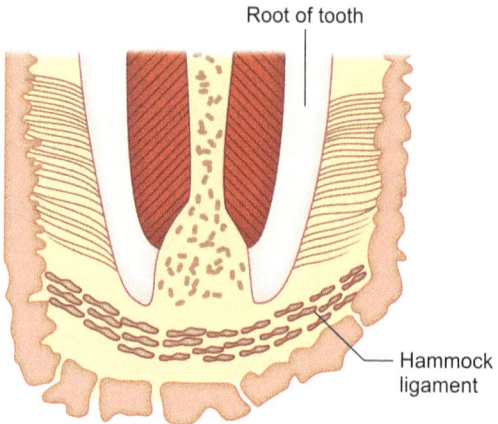

**Fig. 12.8:** Mechanism of eruption—root growth.

passes from one side of bony wall of the socket to the opposite wall. Recent work has shown that this hammock ligament does not extend across the socket, but only separates the pulp from the follicle. It is attached to root only and rootless teeth are seen to erupt also. These make this theory untenable **(Fig. 12.8)**.

### Vascular Pressure

It is known that teeth move in synchrony with the arterial pulse, so local volume changes can produce limited tooth movement. Ground substance can swell by up to 50% with the addition of water and a differential pressure sufficient to cause tooth movement between the tissues below and above an erupting tooth has been reported in the dog.

Again, whether such pressures are the prime movers of teeth is debatable because surgical excision of the root and therefore the local vasculature does not prevent tooth eruption.

### Periodontal Ligament Traction

There is a good deal of evidence that the eruptive force resides in the dental follicle–periodontal ligament complex. The fibroblasts with contractile filaments are in contact with one another to permit summation of contractile forces and exhibit fibronexuses by which such forces can be transmitted to the collagen fiber bundles. These not only remodel but are also inclined at the correct angle to bring about eruptive movement. This angulation of the ligament fiber bundles is a prerequisite for tooth movement and the orientation is believed to be established by the developing root. The follicle, before it becomes periodontal ligament, also plays a role in tooth eruption, even though it may not provide the actual eruptive force.

In summary, eruptive movement is brought about by a combination of events involving a force initiated by the fibroblast. This force is transmitted to the extracellular compartment, via fibronexuses and to collagen fiber bundles, which, aligned in an appropriate inclination brought about by root formation, bring about tooth movement.

In posteruptive tooth movement, the mechanisms for moving the tooth axially during eruption are most likely also used to compensate for occlusal wear. Mesial or proximal drift involves a combination of two separate forces resulting from occlusal contact of teeth and contraction of the transseptal ligaments between teeth.

Running between teeth across the alveolar process is the transseptal ligament and there is evidence that this ligament has a key role in maintaining tooth position. Mesial drift is achieved by contraction of transseptal fibers and enhanced by occlusal forces.

The teeth erupt into oral cavity at different times. A summary of this eruption sequence is as follows **(Fig. 12.9)**.

| *Primary dentition* | *Emergence into oral cavity* |
|---|---|
| *Maxillary* | |
| Central incisor | 7 months |
| Lateral incisor | 9 months |
| Canine | 18 months |
| First molar | 14 months |
| Second molar | 24 months |
| *Mandibular* | |
| Central incisor | 6 months |
| Lateral incisor | 7 months |
| Canine | 16 months |
| First molar | 12 months |
| Second molar | 20 months |

# Eruption and Shedding of Tooth

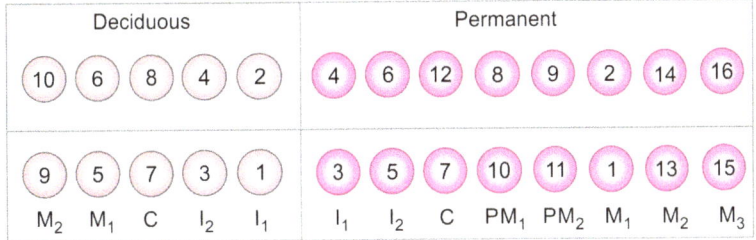

Fig. 12.9: Sequence of eruption of teeth.

*Permanent dentition*
*Maxillary*

| | |
|---|---|
| Central incisor | 7–8 years |
| Lateral incisor | 8–9 years |
| Canine | 11–12 years |
| First premolar | 10–12 years |
| Second premolar | 10–12 years |
| First molar | 6–7 years |
| Second molar | 12–13 years |
| Third molar | 18–25 years |

*Mandibular*

| | |
|---|---|
| Central incisor | 6–7 years |
| Lateral incisor | 7–8 years |
| Canine | 9–10 years |
| First premolar | 10–12 years |
| Second premolar | 11–12 years |
| First molar | 6–7 years |
| Second molar | 11–13 years |
| Third molar | 18–25 years |

Eruption is a multifactorial process and four processes seem to be necessary and they are:
a. There must be the mechanism itself that generates the eruptive forces.
b. There are processes whereby eruptive forces are translated into eruption by movements through the surrounding tissues (e.g. overcoming the resistance of the tissues to eruption).
c. Eruption must be sustained by processes that enable the tooth to be supported in its new position.
d. Eruption occurs alongside a process of remodeling of periodontal tissues to maintain the functional integrity of the system.

## SHEDDING OF THE DECIDUOUS TEETH

### Definition

The physiologic process resulting in the elimination of the deciduous dentition is called shedding or exfoliation.

### Pattern of Shedding

The shedding of deciduous teeth is the result of progressive resorption of the roots of teeth and their supporting tissue, the periodontal ligament. The removal of the dental hard tissues is accomplished by multinuclear odontoclasts **(Fig. 12.10)**.

In general, the pressure generated by the growing and erupting permanent tooth dictates the pattern of deciduous tooth resorption. At first, this pressure is directed against the root surface of the deciduous tooth itself. Because of the developmental position of the permanent incisor and canine tooth germs and their subsequent physiologic movement in an occlusal and vestibular direction, resorption of the roots of the deciduous incisors and canines begins on their lingual surfaces. Later, these developing tooth germs occupy a position directly apical to the deciduous tooth, which permits them to erupt in the position formerly occupied by the deciduous tooth. Frequently, however, in the case of the permanent mandibular incisors, this apical positioning of the tooth germs does not occur and the permanent tooth erupts lingual to the still functioning deciduous tooth.

Resorption of the roots of deciduous molars often first begins on their inner surfaces

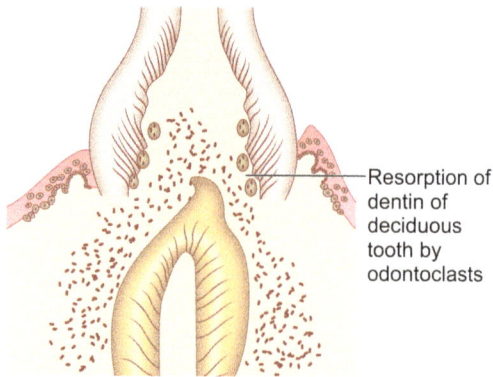

**Fig. 12.10:** Resorption of dental hard tissue by odontoclast.

because the early developing bicuspids are found between them. This resorption occurs long before the deciduous molars are shed and reflects the expansion of their growing permanent successors.

However, as a result of the continued growth of the jaws and occlusal movement of the deciduous molars, the successional tooth germs come to lie apical to the deciduous molars. This change in position provides the growing bicuspids with adequate space for their continued development and also relieves the pressure on the roots of the overlying deciduous molars. The areas of early resorption are repaired by the deposition of a cementum-like tissue. When the bicuspids begin to erupt, resorption of the deciduous molars is again initiated and this time continues until the roots are completely lost and the tooth is shed. The bicuspids thus erupt in the position of deciduous molars.

## Histology of Shedding

The cells responsible for the removal of dental hard tissue are identical to osteoclasts, the highly specialized cells responsible for the removal of bone, and are called odontoclasts. Odontoclasts are readily identifiable in the light microscope as large, multinucleated cells occupying resorption bays on the surface of a dental hard tissue. Their cytoplasm is vacuolated and the surface of the cell adjacent to the resorbing hard tissue forms a "brush" border.

Histochemically, a characteristic feature of the odontoclast is a high level of activity of the enzyme acid phosphatase. These light-microscope observations have been confirmed and extended with the electron microscope. The brush border is resolved as a ruffled border produced by extensive folding of the cell membrane into a series of invaginations 2–3 mm deep, with mineral crystallites within the depths of the invaginations. The cytoplasm of the odontoclast is characterized by an exceptionally high content of mitochondria and many vacuoles, which are especially concentrated adjacent to the ruffled border.

Acid phosphatase activity occurs within these vacuoles **(Fig. 12.11)**.

Odontoclasts are able to resorb all the dental hard tissues including, on occasions, enamel. When dentin is being resorbed, the presence of the tubules provides a pathway for the easy extension of odontoclast processes. Odontoclasts probably have the same origin as osteoclasts. The monocyte, circulating in the blood, originally gives rise to all the different tissue macrophages, including the osteoclast, but what is not certain is whether osteoclasts are further formed from mainly resident tissue macrophages or continuously from circulating monocytes. Odontoclasts are most commonly found on surfaces of the roots in relation to the advancing permanent tooth. However, they have also

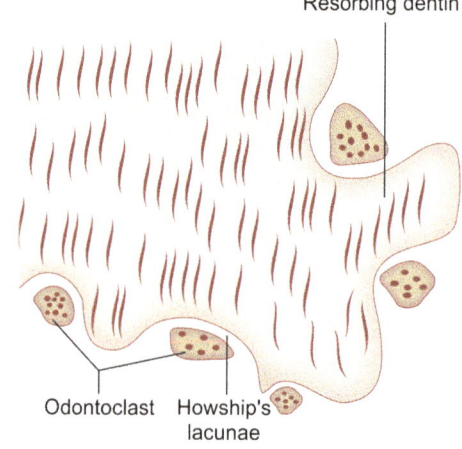

**Fig. 12.11:** Odontoclast activity.

been described in the root canals and pulp chambers of resorbing teeth lying against the predentin surface. Although their location in the pulp chamber has been disputed, the most likely reason is that different patterns of resorption exist for different teeth. For example, single-rooted teeth are usually shed before root resorption is complete; therefore, odontoclasts are not found within the pulp chambers of these teeth and the odontoblast layer remains intact. In molars, however, the roots are usually completely resorbed and the crown is also partially resorbed before exfoliation. When this happens, the odontoblast layer is replaced by odontoclasts, which resorb both primary and secondary dentin. Sometimes all the dentin is removed, and the vascular connective tissue is visible beneath the translucent cap of enamel.

The process of tooth resorption is not continuous, since there are periods of rest and repair; however, in the long term, resorption predominates over repair. Repair is achieved by cells resembling cementoblasts that lay down a dense collagenous matrix in which spotty mineralization occurs. The final repair tissue resembles cellular cementum but is less mineralized.

## Mechanism of Resorption and Shedding

Pressure from the erupting successional tooth plays a key role because the odontoclasts differentiate at predicted sites of pressure. The finding of mineral crystallites in the depths of the ruffled border and the fact that scanning electron microscopy indicates that the collagenous matrix of the dentin becomes exposed during resorption suggest that mineral is removed first. The acid phosphatase content of the vesicles close to the ruffled border suggests that these structures are phagosomes in which breakdown of ingested material is taking place. The most likely sequence of events in resorption of dental hard tissue by the odontoclast is an initial removal of mineral followed by extracellular dissolution of the organic matrix (mainly collagen) to smaller molecules, which are then taken up by the odontoclast and degraded further.

The forces of mastication applied to the deciduous tooth are also capable of initiating the resorption.

## CLINICAL CONSIDERATIONS

### Aberrations in Eruption

**Delayed eruption:** It is caused by local or systemic factors like nutritional, genetic, and endocrine deficiencies.

**Premature eruption:** Sometimes infants are born with erupted lower central incisors which should be extracted as early as possible as they prevent suckling.

### Teething

It is the inflammatory response of an infant as teeth break through oral mucosa. The infant may suffer from some pain, slight fever, and general malaise.

### Remnants of Deciduous Teeth

Sometimes parts of the roots of deciduous teeth are not in the path of erupting permanent teeth and may escape resorption. Such remnants, consisting of dentin and cementum, may remain embedded in the jaw for a considerable time.

### Retained Deciduous Teeth

Deciduous teeth may be retained for a long time beyond their usual shedding schedule. Such teeth are usually without permanent successors or their successors are impacted. They are invariably out of function. Retained deciduous teeth are most often the upper lateral incisor, less frequently the second permanent premolar, especially in the mandible, and rarely the lower central incisor. If a permanent tooth is ankylosed or impacted, its deciduous predecessor may also be retained. This is most frequently seen with the deciduous and permanent canine teeth.

### Submerged Deciduous Teeth

Trauma may result in damage to either the dental follicle or the periodontal ligament. If this happens, the eruption of the tooth ceases and it becomes ankylosed to the bone of the jaw. Because of continued eruption of neighboring teeth and increased height of the alveolar bone, the ankylosed tooth may be either "shortened" or submerged in the alveolar bone. Submerged deciduous teeth prevent the eruption of their permanent successors or force them from their position.

## QUESTIONNAIRE

1. Define eruption of tooth. Describe the types of tooth movement in different phases of eruption.
2. Discuss histology of tooth movement in different phases of eruption.
3. Enumerate the theories of tooth eruption. Discuss the different theories of tooth eruption.
4. Write notes on:
   a. Hammock ligament.
   b. Gubernacular cord.
   c. Fibronexus.
5. Define shedding. What are the factors responsible for shedding?
6. Discuss the pattern of shedding in anterior teeth and posterior teeth. Describe the histology of shedding.
7. Describe the mechanism of resorption and shedding.
8. Write notes on:
   a. Delayed eruption.
   b. Premature eruption.
   c. Retained deciduous teeth.
   d. Submerged deciduous teeth.

## BIBLIOGRAPHY

1. Antonio N. Ten Cate's Oral Histology Development, Structure, and Function, 7th edition. Mosby: Elsevier; 2008.
2. Berkovitz BKB, Holland GR, Moxham BJ. A Colour Atlas and Textbook of Oral Anatomy, Histology and Embryology, 4th edition. Mosby: Elsevier; 2009.
3. Das AK. Dental Anatomy and Oral Histology, 1st edition. West Bengal: Current Books International; 1972.
4. Kumar GS. Orban's Oral Histology and Embryology, 12th edition. Mosby: Elsevier; 2009.

# CHAPTER 13

# Enamel

Enamel is the most highly mineralized tissue, covering the anatomic crown of the tooth.

## PHYSICAL CHARACTERISTICS

### Thickness
The thickness varies over different parts of a tooth and from one type of tooth to another. It is thickest over the cusps of the molars where it measures about 2.5 mm and over incisal edge of incisors where it measures 2 mm. It thins down to knife edge at cervical margin and also thin at fissures and pits.

### Density
It varies from 3.0 g/mL to 2.84 g/mL. The density decreases from surface of enamel to dentinoenamel junction. The permanent teeth have more density than deciduous teeth. The density of enamel increases progressively during development. The final value is reached after eruption and further increases with absorption of mineral from saliva. The permanent upper incisors have the maximum density and premolars and lower incisors have the least.

### Color
Enamel is semitranslucent. The color depends on the thickness. It appears bluish-white or grayish at the thick opaque areas and yellowish-white at the thin areas reflecting underlying dentin. The enamel on deciduous teeth, being more opaque, appears much whiter.

### Hardness
Enamel is the hardest calcified tissue in the human body because of its high content of mineral salts and their crystalline arrangement. The hardness varies from 5 Mohs to 8 Mohs (Dentin 3-4 Mohs, Diamond 10 Mohs). This property enables enamel to withstand the heavy loads of mastication and limit the amount of wear.

### Specific Gravity
The specific gravity of enamel is 2.8-3.1. This fact has been useful when separating enamel from dentin for analytical purposes.

### Permeability
The enamel is selectively permeable. It possesses a submicroscopic pore system in interprismatic and intercrystal spaces, permitting complete or partial passage of certain molecules.

### Solubility
Enamel dissolves in acid media. The solubility rate is influenced by certain ions and molecules such as fluorides, silver nitrate, zinc chloride, etc. The surface enamel is less soluble in acids than deeper enamel.

### Tensile Strength and Compressibility
Enamel has a low tensile strength and has high modulus of elasticity. So, it is rigid in structure but extremely brittle.

### Refractive Index
Enamel is a crystalline material and is birefringent, the crystals refracting light differently in different directions. The tissue has an average refractive index of 1.62.

## CHEMICAL COMPOSITION

Mature enamel consists of mainly inorganic material and only a small amount of organic substance and water. The exact composition varies between teeth, within different parts of the same tooth, and even between the core and periphery of the same prism. An estimate of their composition is as follows:

|  | Weight | Volume |
|---|---|---|
| Organic | 1% | 2% |
| Inorganic | 96% | 89% |
| Water | 3% | 9% |

## Inorganic Composition

The inorganic component is mainly calcium phosphate in the form of hydroxyapatite crystals $[Ca_{10}(PO_4)_6(OH)_2]$. The apatites are variable, depending on the amount and variety of ion content. Fluoride, carbonate, magnesium, potassium, sodium, strontium, radium, and vanadium can replace phosphate to modify the apatite crystal. Fluoride makes enamel more resistant to acid and is anticariogenic.

## Organic Composition

The organic matter increases toward dentinoenamel junction and is least at the surface. The organic content of the deciduous teeth is slightly higher than that of the permanent series. A fine, lacy network of organic material appears between the hydroxyapatite crystals. Two groups of proteins are found in developing enamel and often collectively known as enamelins.

### Amelogenins

These are rich in proline. They are gradually removed during the development of enamel. Mature enamel contains degradation products of amelogenins.

### Nonamelogenins

They are rich in glycine and aspartic acid. They are present in mature enamel.

Enamel proteins do not appear to be fibrous and they form relatively structureless gel. Chemical analyses of the organic matrix of mature enamel indicate that the amino acid composition is not closely related to keratin and is distinctly different from collagen. Roentgen ray diffraction studies reveal that the molecular structure is typical of the group of proteins called cross-β-proteins. Histochemical reactions have suggested that the enamel-forming cells of developing teeth contain a polysaccharide-protein complex. The presence of other organic elements such as lipids is controversial.

## STRUCTURE OF ENAMEL

Enamel, having high mineral content, is studied in prepared ground section and under light microscope by means of transmitted light. Enamel is composed of the following:
1. Enamel rods (prisms)
2. Rod sheaths
3. Cementing interrod substance.

### Enamel Rods

#### Under Light Microscope

In longitudinal section under light microscope, the basic structural unit of enamel, the rods, are aligned perpendicularly to dentinoenamel junction, follow wavy course through one-third of enamel, and then follow a direct path to the external surface of enamel **(Figs. 13.1A and B)**. The number of enamel rods has been estimated as ranging from 5 million in lower lateral incisors to 12 million in the upper first molars. The length of most rods is greater than the thickness of enamel because of oblique direction and wavy course of the rods. The rods located in the cusps, the thickest part of enamel, are longer than those at cervical areas of the teeth. The diameter of the rods increases from the dentinoenamel junction toward the surface of the enamel at a ratio of about 1:2, the average diameter being 4 μm.

In cross section under light microscope, the rods appear hexagonal. They may resemble fish scale or keyhole. Indeed, three shapes are commonly seen **(Fig. 13.2)**.

Pattern 1—prisms appear completely circular, found near dentinoenamel junction.

Pattern 2—prisms are arranged in longitudinal rows.

# Enamel

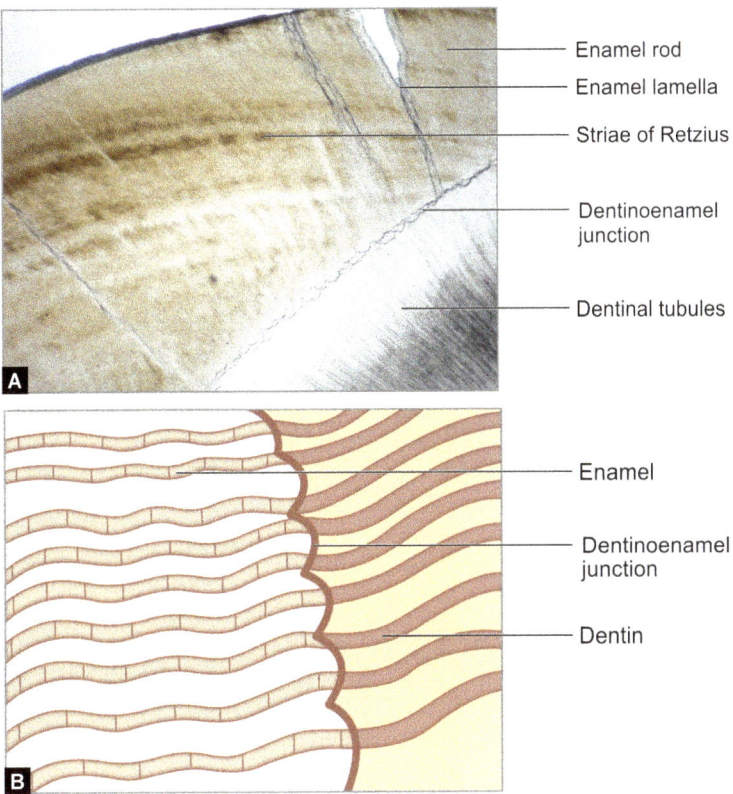

**Figs. 13.1A and B:** Enamel rods. Under light microscope (longitudinal section).

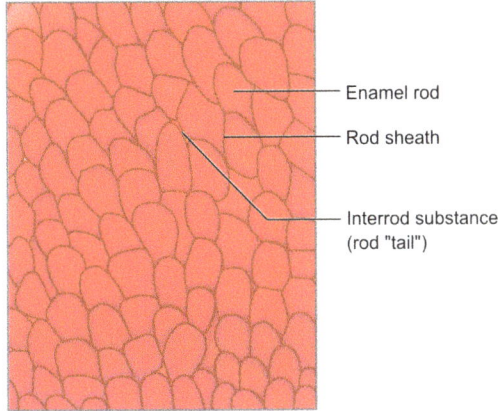

**Fig. 13.2:** Enamel rods in cross section.

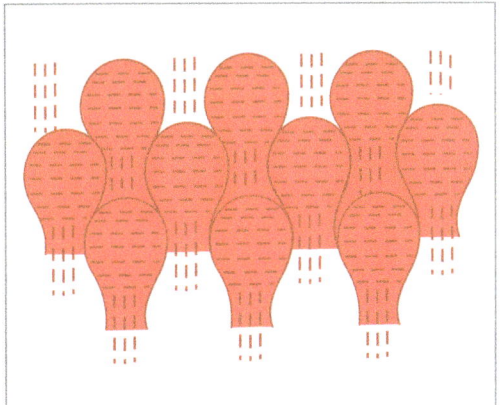

**Fig. 13.3:** Keyhole appearance of rods.

Pattern 3—prisms are arranged in rows but are staggered to give the keyhole shape.

## Under Electron Microscope

Enamel rod is shaped somewhat like a cylinder and measures about 5 µm in breadth and 9 µm in length. The rods on cross section look like keyholes **(Fig. 13.3)**. The rounded portion of each rod lies between the tails of two adjacent rods.

Such interlocking arrangement provides enamel with additional strength and stability.

The rod is so oriented that rounded portion points toward occlusal direction and the tail end is oriented toward cervical region.

Each enamel rod is tightly packed with crystallites which vary in shape and size. The mature crystals are ribbon-like or hexagonal having an average size of 1,600 Å (length) × 300 Å (thickness) × 900 Å (width) (1 nanometer = 10 angstrom units). The crystals are arranged parallel to the long axes of the rods in round part and deviate about 65° in tail part of the rod **(Fig. 13.4)**.

The organic matrix forms an envelope surrounding each apatite crystal. The surfaces of rods are visible because of abrupt changes in crystal orientation from one rod to another. For this reason, the crystals are not tightly packed and there may be more space for organic matrix at these surfaces. This accounts for the rod sheath visible in the light microscope.

### Striations

Each enamel rod is built up of segments separated by dark lines or transverse striations at 4 µm interval. The reasons for the striations may be:
1. Enamel matrix is formed in rhythmic fashion and the cross striations are the boundaries of daily matrix deposition.
2. They are the areas of disturbed calcification.
3. They are optical effect due to orientation of the crystals.
4. A tertiary curvature or undulation with a periodicity of 4 µm.

### Direction of Enamel Rods

The enamel rods are aligned in planes best suited to withstand the masticatory forces. So, there are variations in rod orientation in different areas. Usually, rods are oriented at right angles to the dentin surface as well as they end perpendicular to tooth surface. But they follow a wavy course in between.

In deciduous teeth, the rods are perpendicular to the dentinoenamel junction. In cervical and central parts of the crown, the rods are horizontal. Near the incisal edge or tip of the cusps, they change gradually to an increasingly oblique direction until they are almost vertical **(Fig. 13.5A)**. In permanent teeth, the arrangement of the rods is similar in the occlusal two-thirds of the crown.

In the cervical region, the rods deviate from the horizontal in an apical direction and at acute angle with the dentinoenamel junction **(Fig. 13.5B)**.

The enamel rods are divergent at the cuspal eminences while they are convergent in pits and fissure areas **(Fig. 13.6)**.

Groups of rods after leaving dentinoenamel junction curve gently to the right (dextroflexion) and then pursue a straight course for a distance and again curve gently to the left (sinistroflexion), forming an arc **(Fig. 13.7)**.

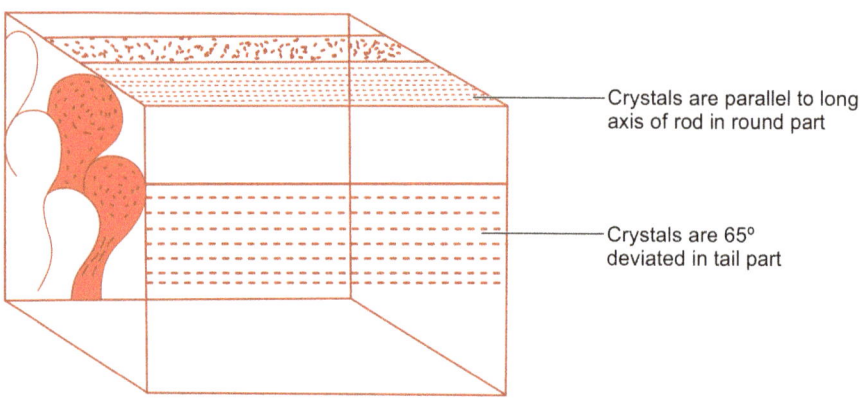

**Fig. 13.4:** Arrangement of crystals in enamel rod.

# Enamel

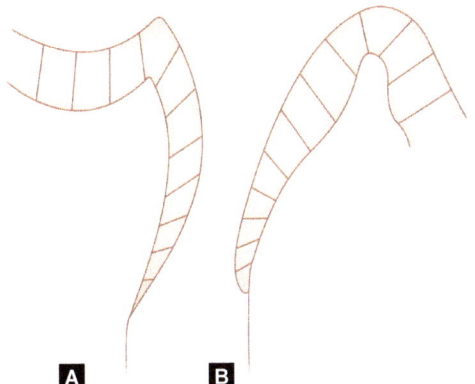

**Figs. 13.5A and B:** (A) Direction of rods in deciduous tooth; (B) Direction of rods in permanent tooth.

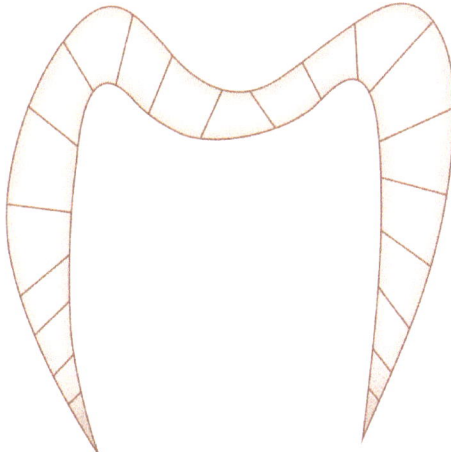

**Fig. 13.6:** Enamel rods in cuspal eminence and in pits and fissure areas.

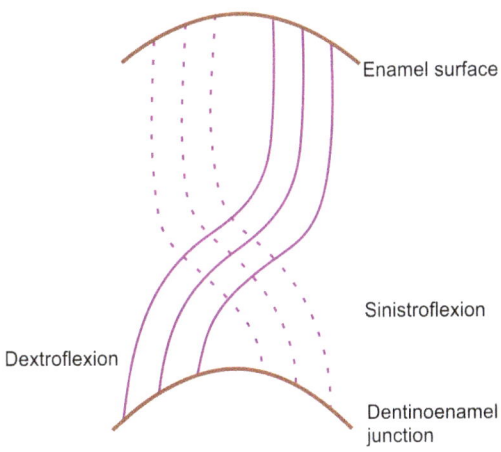

**Fig. 13.7:** Curvature of enamel rod.

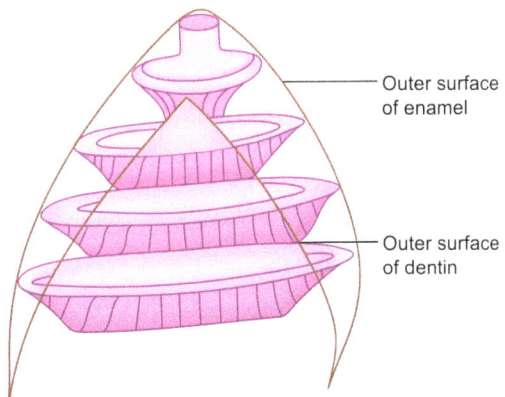

**Fig. 13.8:** Alternate deviation of enamel rod.

If the middle part of the crown is divided into thin horizontal disks, the enamel rods bend toward the right in one disk and then bend toward the left in the adjacent disk **(Fig. 13.8)**.

This alternating clockwise and counter-clockwise deviation of the rods can be observed at all levels of the crown if the disks are cut in the planes of rod direction.

## Gnarled Enamel

If the section of the enamel cut in an oblique plane is examined, under the microscope, the enamel rods appear twisted around each other in the region of cusps and incisal edge near dentin.

The alternate right and left deviation of the rods becomes more complicated in an oblique plane. The bundles of rods appear to intertwine more irregularly. This optical appearance of the enamel is called gnarled enamel **(Figs. 13.9A and B)**. This is associated with an increased strength of the enamel.

## Rod Sheath

Under light microscope, rod sheath appears as distinct thin layer peripheral to the rods. The characteristic features of rod sheath are:
a. It has a different refractive index.
b. It stains darker and is more acid resistant than the rods.
c. It is less calcified and contains more organic substance.

# Enamel

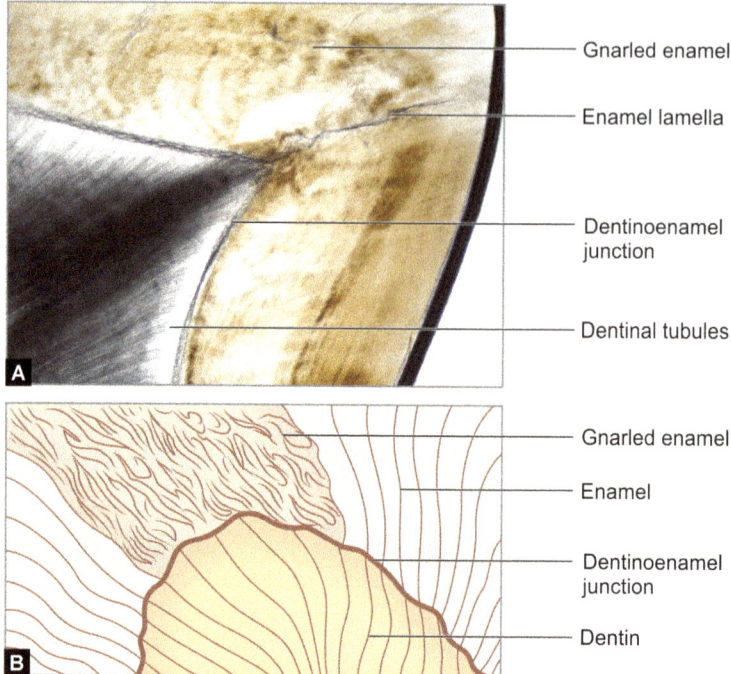

**Figs. 13.9A and B:** Gnarled enamel.

Under electron microscope, the rod sheath is not a discrete structural entity but an organically rich interrod space devoid of apatite crystals.

## Interrod Substance

The light microscope reveals that the rods are cemented together by interred substance which has a slightly higher refractive index than the rods.

Electron microscopic studies reveal that the enamel prism has a keyhole or fish scale shape. The so-called interrod cement substance is an extension or the tail of the adjacent rod. The crystallites at this region have a different orientation than the rounded part which gives optical illusion of a separate cement substance. It contains more organic substance.

## Incremental Lines of Retzius

The incremental lines of Retzius or striea of Retzius **(Figs. 13.10A to C)** are a series of irregularly spaced concentric brown lines seen running obliquely across the enamel rods, when a longitudinal ground section of a tooth is examined under the microscope by transmitted light. In cuspal or incisal region, they form concentric arcs and terminate at dentinoenamel junction. Near the middle-third and cervical region, these parallel lines fan out toward the enamel surface and do not complete the arc.

As the lines of Retzius proceed toward the enamel surface, some reach up to enamel and some are falling short of the enamel surface. As a result of this, there are transverse, wave-like grooves present on the surface of the tooth as external manifestations of Striae of Retzius. They are continuous around a tooth and lie parallel to each other and to the cementoenamel junction. They are known as perikymata **(Fig. 13.11)**. There are around 30 perikymata per mm in the region of the cementoenamel junction and 10 per mm near occlusal or incisal edge of a surface. In transverse section, the lines of Retzius encircle the enamel in the same manner as the annual growth rings of the tree.

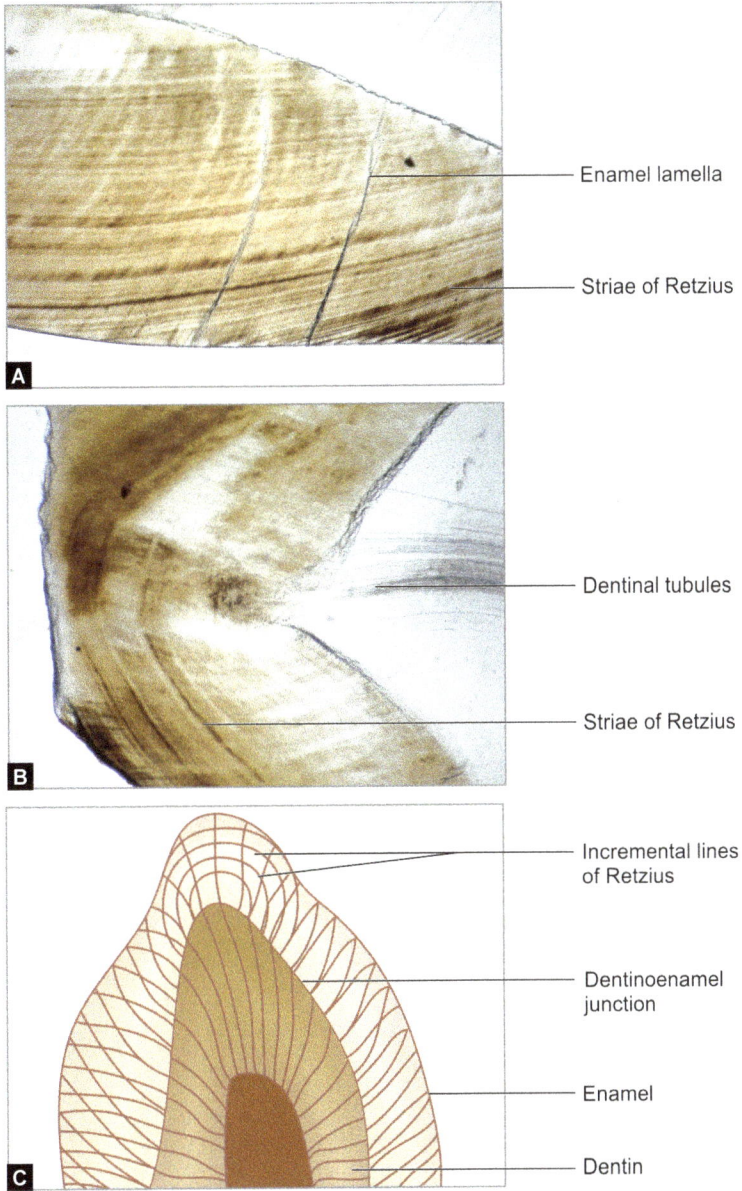

**Figs. 13.10A to C:** Incremental lines of Retzius (Striae of Retzius).

***Significance of lines of Retzius (different views)***

1. They signify the incremental pattern of enamel deposition. After 16 µm interval, there is a rest period of deposition which is illustrated as Striae of Retzius. They are rich in organic content.
2. Incremental lines have been attributed to periodic bending of the enamel rods.
3. Variation in basic organic structure.
4. Physiologic calcification rhythm.
5. It is a secondary curvature of prism with a periodicity of 16–100 µm.

Incremental lines are accentuated due to metabolic disturbances, infections (conditions disturbing amelogenesis) causing the rest periods to be the unduly prolonged.

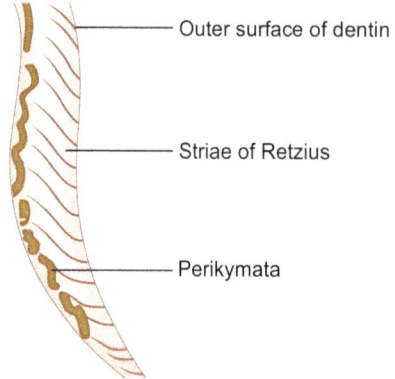

Fig. 13.11: Perikymata.

## Neonatal Line

The deposition of prenatal and postnatal enamel is demarcated by an accentuated line of Retzius, the neonatal line **(Figs. 13.12A and B)**. The disturbance of birth like abrupt change in the environment and nutrition of the newborn infant results in the formation of neonatal line. Since these lines are seen in all enamel forming at the time of birth, they are found in all the deciduous teeth and in the larger cusps of the permanent first molars.

The prenatal enamel is usually better developed than the postnatal enamel as the fetus develops in a well-protected environment with an adequate supply of all the essential materials, even at the expense of the mother. Because of the undisturbed and even development of the enamel prior to birth, perikymata are absent in the occlusal parts of the deciduous teeth, whereas they are present in the postnatal cervical parts.

## Hunter-Schreger Bands

When a longitudinal ground section of tooth is seen in oblique reflected light (light will fall directly on object), a series of alternating

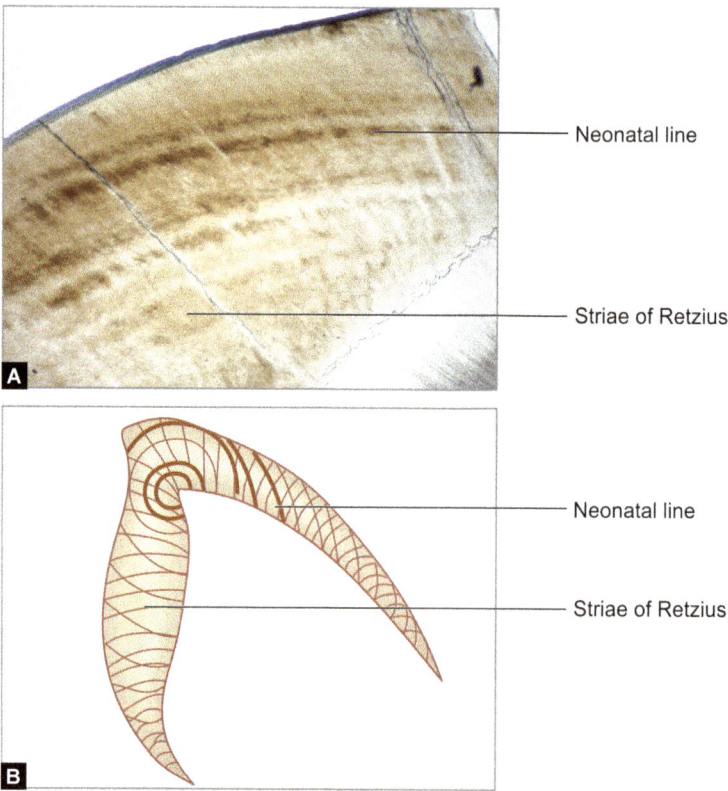

**Figs. 13.12A and B:** Neonatal line.

# Enamel

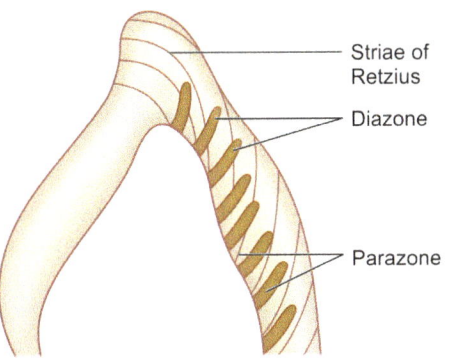

Fig. 13.13: Hunter-Schreger bands.

dark and light bands are seen in enamel and they are known as Hunter-Schreger bands (**Fig. 13.13**). They start at the dentinoenamel junction and run perpendicular to the Striae of Retzius. These bands are more prominent near dentinoenamel junction and become indistinguishable toward periphery. The dark bands are referred to as diazones and the light bands are called parazones.

### Significance of Hunter-Schreger bands (different views)

1. It is an optical phenomenon. The change in direction of rods either absorbs or reflects light giving rise to dark and light bands.
2. There are variations in calcification of the enamel that coincide with the distribution of the bands of Hunter-Schreger.
3. They are composed of alternate zones having a slightly different permeability and a different content of organic material.
4. It is a primary curvature of prism at a periodicity of about 1,000 µm.

### Enamel Tufts

In transverse ground section, tasseled or unbraided projections are seen.

They are known as enamel tufts as they look like a tuft of grass projecting into enamel (**Figs. 13.14A and B**). The tuft is a narrow, ribbon-like structure, the inner end of which projects into dentin. They follow the direction of enamel rods. It is controversial whether

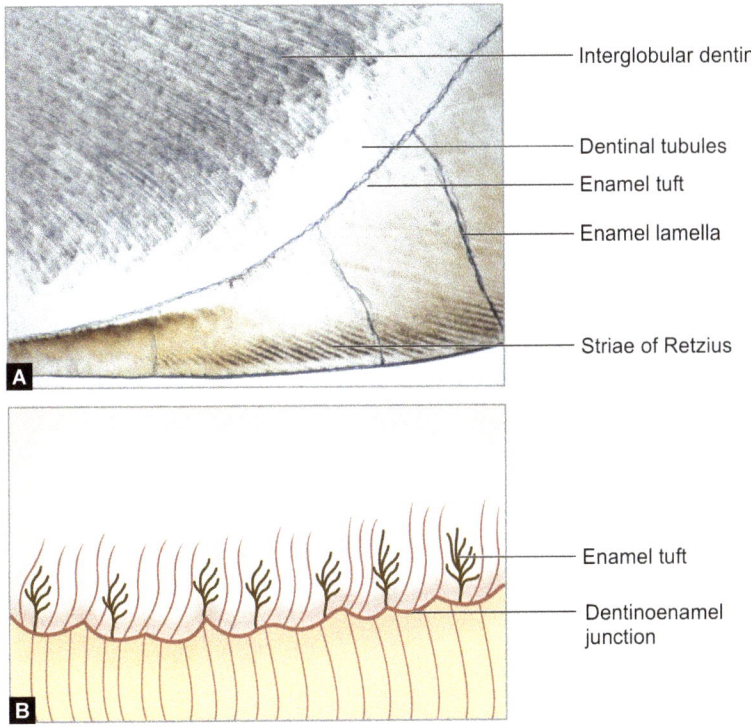

Figs. 13.14A and B: Enamel tufts.

the enamel tufts are composed of rods, rod sheaths, or interrod substance. They are hypocalcified structures rich in organic matter and are more permeable. According to one school of thought, when a substance changes from the liquid to the solid state, contractions occur. In enamel, hydroxyapatite changes from the ionic (liquid) state in the ameloblast secretions to the solid state in the enamel crystallites.

With the change of state, contractions will be expected and it is possible that these contractions could lead to widening of prism sheaths which correspond with the enamel tuft.

### Enamel Spindles

The odontoblastic processes of dentin may cross the dentinoenamel junction and project into the enamel. They are thickened at their end and are termed enamel spindle **(Figs. 13.15A and B)**.

They project at right angles to dentino-enamel junction and correspond to the original direction of the ameloblasts. Since the enamel rods are formed at an angle to the axis of the ameloblasts, the direction of spindles and rods is divergent. They make the area hypersensitive to pain. In ground sections of dried teeth, the organic content of the spindles disintegrates and is replaced by air, and the spaces appear dark in transmitted light.

### Enamel Lamellae

Enamel lamellae **(Fig. 13.16)** are thin, leaf-like structures that extend from the enamel surface toward the dentinoenamel junction. They may extend to and sometimes penetrate into the dentin. They consist of organic material and little mineral. They may be formed before or after eruption. They may develop in planes of tension. When rods cross such a plane, a short segment of rod may not fully calcify.

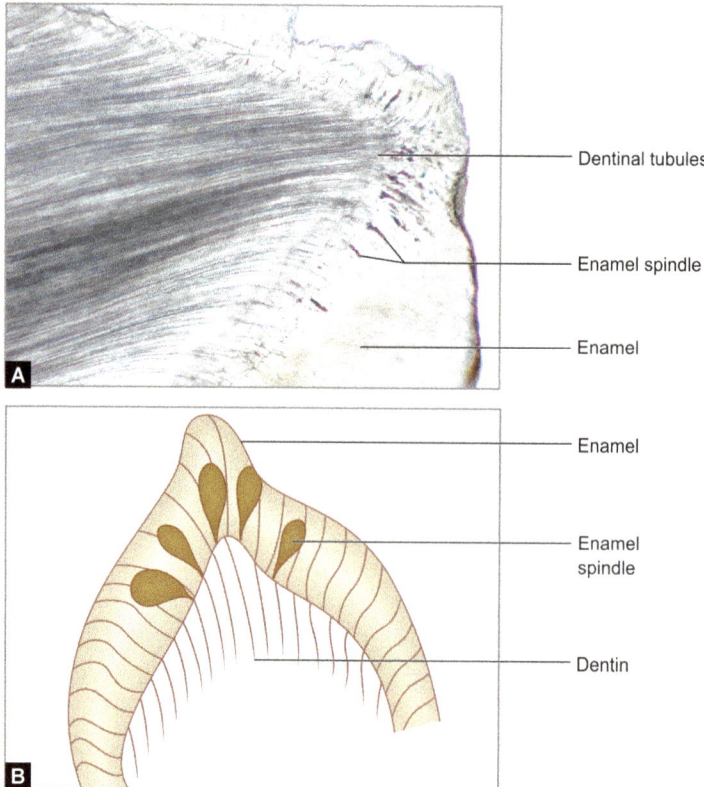

**Figs. 13.15A and B:** Enamel spindles.

# Enamel

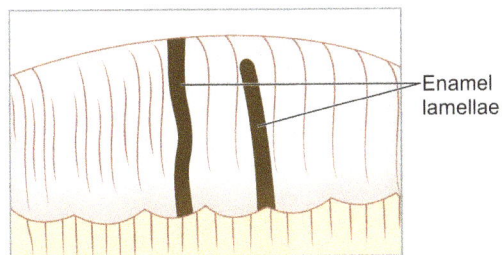

Fig. 13.16: Enamel lamellae.

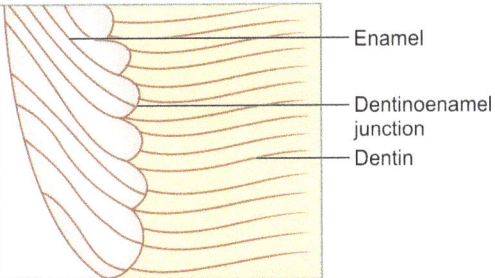

Fig. 13.17: Dentinoenamel junction.

The enamel lamellae are hypomineralized areas containing cellular debris and stain readily with organic dyes. Enamel lamellae are generally seen in cervical region and below pits and fissures in posterior teeth.

*Enamel lamellae may be of three types:*
*Type A:* Lamellae composed of poorly calcified rod segments.
*Type B:* Lamellae consisting of degenerated cells.
*Type C:* Lamellae arising in erupted teeth where the cracks are filled with organic matter, presumably originating from saliva. This is the most common type of lamella.

Type A lamellae are restricted to the enamel; those of types B and C may reach into dentin. Enamel lamellae represent a defect on the enamel surface and may form a pathway for bacteria and initiation of caries.

> In ground section, enamel lamellae may be confused with cracks caused by grinding of specimen. Careful decalcification of ground sections of enamel makes possible the distinction between cracks and enamel lamellae.

## Dentinoenamel Junction

The region of the tooth where dentin meets the enamel is dentinoenamel junction. In a ground section, the dentin at the dentinoenamel junction is pitted. The rounded projections of the enamel are fitted into the pits of dentin. As a result, the junction can be easily seen as a series of scallops (**Fig. 13.17**) and convexity of the scallops are directed toward dentin. This causes a firm bondage between these two structures.

In demineralized section, where the enamel has been removed, the scalloped nature of the junction can be clearly seen. The electron microscope reveals that the crystals of dentin and enamel intermix. The scanning electron microscope reveals the junction to be a series of ridges rather than spikes, which arrangement probably increases the adherence between dentin and enamel. The ridging is most pronounced in coronal dentin, where occlusal stresses are the greatest. The shape and nature of the junction prevent shearing of the enamel during function.

## Cementoenamel Junction

It is the region of the tooth where enamel meets the cementum at the cervical line (**Fig. 13.18**).

Three possible variations may exist at the cementoenamel junction.
1. The cervical enamel is covered by cementum for a short distance (**Figs. 13.19AI and II**). It occurs in 60% of the teeth. This occurs when the enamel epithelium degenerates at its cervical

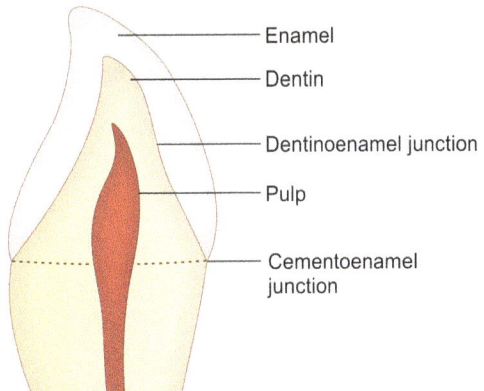

Fig. 13.18: Cementoenamel junction.

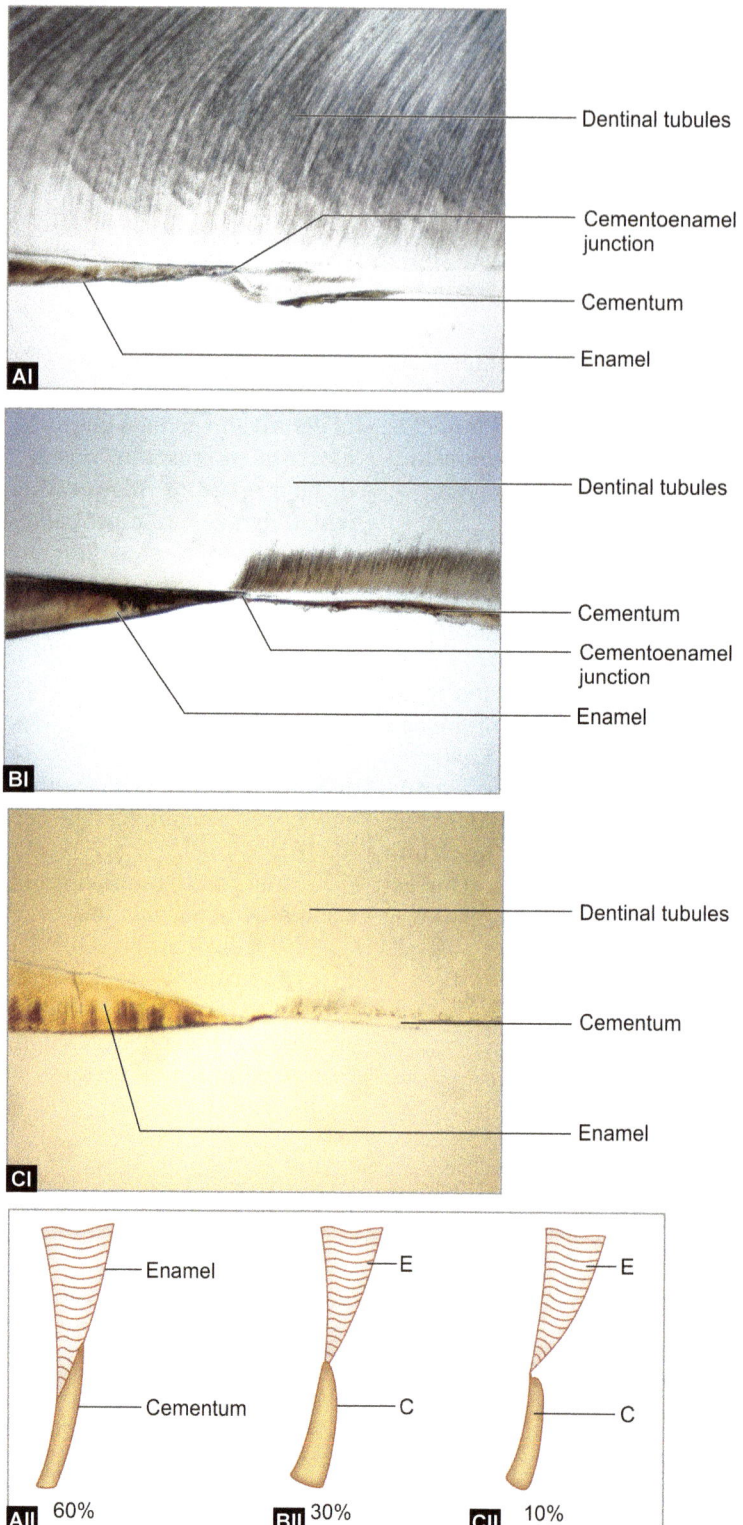

**Figs. 13.19A to C:** Variations of cementoenamel junction: **(AI and II)** Enamel covered by cementum; **(BI and II)** Enamel meets cementum; **(CI and II)** Enamel and cementum do not meet.

termination, permitting connective tissue to come in direct contact with enamel surface.
2. In approximately 30% of all teeth, cementum meets the cervical end of enamel in a relatively sharp line **(Figs. 13.19BI and II)**.
3. In about 10% of the teeth, enamel and cementum do not meet **(Figs. 13.19CI and II)**. This occurs when enamel epithelium in the cervical portion of the root is delayed in its separation from dentin. In such case, there is no cementoenamel junction. Instead, a zone of the root is devoid of cementum and for the time being covered by reduced enamel epithelium.

**Surface structures:** A relatively structureless layer of enamel, approximately 30 µm thick has been described in 70% of permanent teeth and all deciduous teeth. This enamel is mostly found in the cervical region.

This part is heavily mineralized than the bulk of the enamel beneath it.

## Enamel Cuticle

The crown of a newly erupted tooth is covered by a delicate membrane known as primary enamel cuticle. It is the last secretory product of ameloblast after the enamel is laid down.

The primary enamel cuticle and reduced enamel epithelium (formed by condensation of outer enamel epithelium, inner enamel epithelium, and stratum intermedium) combined are known as Nasmyth's membrane.

Under the electron microscope, the primary enamel cuticle is 200 angstrom thick and structurally it is atypical basal lamina found beneath most epithelia. It is organically connected to both enamel matrix and ameloblast. Like the basement membrane, the cuticle also perhaps controls the ionic character of enamel rods by controlling selection and rate of ionic or molecular exchange. This layer is more resistant to acids and alkalies than the enamel. Mastication and brushing wear away the enamel cuticle after eruption. Secondary cuticle is the acellular keratinized layer produced by the reduced enamel epithelium after tooth eruption. It covers not only enamel, but also a part of the cementum. It is about 10 µm in thickness.

## Pellicle

Enamel is covered by pellicle, the salivary glycoprotein, immediately after eruption. The pellicle reforms within hours after the enamel surface is mechanically cleaned.

## Plaque

Within a day or two after the pellicle has formed, it becomes colonized by micro-organisms to form bacterial plaque.

## AGE CHANGES OF ENAMEL

1. Attrition or wear of the occlusal surfaces or proximal contact points as a result of mastication leads to loss of vertical dimension of crown and flattening of the proximal contour.
2. Total amount of organic matrix increases.
3. Superficial enamel layer becomes rich in nitrogen and fluorine due to continuous uptake and becomes resistant to decay.
4. Permeability to fluid is reduced due to age change process.

## CLINICAL CONSIDERATIONS

1. Enamel cannot be repaired in case of damage in attrition due to mastication, abrasion due to abnormal brushing, and erosion due to chemicals as ameloblasts undergo degeneration after formation of enamel.
2. Presence of pits and fissures and enamel lamellae are the potential locations for the initiation and propagation of dental caries.
3. Incorporation of fluorine in apatite crystals of enamel by topical application of sodium or stannous fluoride, use of fluoride-containing dentifrice, and adjustment of fluoride level in communal water supply to 1 part per million forms fluorapatite which makes the tooth resistant against caries.
4. Direction of rods at cervical region is different in deciduous and permanent teeth. The course of enamel rods is of importance in cavity preparation.

## QUESTIONNAIRE

1. What is enamel? What are the physical characteristics and chemical composition of enamel?
2. What are the structural components of enamel? Discuss the light microscopic and electron microscopic features of enamel rod? Describe the course of enamel rod.
3. Write notes on:
    a. Gnarled enamel.
    b. Incremental lines of Retzius.
    c. Neonatal line.
    d. Hunter-Schreger bands.
    e. Enamel tufts.
    f. Enamel lamellae.
    g. Enamel spindles.
    h. Dentinoenamel junction.
    i. Cementoenamel junction.
    j. Perikymata.
    k. Enamel cuticle.
4. Discuss the age changes in enamel.

## BIBLIOGRAPHY

1. Antonio N. Ten Cate's Oral Histology Development, Structure, and Function, 7th edition. Mosby: Elsevier; 2008.
2. Berkovitz BKB, Holland GR, Moxham BJ. A Colour Atlas and Textbook of Oral Anatomy, Histology and Embryology, 4th edition. Mosby: Elsevier; 2009.
3. Das AK. Dental Anatomy and Oral Histology, 1st edition. West Bengal: Current Books International; 1972.
4. Gaunt WA, Osborn JW, Ten Cate AR. Advances in Dental Histology. Bristol: John Wright and Sons Ltd.; 1967.
5. Kumar GS. Orban's Oral Histology and Embryology, 12th edition. Mosby: Elsevier; 2009.
6. Osborn JW, Ten Cate AR. Advanced Dental Histology, 3rd edition. Bristol: John Wright and Sons Ltd.; 1976.

# CHAPTER 14

# Dentin

The dentin is the mineralized tissue forming the main bulk of the tooth. In the coronal part of the tooth, it is covered by the enamel and in the radicular portion by the cementum.

## PHYSICAL CHARACTERISTICS

### Color

The color varies from light yellow in deciduous teeth to yellow in permanent dentition. The color becomes darker with age. As the enamel is semitranslucent, dentin gives its color to the crown of the tooth.

### Hardness

It is softer than enamel but harder than bone and cementum. The hardness varies in different areas of dentin. The highest microhardness is seen in areas about 450 µm from dentinoenamel junction with an average 70 KHN (Knoop hardness number: enamel-300 KHN). The lowest value (20 KHN) is found in about 100 µm from the dentinoenamel junction.

Hardness increases with age.

### Permeability

It is highly permeable because of dentinal tubules. Permeability decreases with advancing age.

### Tensile Strength and Compressibility

It is highly elastic. This property is essential for the support of nonresilient enamel. Dentin has greater compressive and tensile strengths than enamel.

It is semitransparent and more so in deciduous teeth.

### Radio Density

It is less mineralized than enamel and is therefore less radiopaque than enamel.

It shows positive birefringence under polarized light.

### Specific Gravity

The specific gravity of dentin is approximately 2.1.

## CHEMICAL COMPOSITION

|           | Weight | Volume |
|-----------|--------|--------|
| Organic   | 70%    | 47%    |
| Inorganic | 20%    | 32%    |
| Water     | 10%    | 21%    |

The inorganic component consists of hydroxyapatite crystals, $3Ca_3(PO_4)_2\, Ca(OH)_2$. The crystals are plate-shaped and much smaller than the hydroxyapatite crystals in enamel. Dentin also contains small amounts of fluoride, phosphates, carbonates, and sulfates.

The organic substance consists of collagenous fibril (Type 1 collagen, 90% of matrix) and a ground substance of mucopolysaccharides (proteoglycans and glycosaminoglycans), phosphoprotein, and 1.7% lipid.

## STRUCTURE OF DENTIN

The dentin is composed of the following:
1. The dentinal tubules containing the protoplasmic processes of odontoblasts.
2. Dentinal matrix.

The cell bodies of the odontoblasts are arranged in a layer on the pulpal surface of the dentin (**Fig. 14.1**) and only their cytoplasmic

# Dentin

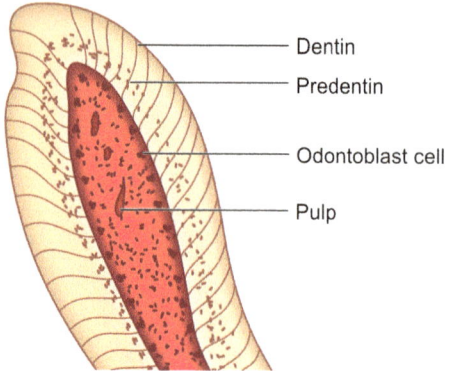

Fig. 14.1: Odontoblast cell.

processes are included in the tubules in the mineralized matrix. Each cell gives rise to one process, which traverses the predentin and calcified dentin within one tubule and terminates in a branching network at the junction with enamel and cementum. Tubules are found throughout normal dentin.

## Dentinal Tubules

The dentinal tubules follow an S-shaped curvature which is more pronounced in crown and less in root. Starting at the right angle from the pulpal surface, the first convexity is directed toward the apex of the tooth **(Figs. 14.2A and B)**.

These tubules end perpendicular to the dentinoenamel and dentinocemental junctions. Near the root tip and along the incisal edges and cusps, the tubules are almost straight. Over their entire lengths, the tubules exhibit minute, relatively regular secondary curvatures that are sinusoidal in shape.

The ratio between the outer and inner surfaces of dentin is about 5:1. So the tubules are wide apart in periphery and more closely packed near the pulp. The tubules are larger in diameter near the pulpal cavity (3–4 μm) and smaller at their outer ends (1 μm). The ratio between the number of tubules per unit

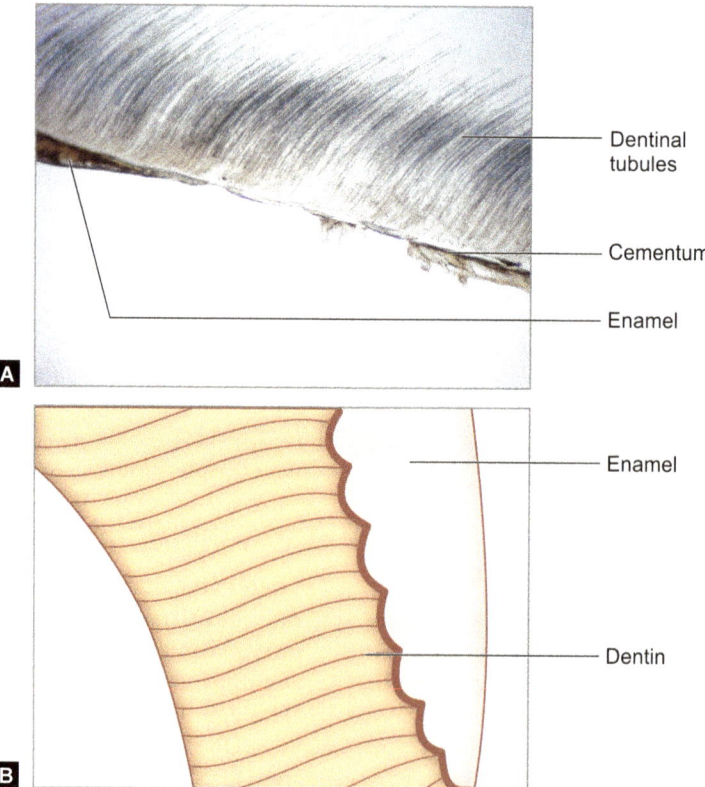

**Figs. 14.2A and B:** S-shaped curvature of dentinal tubules.

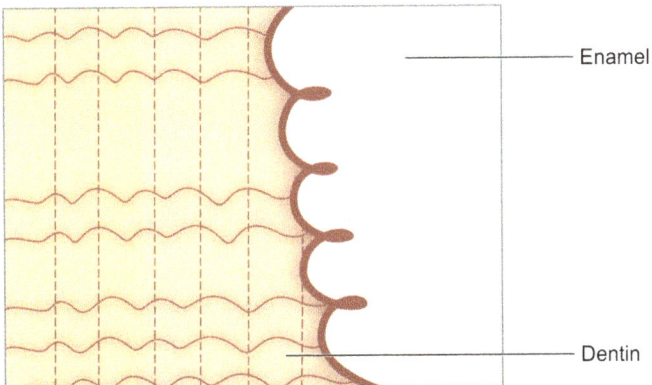

**Fig. 14.3:** Secondary curves and lateral branches of dentinal tubules.

area on the pulpal and outer surfaces of the dentin is about 4:1. Near the pulpal surface of the dentin, the number of tubules per square millimeter varies between 50,000 and 90,000. There are more tubules per unit area in the crown than in the root. The dentinal tubules have lateral branches throughout dentin (**Fig. 14.3**). They are termed canaliculi or microtubules. These canaliculi are 1 μm or less in diameter and originate more or less at right angle to the main tubule. Some of them enter adjacent or distant tubules while others end in the intertubular dentin. Occasionally odontoblast processes pass across the dentinoenamel junction into enamel. Many of them are thickened at the end and are termed enamel spindles. They seem to originate from the processes of odontoblasts that extend into ameloblast layer before enamel forms. As enamel formation begins, they are entrapped in enamel.

## PERITUBULAR (INTRATUBULAR) DENTIN

The hypermineralized dentin surrounding the dentinal tubules is termed peritubular dentin (**Fig. 14.4**). It is 9% more mineralized than intertubular dentin. It is roughly 44 nm wide near the pulp end, 750 nm wide near the dentinoenamel junction, and sharply demarcated from the intertubular dentin. By its growth, it constricts the dentinal tubule to a diameter of 1 μm near dentinoenamel junction. After decalcification, the odontoblast process appears to be surrounded by an empty space due to demineralization of hypercalcified area. According to some investigators, the calcified tubule wall has an inner organic lining termed the lamina limitans which is rich in glycosaminoglycan.

> Anatomically, however, the term peritubular dentin is incorrect because this dentin forms within the dentinal tubule (not around it), narrowing the tubular lumen. So it is more accurately intratubular rather than peritubular dentin.

## INTERTUBULAR DENTIN

It is located between the zones of peritubular dentin (**Fig. 14.4**) and forms the main bulk of dentin. Organic matrix is half of its volume and collagen fibers are oriented around the dentinal tubules.

The fibrils range from 0.5 μm to 0.2 μm in diameter and exhibit cross banding at 64 nm (640 angstrom) intervals, which is typical for collagen. Hydroxyapatite crystals, which are averagely 0.1 μm in length, are formed along

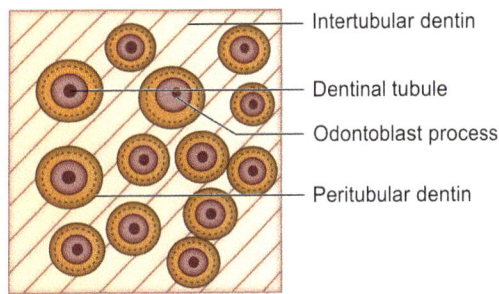

**Fig. 14.4:** Peritubular and intertubular dentin.

the fibers with their long axes oriented parallel to collagen fibers.

## PREDENTIN

The predentin is the unmineralized matrix of dentin, adjacent to the pulp tissue, and is 2–6 μm wide, depending on the activity of the odontoblast (**Fig. 14.5**). It consists principally of collagen, glycoproteins, and proteoglycans. This layer of predentin is always present as deposition of mineral lags behind the formation of organic matrix of dentin. As the collagen fibers undergo mineralization at the predentin-dentin front, the predentin then becomes dentin and a new layer of predentin forms circumpulpally. The rate of deposition of predentin diminishes with advancing age.

## ODONTOBLAST PROCESS

The odontoblast processes are the cytoplasmic extensions of the odontoblasts. The odontoblasts reside in the peripheral pulp at the pulp–predentin border and their processes extend into the dentinal tubules (**Fig. 14.6**). The processes are largest in diameter near pulp (3–4 μm) and taper to approximately 1 μm further into dentin.

They are closely packed near pulp (around 75,000/mm²) and spread widely at periphery (30,000/mm²). These processes give off lateral branches that radiate diagonally toward the outer dentinal surface and extend laterally into adjacent tubule. The processes end in several terminal branches that extend up to dentinoenamel and dentinocemental junction. A few tubules may extend beyond the dentinoenamel junction into the enamel and are known as enamel spindles.

The odontoblastic process (**Fig. 14.7**) lies within a cell membrane. The process is composed of microtubules of 20 μm in diameter and small filaments 5–7.5 μm in diameter. Occasionally, mitochondria, lysosomes, microvesicles, and coated vesicles that may open to the extracellular space are also seen.

Different opinions of investigators whether the odontoblast processes extend through the thickness of mature human dentin:
a. Transmission electron microscopy shows that the dentinal tubules contain odontoblast process up to 200–300 μm from the pulp.
b. Scanning electron microscopy shows the presence of odontoblastic process at dentinoenamel junction. Some investigators believe that it is not the living process of the odontoblast but the organic lining membrane of the tubule (lamina limitans).
c. Cryofractured human teeth reveal the odontoblast process to extend to the dentinoenamel junction.
d. Immunofluorescent technique reveals tubulin (as intracellular protein of microtubules) throughout the thickness of dentin.
From different opinions, it is appropriate to consider that some odontoblast processes traverse the thickness of dentin. In other areas, a shortened process may be characteristic in tubules that are narrow or obliterated by mineral deposit.

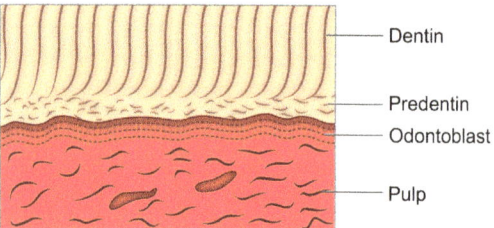

Fig. 14.5: Predentin.

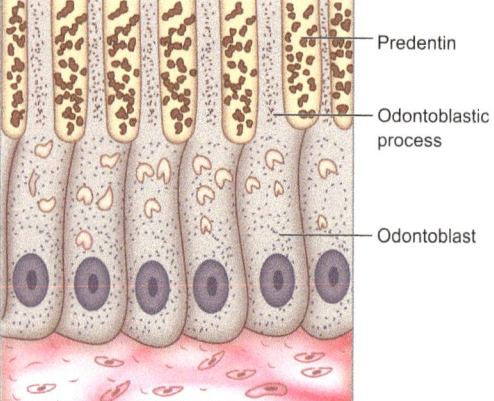

Fig. 14.6: Odontoblast process.

## DIFFERENT FORMS OF DENTIN

Dentin formation is a continuous process and three different types of dentin are recognized.

### Primary Dentin

It is the dentin formed from initial phase up to the completion of root.

### Mantle Dentin

It is the first-formed dentin in the crown underlying the dentinoenamel junction.

# Dentin

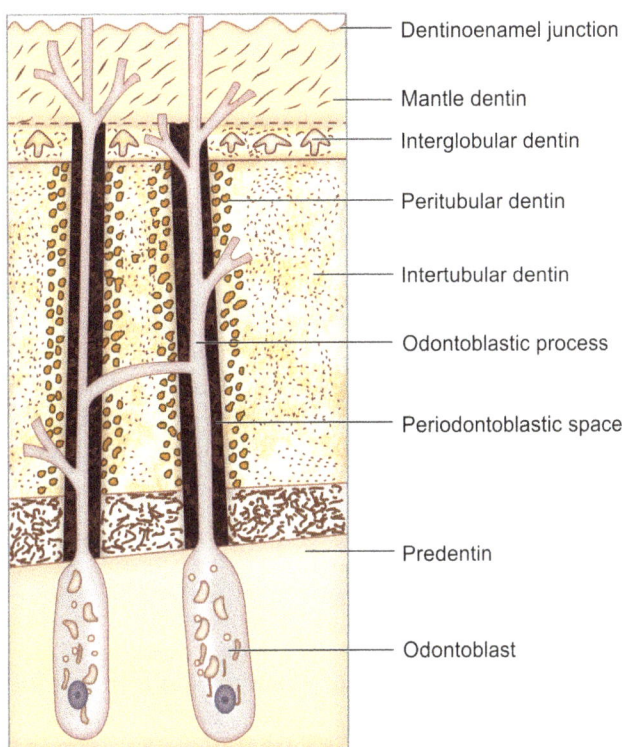

Fig. 14.7: Odontoblast and its process in the dentinal tubule.

It is thus the outer or most peripheral part of the primary dentin and is about 20 μm thick. The collagen fibers of mantle dentin are perpendicular to the enamel-dentin junction and it is hypomineralized compared to circumpulpal dentin. The dentinal tubule in mantle dentin branch more profusely than those in circumpulpal dentin.

## Circumpulpal Dentin

It forms the remaining primary dentin or bulk of the tooth. It represents all of the dentin formed prior to root completion. The collagen fibers are much smaller in diameter (0.05 μm) and are more closely packed together. They are parallel to the dentinoenamel junction. The circumpulpal dentin may contain slightly more mineral than mantle dentin.

## Secondary Dentin (Physiologic Secondary Dentin)

It is a narrow band of dentin bordering the pulp and representing that dentin formed after root completion. This dentin contains fewer tubules than primary dentin. There is usually a bend in the tubules where primary and secondary dentin interface (**Fig. 14.8**).

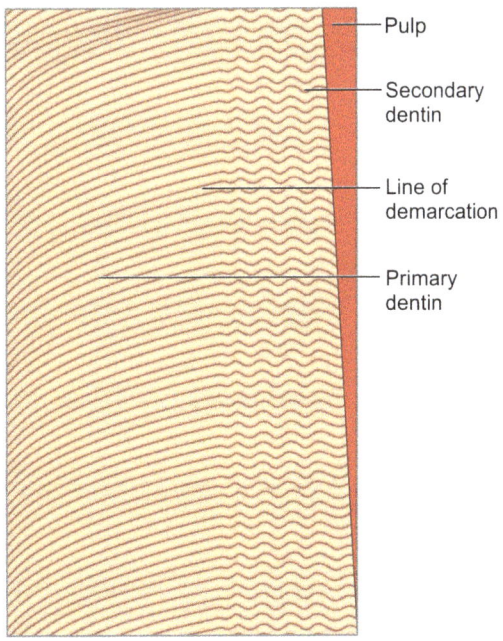

Fig. 14.8: Secondary dentin.

## Tertiary Dentin (Reactive, Reparative, or Irregular Secondary Dentin)

It is produced in reaction to various stimuli, such as attrition, caries, or a restorative dental procedure. It is produced only by cells directly affected by the stimulus. The quality and quantity of tertiary dentin produced are related to the cellular response initiated, which depends on the intensity and duration of the stimulus. The dentin contains regularly or irregularly arranged tubules which are sparse in number. The cells forming tertiary dentin either line its surface or are included in the dentin and in the latter case, the dentin is referred to as osteodentin.

### Incremental Lines of Von Ebner

The incremental lines of Von Ebner or imbrication lines **(Fig. 14.9)** appear as fine lines or striations in dentin. They reflect the daily rhythmic, recurrent deposition of dentin matrix and period of rest between daily increments. The distance between lines varies from 4 μm to 8 μm in the crown and much less in the root. The daily increment decreases after a tooth reaches functional occlusion. The course of the lines indicates the growth pattern of the dentin. These fine lines run at right angles to the dentinal tubules.

Some incremental lines are accentuated because of disturbances in the matrix and mineralization process. These are hypocalcified bands and are known as *contour lines of Owen*.

### Neonatal Line

This is an accentuated, hypocalcified contour line separating the prenatal and postnatal dentin **(Fig. 14.9)**. The line reflects the abrupt change in environment that occurs at birth. There is interruption of growth due to metabolic adjustment. The dentin matrix formed prior to birth is usually of better quality than that formed after birth. These lines are seen in the deciduous teeth and permanent first molar.

### Interglobular Dentin

Sometimes mineralization of dentin begins in small globular areas that fail to fuse into a homogenous mass. This results in zones of hypomineralization between the globules. These zones are known as interglobular dentin **(Figs. 14.10A and B)**.

These are seen in the crown of the teeth in circumpulpal dentin just below the mantle dentin and it follows the incremental pattern. The dentinal tubules pass uninterrupted through interglobular dentin. Thus, it reveals a defect of mineralization and not matrix formation.

### Granular Layer of Tomes

When dry ground sections of the root dentin are examined under the microscope in transmitted light, a thin granular layer is visible in dentin adjacent to cementodentinal junction. This layer is known as Tomes' granular layer **(Figs. 14.11A and B)**. This zone increases slightly in amount from the cementoenamel junction to the root apex. It is caused by a coalescing and looping of the terminal portions of the dentinal tubules.

### Dentinocemental Junction

This is a thin smooth boundary line between dentin and cementum in permanent tooth and scalloped in deciduous tooth. The attachment is firm in both sets of dentitions.

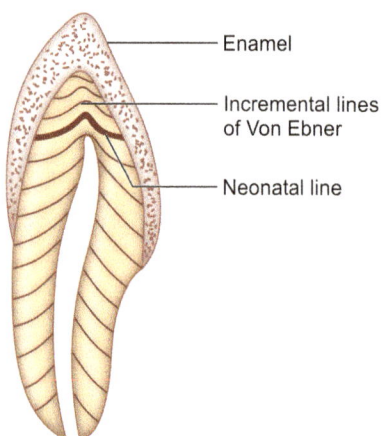

**Fig. 14.9:** Incremental lines of Von Ebner and neonatal line.

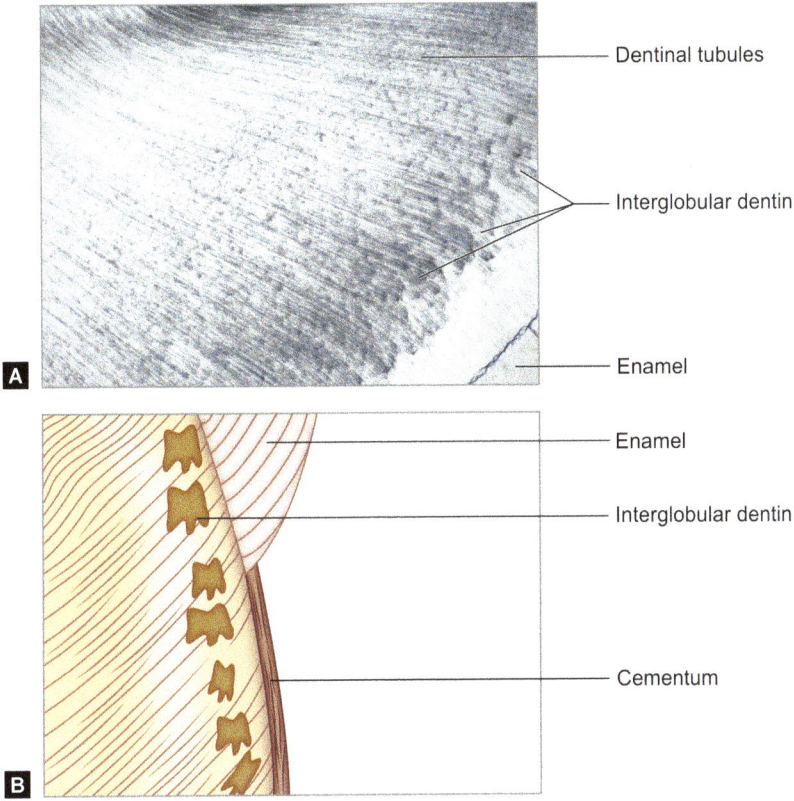

**Figs. 14.10A and B:** Interglobular dentin.

It is peripheral to Tomes' granular layer. It is debatable whether this layer is a form of dentin or a distinct tissue forming part of the tooth's attachment apparatus and cementing cementum to dentin **(Fig. 14.11B)**.

### Innervation of Dentin

Dentin is a highly sensitive tissue. The anatomic basis and mechanism for this sensitivity is highly controversial. The myelinated nerve fibers of pulp lose their myelin sheath in subodontoblastic layer and traverse up to odontoblast layer. Some of the fibers end in predentin and inner dentin up to 100–150 μm from the pulp. Most of these small vesiculated endings are located in tubules in coronal part of tooth, especially in the pulp horn. The nerves and their terminals are found in close association with the odontoblast process within the tubule. The primary afferent somatosensory nerves of the dentin and pulp project to the main sensory nucleus of the midbrain.

## THEORIES OF PAIN TRANSMISSION THROUGH DENTIN

There are three basic theories of pain conduction through dentin:

### Direct Neural Stimulation

The stimuli in some manner as yet unknown reach the nerve ending of inner dentin. The theory is not widely accepted.

### Hydrodynamic Theory

Various stimuli such as heat, cold, airblast desiccation, or mechanical pressure affect fluid movement in the dentinal tubules. This fluid movement, either inward or outward, stimulates the pain mechanism in the tubules by mechanical disturbance of the nerves

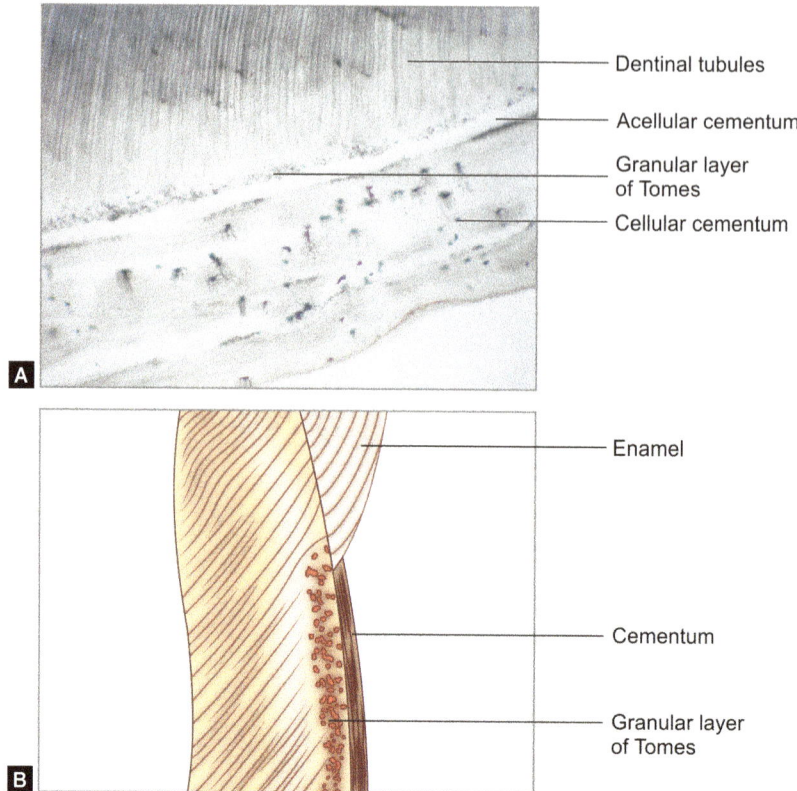

**Figs. 14.11A and B:** Granular layer of Tomes and dentinocemental junction.

closely associated with the odontoblast and its process. This is the most popular theory.

### Transduction Theory

According to this theory, the odontoblast process is the primary structure excited by the stimulus and that the impulse is transmitted to the nerve endings in the inner dentin. This is also not well-accepted theory as there are no neurotransmitter vesicles in the odontoblast process to facilitate the synapse.

## AGE AND FUNCTIONAL CHANGES

### Vitality of Dentin

Dentin is a vital tissue and it reacts to physiologic stimuli. Though the dentin is laid down throughout the life of tooth, after eruption, dentinogenesis slows down. Dentin reacts differently to mechanical, bacterial (dental caries), thermal, chemical, and electrical stimulation depending upon the intensity of the stimulus.

### Reparative Dentin

It is a localized deposit of dentin on the wall of the pulp cavity as a reparative process, when odontoblast cells are damaged due to external stimulation like attrition, abrasion, erosion, and dental caries **(Figs. 14.12A to D)**. The majority of odontoblasts degenerate and are replaced by the migration of undifferentiated perivascular cells from deeper region of pulp. Both damaged odontoblasts and newly differentiated odontoblasts begin deposition of reparative dentin to seal off the zone of injury.

Reparative dentin is characterized by fewer and more twisted tubules and less mucopolysaccharide than normal dentin. Dentin-forming cells are often included in the matrix-forming osteodentin. As tubules are sparse and there is irregular, dense

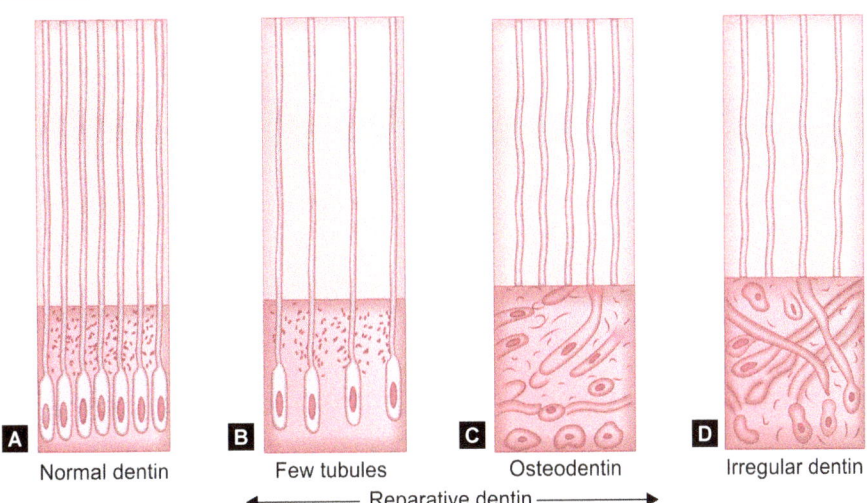

Figs. 14.12A to D: Normal and reparative dentin.

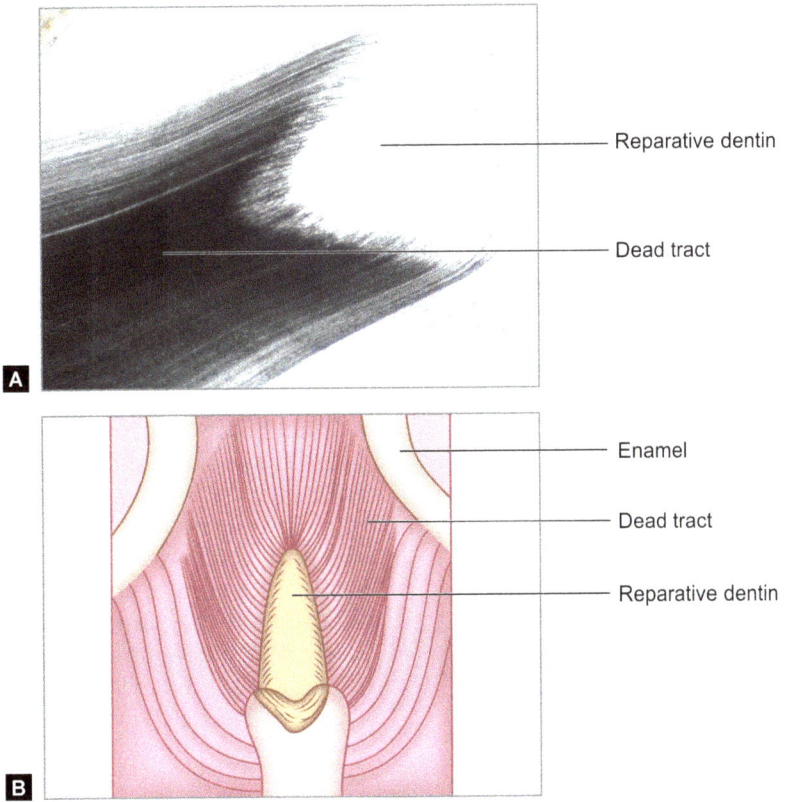

Figs. 14.13A and B: Reparative dentin.

calcification, the reparative dentin appears white in transmitted light and dark in reflected light **(Figs. 14.13A and B)**.

### Dead tracts

These are groups of dark lines that follow the course of dentinal tubules, visible when

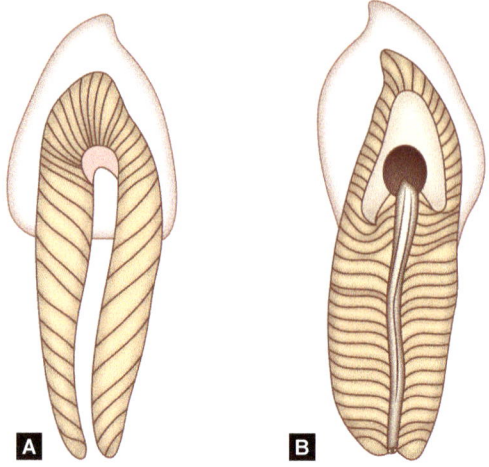

**Figs. 14.14A and B:** Dead tract: (A) Black in transmitted light; (B) White in reflected light.

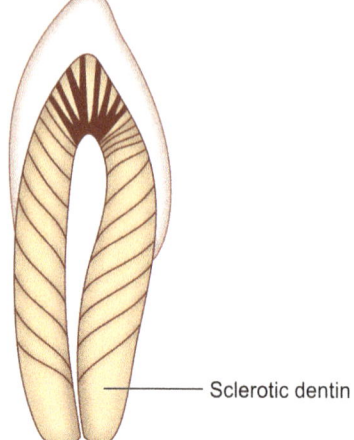

**Fig. 14.15:** Sclerotic dentin.

ground section of dentin is examined under transmitted light.

They appear white under reflected light **(Figs. 14.14A and B)**. The reasons for the formation of the dead tracts are that the odontoblast cells may die or may be injured due to (1) violent stimuli like—(a) bacterial (caries), (b) mechanical (wearing down of tooth due to attrition, abrasion, erosion or cavity preparation), (c) thermal, chemical, electrical (from improper restoration of tooth) or due to (2) overcrowding of odontoblasts (near the area of narrow pulpal horn). As a result, there is either degeneration or retraction of odontoblast process and the dentinal tubules are filled with fluid or gaseous substances which appear black in transmitted light and white in reflected light.

The areas of dead tracts demonstrate decreased sensitivity and appear to a greater extent in older teeth.

### Sclerotic Dentin (Transparent Dentin)

It is hypermineralized dentin which appears white or transparent when a ground section of dentin is examined under transmitted light and dark in reflected light **(Fig. 14.15)**.

Instead of forming reparative dentin or dead tracts, external stimulation (mechanical, thermal, chemical, electrical, and bacterial) may lead to protective changes in the dentin itself. Sometimes, external stimulation may lead to the appearance of collagen fibers and apatite crystals in the dentinal tubules. Gradually, the tubule lumen is obliterated with mineral and the refractive index equalizes with adjacent dentin. When this occurs in several tubules in the same area, the dentin assumes a glassy appearance and becomes translucent. The amount of sclerotic dentin is increased with age and is most common in the apical third of the root and in the crown midway between the dentinoenamel junction and the surface of the pulp.

Because sclerosis reduces the permeability of dentin, it may help to prolong pulp vitality.

Sclerosis of radicular dentin tends to make the roots brittle and they may fracture during extraction. It is also associated with increasing translucency of the root. This starts at the apex in the peripheral dentin just beneath the cementum and extends inward and coronally with increasing age. The length of root affected by translucency is used in forensic dentistry as one method of age estimation.

### CLINICAL CONSIDERATIONS

1. Exposed dentin surface should be sealed with a nonirritating, insulating substance as exposure of 1 mm$^2$ of dentin to noxious stimuli leads to damage of about 30,000 living cells.

2. Tubular configuration of dentin causes rapid penetration and spread of dental caries, pulpitis, and toothache.
3. Being elastic, dentin supports the overlying enamel and the base of cavity preparations is always placed in dentin.

## QUESTIONNAIRE

1. What is dentin? Discuss physical characteristics and chemical composition of dentin.
2. Describe the microscopic structure of dentin with diagram.
3. Differentiate between primary dentin, secondary dentin, and tertiary dentin.
4. What do you mean by mantle dentin, circumpulpal dentin, predentin, peritubular dentin, and intertubular dentin?
5. Write notes on:
   a. Incremental lines of Von Ebnar.
   b. Neonatal line.
   c. Interglobular dentin.
   d. Granular layer of Tomes.
   e. Reparative dentin.
   f. Dead tracts.
   g. Sclerotic dentin.
6. Discuss the theories of pain transmission through dentin.
7. Discuss the age changes and functional changes in dentin.

## BIBLIOGRAPHY

1. Anderson DJ. Sensory Mechanisms in Dentin. Oxford: Pergamon Press; 1963.
2. Antonio N. Ten Cate's Oral Histology Development, Structure, and Function, 7th edition. Mosby: Elsevier; 2008.
3. Berkovitz BKB, Holland GR, Moxham BJ. A Colour Atlas and Textbook of Oral Anatomy, Histology and Embryology, 4th edition. Mosby: Elsevier; 2009.
4. Das AK. Dental Anatomy and Oral Histology, 1st edition. West Bengal: Current Books International; 1972.
5. Gaunt WA, Osborn JW, Ten Cate AR. Advances in Dental Histology. Bristol: John Wright and Sons Ltd.; 1967.
6. Kumar GS. Orban's Oral Histology and Embryology, 12th edition. Mosby: Elsevier; 2009.
7. Osborn JW, Ten Cate AR. Advanced Dental Histology, 3rd edition. Bristol: John Wright and Sons Ltd.; 1976.

# CHAPTER 15

# Pulp

The pulp is a delicate mesenchymal connective tissue that occupies the pulp cavity in the central part of tooth. It is surrounded by dentin on all sides except at the apical foramen and accessory pulp canal openings where it is in communication with periodontal soft tissue. Every person normally has a total of 52 pulp organs, 32 in the permanent and 20 in the primary teeth. The total volume of all permanent teeth pulp organs is 0.38 cc and the mean volume of a single adult human pulp is 0.02 cc. Molar pulps are three to four times larger than incisor pulps.

## FUNCTIONS

### Inductive

The first role of the pulp anlage is to induce oral epithelial differentiation into dental lamina and enamel organ formation. The pulp anlage also induces the developing enamel organ to become a particular type of tooth.

### Formative

The main function of pulp is formation of dentin, as odontoblasts, the dentin-forming cells are present bordering the pulp tissue.

### Nutritive

It supplies nutrition to the dentin through blood vessels and odontoblastic processes and maintains vitality of tooth.

### Sensory

The sensory nerves in the pulp respond with pain to all stimuli such as heat, cold, pressure, operating cutting procedures, and chemical agents. The nerves also initiate reflexes that control circulation in the pulp.

### Defensive

The pulp is an organ with remarkable reparative abilities. It responds to irritation like mechanical, thermal, chemical, or bacterial and it protects itself and the vitality of the tooth by producing reparative dentin and mineralizing any affected dentinal tubule.

## ANATOMY

The pulp cavity is divided into :
1. Pulp chamber (coronal pulp).
2. Root canal (radicular pulp).

### Pulp Chamber (Coronal Pulp)

In young teeth, the shape of the pulp chamber is the same as the outline of outer surface of dentin. The extension of the pulp chamber into the cusps of tooth is called pulpal horns. The pulp chamber is large at the time of eruption but becomes smaller with advancing age due to deposition of secondary dentin.

### Root Canal (Radicular Pulp)

It extends from cervical region of the crown to the root apex. In the anterior teeth, the radicular pulps are single and in posterior ones multiple. The shape of the radicular pulp is tubular. It is continuous with periapical connective tissues through apical foramen.

### Apical Foramen

The location, shape, size, and number of the apical foramen vary. The opening may be bounded by dentin or by cementum. The average size of the apical foramen of maxillary teeth in adult is 0.4 mm. In mandibular teeth, it is slightly smaller, being 0.3 mm in diameter.

Shape of coronal and radicular pulp and volume of pulp are variable in different

# Pulp

**TABLE 15.1:** Pulp cavity of different teeth (permanent series).

| Maxillary teeth | Coronal pulp | Radicular pulp | Volume of pulp |
|---|---|---|---|
| Central incisor | Shovel-shaped, three short horns | Triangular in cross-section with point of triangle pointing lingually | 0.012 cc |
| Lateral incisor | Spoon-shaped | Round in cross-section evenly tapered to apex | 0.011 cc |
| Canine | Longest pulp, elliptical in cross-section | Distally inclined apex | 0.015 cc |
| First premolar | Large occluso-cervical pulp organ | Two smooth funnel-shaped radicular pulps | 0.018 cc |
| Second premolar | Same | One root | 0.017 cc |
| First molar | Roughly rectangular cervical cross-section with the greatest dimension buccolingually with mesiobuccal prominence | Three radicular pulps, lingual is longest | 0.068 cc |
| Second molar | Same | Same | 0.044 cc |
| Third molar | Same | Same | 0.023 cc |
| Central incisor | Smallest pulp organ, long, narrow with a flattened elliptical shape in cross-section buccolingually | Single, narrow radicular pulp | 0.006 cc |
| Lateral incisor | Same as central only smaller in all dimensions | Same | 0.007 cc |
| Canine | Similar to but shorter than maxillary canine | Radicular pulp begins tapering at midpoint, ending in a distally inclined apex | 0.014 cc |
| First premolar | Similar to mandibular canine but missing lingual pulp horn | Single radicular pulp | 0.015 cc |
| Second premolar | Similar to mandibular canine, lingual horn smaller | Single and triangular in cross-section | 0.015 cc |
| First molar | Coronal cross-section is rectangular with the mesiodistal dimension greatest. It shows mesiobuccal prominence with highest mesiobuccal horn | Two radicular pulps, distal being shorter, straighter, and singular. Mesial is longer, curved, and doubled | 0.053 cc |
| Second molar | Same | Same | 0.032 cc |
| Third molar | Same | Same | 0.031 cc |

maxillary and mandibular teeth. Shape of coronal and radicular pulp and volume of pulp of different permanent maxillary and mandibular teeth are given in tabular form (Table 15.1).

## Accessory Canals

Accessory canals leading from the radicular pulp laterally through the root dentin to the periodontal tissue may be seen anywhere along the root but are particularly numerous in the apical third of the root. It is formed maybe due to premature loss of root sheath cells and subsequent failure of dentin formation in a localized region. Accessory canals may also occur where developing root encounters a blood vessel. If the vessel is located in the area where dentin is forming, the hard tissue may develop around it, making a lateral canal from the radicular pulp.

## DEVELOPMENT

The tooth pulp is initially called dental papilla. It is designated as pulp only after dentin forms around it. In the earliest stages of tooth development, it is the area of the proliferating future papilla that causes the oral epithelium to invaginate and form the enamel organs. These organs then enlarge to enclose the dental papillae in their central portions. The dental papilla further controls whether the forming enamel organ is to be an incisor or a molar.

The young dental papilla is highly vascularized, and a well-organized network of vessels appears by the time dentin formation begins. The cells of the dental papilla appear as undifferentiated mesenchymal cells which differentiate into stellate-shaped fibroblasts.

Ameloblasts are differentiated from inner enamel epithelium and the odontoblasts are differentiated from peripheral cells of the dental papilla. As dentinogenesis begins, the dental papilla is designated as pulp organ.

Few large myelinated nerves are found in the pulp until the dentin of the crown is well-advanced. At that time, nerves reach the odontoblastic zone in the pulp horns. The sympathetic nerves, however, follow the blood vessels as the pulp begins to organize.

## STRUCTURAL FEATURES

The pulp consists of (1) cells and (2) intercellular substance.

| PULP | |
|---|---|
| **Cells** | **Intercellular substance** |
| a. Odontoblasts | a. Fibers |
| b. Fibroblast | b. Vessels |
| c. Defense cells | c. Nerve fibers |
| | d. Ground substance |

From periphery to the center, the different zones are **(Figs. 15.1A to C)**:
1. The odontoblast cell layer
2. The cell-free zone (Weil's zone)
3. The cell-rich zone.

### Cells

### Odontoblasts

The odontoblasts are highly differentiated connective tissue cells. They lie in a continuous row near the dentinal end of the pulp and their protoplasmic processes project through the dentinal tubules. They are tall columnar in the crown **(Fig. 15.2)**, cuboidal in the middle of the root, and flat, spindle-shaped near the apex of tooth. They are approximately 25–40 μm in length and 5–7 μm in diameter.

The cell contains a large oval nucleus which fills the basal part of the cells. The nuclei are placed at different levels and therefore the cells appear to be stratified. The cells in the odontoblastic row lie very close to each other and the plasma membranes of adjacent cells exhibit junctional complexes.

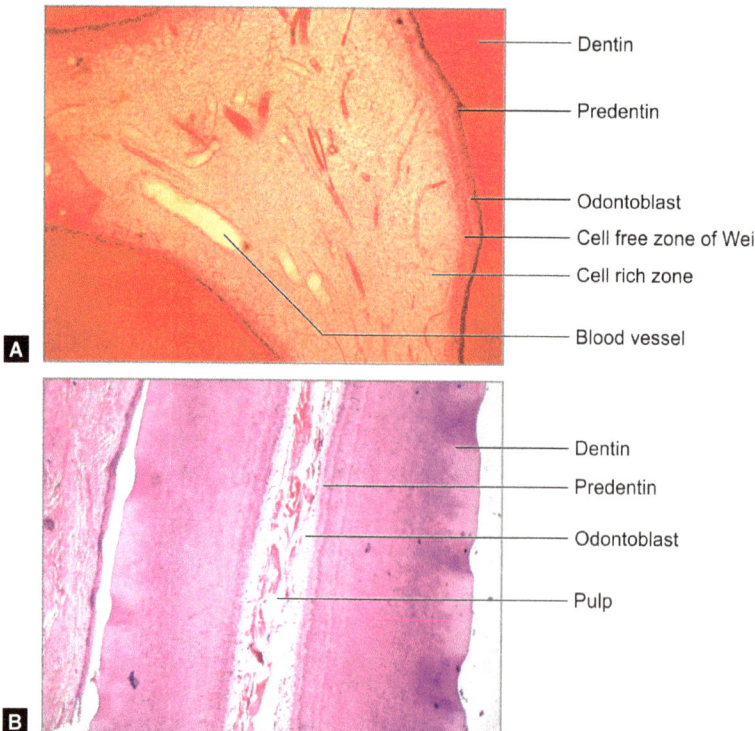

**Figs. 15.1A and B:** Photomicrograph of histology of pulp.

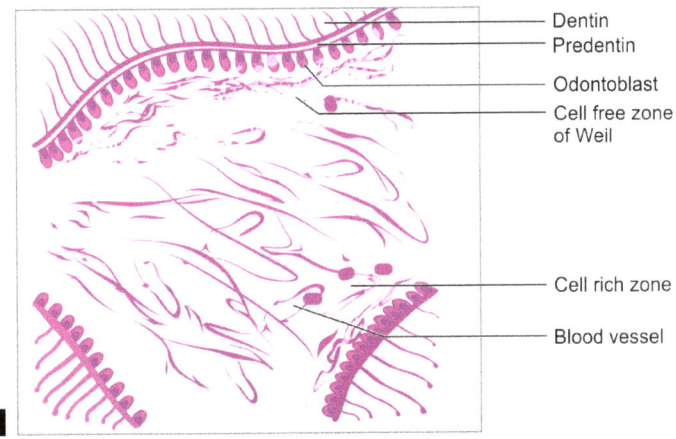

**Fig. 15.1C:** Schematic diagram of histology of pulp.

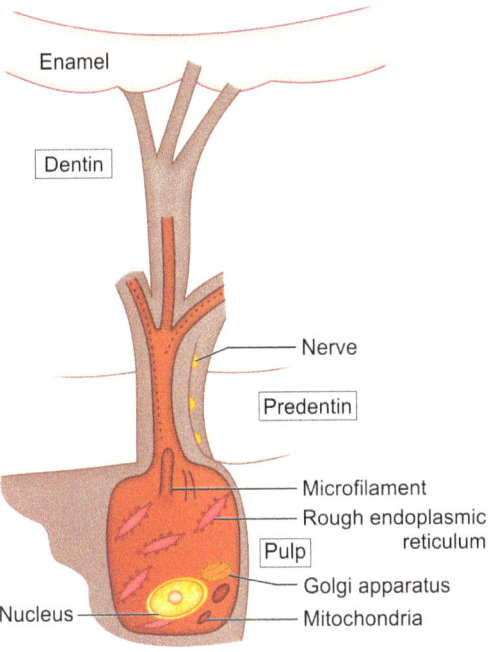

**Fig. 15.2:** Odontoblast.

Immediately adjacent to the nucleus, basally there are rough endoplasmic reticulum and the Golgi apparatus. Further toward the apex of the cell appears an abundance of rough surfaced endoplasmic reticulum. There is a striking difference in the cytoplasm of the young cell body, active in dentinogenesis, and the older cell.

During the early active phase, the Golgi apparatus is more prominent, the rough endoplasmic reticulum is more abundant, and numerous mitochondria appear throughout the odontoblast. Near the pulpal predentin junction, the cell cytoplasm is devoid of organelles. The clear terminal part of the cell body and the adjacent intercellular junction is known as the terminal bar apparatus of the odontoblast. At this zone, the cell constricts to a diameter of 3–4 µm where the cell process enters the predentinal tubule. The process of the cell contains no endoplasmic reticulum except at the early period of active dentinogenesis when it contains occasional mitochondria and a great number of vesicles. There is evidence of protein synthesis along the tubule wall. The main process of odontoblast cell is known as Tomes' process.

***Function: Formation of dentin***

In the crown, just deep to the odontoblast layer, a zone is seen which is comparatively devoid of cells. It is known as cell-free zone (zone of Weil or subodontoblastic layer). It contains a network of nerve fibers, the subodontoblastic plexus, or plexus of Raschkow. In zone of Weil, though cells are very few in number, fibroblasts and mesenchymal cells in this zone may differentiate to odontoblast on demand. Nerves and blood vessels pass through zone of Weil to arrive at odontoblast and predentin. This zone is generally not seen in young teeth and therefore may be an artifact (a defect during tissue processing). Deeper to the cell-free zone, there is a narrow zone of pulp tissue in which the cells are more numerous than elsewhere in the pulp. This zone has a rich capillary network. This cell rich zone is also present in root but not conspicuous.

## Fibroblasts

The fibroblasts are the most numerous cell types in the pulp. They have typical stellate shape and extensive processes are joined by intercellular junctions to the processes of other fibroblasts. Under light microscope, the fibroblast nuclei stain deeply with basic dyes (hematoxylin) and cytoplasm is lighter stained and appears homogeneous.

Electron microscope reveals abundant rough-surfaced endoplasmic reticulum, mitochondria, and other organelles in the fibroblast cytoplasm. This indicates that these cells are active in pulpal collagen production and are seen in young pulp.

In older pulp, they appear rounded or spindle-shaped with short processes and exhibit fewer intracellular organelles. They are termed fibrocytes.

### Functions
1. Synthesis of collagen fiber throughout the pulp matrix during the life of the tooth.
2. Capable of ingesting and degrading the same matrix.

## Defense Cells

The cells which are important to the defense of the pulp are the histiocytes or macrophage, mast cells, and the plasma cells **(Fig. 15.3)**. In addition, there are cells from blood vascular elements such as the neutrophils, eosinophils, basophils, lymphocytes, and monocytes.

- **Histiocyte:** The histiocyte or macrophage is an irregularly shaped cell with short blunt processes. In the light microscope, the nucleus is somewhat smaller, more rounded, and darker staining than that of fibroblasts and it exhibits granular cytoplasm. These cells are usually associated with small blood vessels and capillaries.

  Ultrastructurally, the macrophage exhibits a rounded outline with short, blunt processes and contains mitochondria, rough surfaced endoplasmic reticulum, free ribosomes, and also a moderately dense nucleus.

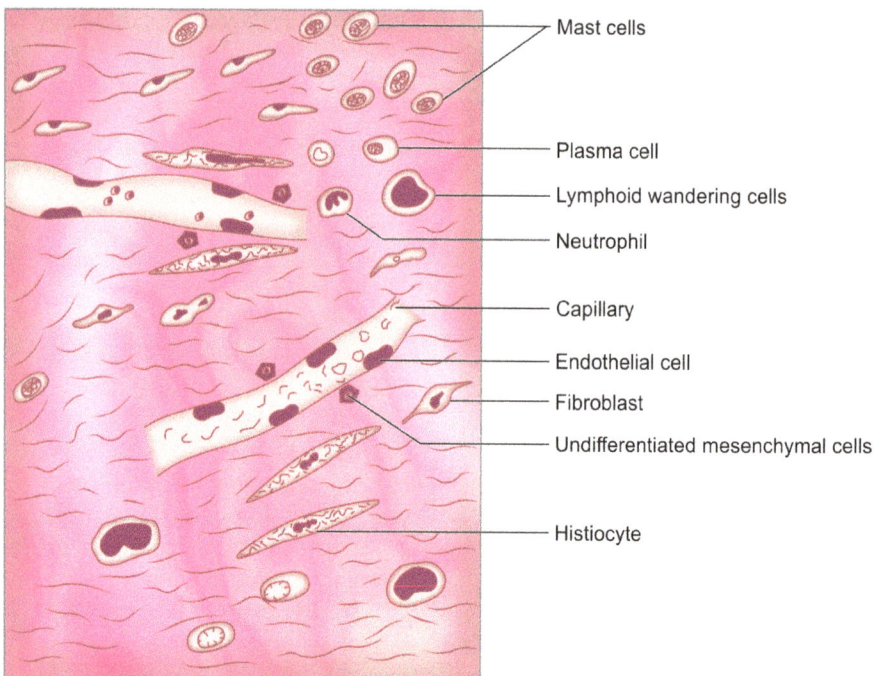

**Fig. 15.3:** Defense cells of pulp.

There are aggregates of vesicles, or phagosomes, which contain phagocytized dense irregular bodies.
- **Lymphocytes and eosinophils:** They are found extravascularly in the normal pulp but during inflammation, they increase in number.
- **Mast cells:** They are seen along the vessels in the inflamed pulp. They have a round nucleus and contain many dark-staining granules in the cytoplasm.
- **Plasma cells:** They are seen during inflammation of the pulp. With the light microscope, the plasma cell nucleus appears small and concentric in the cytoplasm. The chromatin of the nucleus is adherent to the nuclear membrane and gives the cell a cartwheel appearance. The cytoplasm is basophilic with a light stained Golgi zone adjacent to nucleus. Under electron microscope, the cell has a densely packed, rough surfaced endoplasmic reticulum.

*Function*
**Production of antibodies:** Lymphoid wandering cells originate in the bloodstream and can act as macrophage.

## Undifferentiated Mesenchymal Cells

These cells are seen in very young pulp but only a few are seen in the pulps after root completion. They are polyhedral in shape with peripheral processes and contain large oval nuclei. They are found along pulp vessels, in the cell rich zone, and scattered throughout central pulp. They are totipotent cell and on demand they may become odontoblast, fibroblast, or macrophages.

## Intercellular Substance

It is a dense, gel-like substance, composed of:
a. Acid mucopolysaccharides.
b. Protein polysaccharide (glycosaminoglycans and proteoglycans).
c. Chondroitin A.
d. Chondroitin B.
e. Hyaluronic acid.
f. Glycoprotein.

*Functions*
1. It lends support to the cells of the pulp.
2. It serves as a means for transport of nutrients from the blood vessels to the cells.
3. It also serves as a transport of metabolites from cells to the blood vessels.

## Fibers

The collagen fibers in pulp exhibit typical cross-striation and at 64 nm (640 angstrom) and range in length from 10 to 100 nm or more. In young pulp, fibers ranging in diameter from 10 nm to 12 nm have been observed. Fibers may appear scattered throughout the coronal or radicular pulp and these are termed diffuse collagen or they may appear in bundles and are termed bundle collagen. Fiber bundles are more prevalent in root canals, especially near apical region. After root completion, the pulp matures and bundles of collagen fibers increase in number.

## Blood Vessels

The pulp organ is highly vascularized. Blood vessels arise from the inferior or superior alveolar artery and also drain by the same veins in both the mandibular and maxillary regions. The pulp vessels communicate with the vessels of periodontium through apical foramen and also through accessory canals. Small arteries and arterioles enter the apical canal and pursue a direct route to the coronal pulp. Along their course, they give off numerous branches in the radicular pulp that pass peripherally to form plexus in the odontogenic region. The capillaries form loops close to odontoblast and form a plexus in subodontoblastic zone. From this plexus, branches pass between the odontoblasts toward predentin and may form a plexus near it. Pulpal blood flow is more rapid than in most areas of the body as pulpal pressure is among the highest of body tissues. Veins and venules that are larger than the arteries also appear in the central region of the root pulp. They exhibit much thinner walls in relation to the size of the lumen. Both venous-venous anastomosis and arteriole-venous anastomosis occur in the pulp. The arteriole-venous shunts may have an important role in regulation of pulpal blood flow. Frequently arteriole or precapillary loops with capillaries are found underlying the odontogenic zone in the coronal pulp.

The terminal network of capillaries in the coronal pulp appears nearly perpendicular to the main trunks. A few peripheral capillaries found among the odontoblasts have fenestrations in the endothelial cells. These fenestrated capillaries are assumed to be involved in rapid transport of metabolites at a time when the odontoblasts are active in the process of dentinal matrix formation and its subsequent calcification.

## Lymph Vessels

The presence of lymph vessels in the dental pulp is controversial. Lymph vessels draining the pulp and periodontal ligament have a common outlet. Those draining the anterior teeth pass to the submental lymph nodes; those of the posterior teeth pass to the submandibular and deep cervical lymph nodes.

## Nerves

The abundant nerve supply in the pulp follows the distribution of the blood vessels. There are two types of nerve fibers:
- **Nonmyelinated (sympathetic nerves):** They are found in close association with the blood vessels of the pulp. They have terminals on the muscle cells of the larger vessels and function in vasoconstriction.
- **Myelinated (sensory):** They are sensory nerves. Whatever be the nature of stimulation, the only sensation felt by pulpal nerves is that of pain. It cannot differentiate between heat, cold, touch, pressure, or chemicals. It is due to the free nerve endings which are specific for pain. Pulpal nerve cannot also localize the pain as it does not have the receptors for proprioception. The nerve fibers divide and redivide into smaller branches as they migrate coronally. They lose their myelin sheath and form a rich plexus in subodontoblastic zone. From this plexus, nerves pass to odontoblastic layer, dentinal tubules, and predentin.

## Regressive Changes
### Cellular Change

In aging pulp, the cells are characterized by a decrease in size and number of cytoplasmic organelles. The number of cells also becomes fewer.

### Fibrosis

In aging pulp, accumulations of both diffuse fibrillar components and bundles of collagen fibers usually appear. There is sclerosis of vessels.

### Pulp Stone (Denticles)

These are nodular, calcified masses in either or both coronal or root portion of the pulp organ.
A. Classification of pulp stone according to their structure **(Figs. 15.4A to C)**:
   - **True denticles:** They are localized masses of calcified tissue, resembling dentin because of their tubular structure. They are very rare and located close to apical foramen. They are formed due to inclusion of epithelial root sheath in pulp followed by differentiation of odontoblast from pulp cell and formation of masses of dentin. They bear greater resemblance to secondary dentin than primary dentin since tubules are irregular in number.
   - **False denticles:** They do not contain dentinal tubules. They are concentric layers of calcified tissue with a remnant of necrotic cell in the center. Calcification of thrombi in blood vessel may also serve as nidus for false denticle.
   - **Diffuse calcifications:** These are irregular, calcific deposits in the pulpal tissue, usually following collagenous fiber bundles or blood vessels. Mostly, they are found in the root canal.

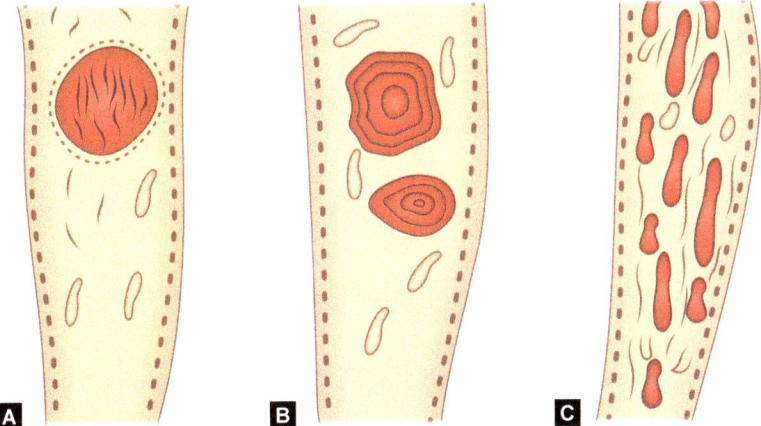

**Figs. 15.4A to C:** (A) True denticles; (B) False denticles; (C) Diffuse calcification.

B. Classification of pulp stone according to location **(Figs. 15.5A to C)**:
- **Free denticles:** They are entirely surrounded by pulp tissue.
- **Attached denticles:** They are partly fused with dentinal wall.
- **Embedded denticles:** They are completely embedded in dentin.

Pulp stones may appear close to blood vessels and nerve trunks. The incidence as well as the size of pulp stones increases with age.

## CLINICAL CONSIDERATIONS

1. For all operative procedures, the shape of the pulp chamber and its extensions into the cusps, the pulp horns, are important to remember.
2. While performing root canal treatment, the size, shape, number, and direction of pulp chamber, root canals, and apical foramen must be kept in mind for successful treatment. Presence of pulp calcifications causes obstruction to root canal treatment.

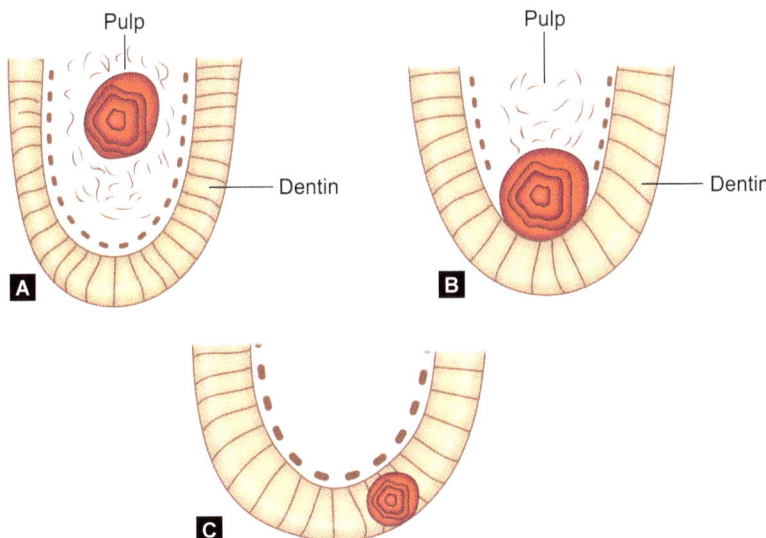

**Figs. 15.5A to C:** (A) Free denticle; (B) Attached denticle; (C) Embedded denticle.

3. The pulp is highly responsive to stimuli. Even a slight stimulus will cause inflammatory cell infiltration. A severe reaction is characterized as one with increased inflammatory cell infiltration adjacent to the cavity site, hyperemia, or localized abscesses.

## QUESTIONNAIRE

1. What is pulp? What are the functions of pulp?
2. What are the different parts of pulp? Differentiate between coronal and radicular pulp.
3. What are the structural components of pulp? Describe in detail about the cells of pulp with diagram.
4. Discuss the vasculature and innervation of pulp.
5. What are the regressive changes in pulp?
6. Write notes on:
   A. Apical foramen.
   B. Accessary canal.
   C. Pulp stone.

## BIBLIOGRAPHY

1. Antonio N. Ten Cate's Oral Histology Development, Structure, and Function, 7th edition. Mosby; 2008.
2. Berkovitz BKB, Holland GR, Moxham BJ. A Colour Atlas and Textbook of Oral Anatomy, Histology and Embryology, 4th edition. Mosby: Elsevier; 2009.
3. Das AK. Dental Anatomy and Oral Histology, 1st edition. Current Publishers; 1972.
4. Gaunt WA, Osborn JW, Ten Cate AR. Advances in Dental Histology. Bristol: John Wright and Sons Ltd.; 1967.
5. Kumar GS. Orban's Oral Histology and Embryology, 12th edition. Mosby; 2009.
6. Osborn JW, Ten Cate AR. Advanced Dental Histology, 3rd edition. Bristol: John Wright and Sons Ltd.; 1976.
7. Seltzer S, Bender IB. The Dental Pulp. Philadelphia: JB Lippincott Co.; 1965.

# CHAPTER 16

# Cementum

Cementum is a mineralized avascular connective tissue that covers the anatomic roots of teeth. It begins at the cervical portion of the tooth at the cementoenamel junction and continues to the apex **(Fig. 16.1)**. Cementum is a medium for the attachment of collagen fibers that bind the tooth to surrounding structures. It is a specialized connective tissue that shares some physical, chemical, and structural characteristics with compact bone. But unlike bone, it is avascular and has no innervation.

## PHYSICAL CHARACTERISTICS

### Hardness
The hardness of fully mineralized cementum is less than dentin.

### Color
Light yellow in color. It can be distinguished from enamel by its lack of luster and darker hue. It is lighter in color than dentin.

### Permeability
It is permeable to a variety of materials. The cellular type is more permeable than acellular type. Permeability decreases with age.

## CHEMICAL COMPOSITION

|           | Weight | Volume |
|-----------|--------|--------|
| Organic   | 65%    | 45%    |
| Inorganic | 23%    | 33%    |
| Water     | 12%    | 22%    |

The inorganic portion consists mainly of calcium and phosphate in the form of hydroxyapatite. Numerous trace elements are found in cementum in varying amounts.

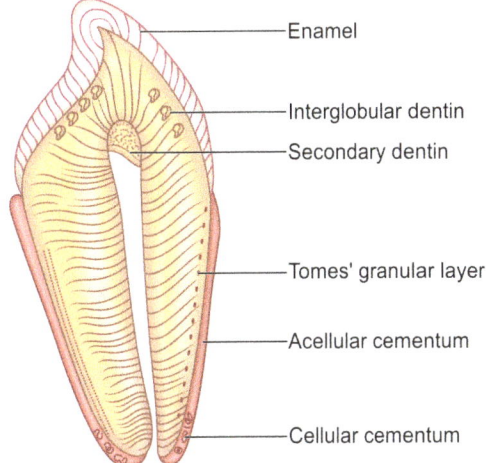

Fig. 16.1: Cementum.

Cementum has the highest fluoride content of all the mineralized tissues. The organic portion of cementum consists primarily of Type I collagen and protein polysaccharides (proteoglycans).

## FUNCTION

- **Attachment:** The primary function of cementum is to furnish a medium for the attachment of collagen fibers that bind the tooth to alveolar bone.
- **Protection:** It protects the root surface from injury and resorption by continuous deposition.
- **Reparative:** Damage to roots such as fractures and resorptions can be repaired by deposition of new cementum.
- **Functional adaptation:** Cementum makes functional adaptation of teeth possible by deposition of cementum in an apical area and thus can compensate for the loss of tooth substance from occlusal wear.

## Cementum

- It helps eruption by apposition at apical end.
- It helps to maintain the width of periodontal ligament.

### STRUCTURE

With the light microscope, two types of cementum can be differentiated. The classification is based on the presence or absence of cells.

1. Acellular
2. Cellular.

### Acellular Cementum

It is a type of cementum that does not incorporate cells, the spider-like cementocytes **(Figs. 16.2A to C)**. It is the first formed cementum and the rate of development is relatively slow. It covers the root and extended from cementoenamel junction to the apex,

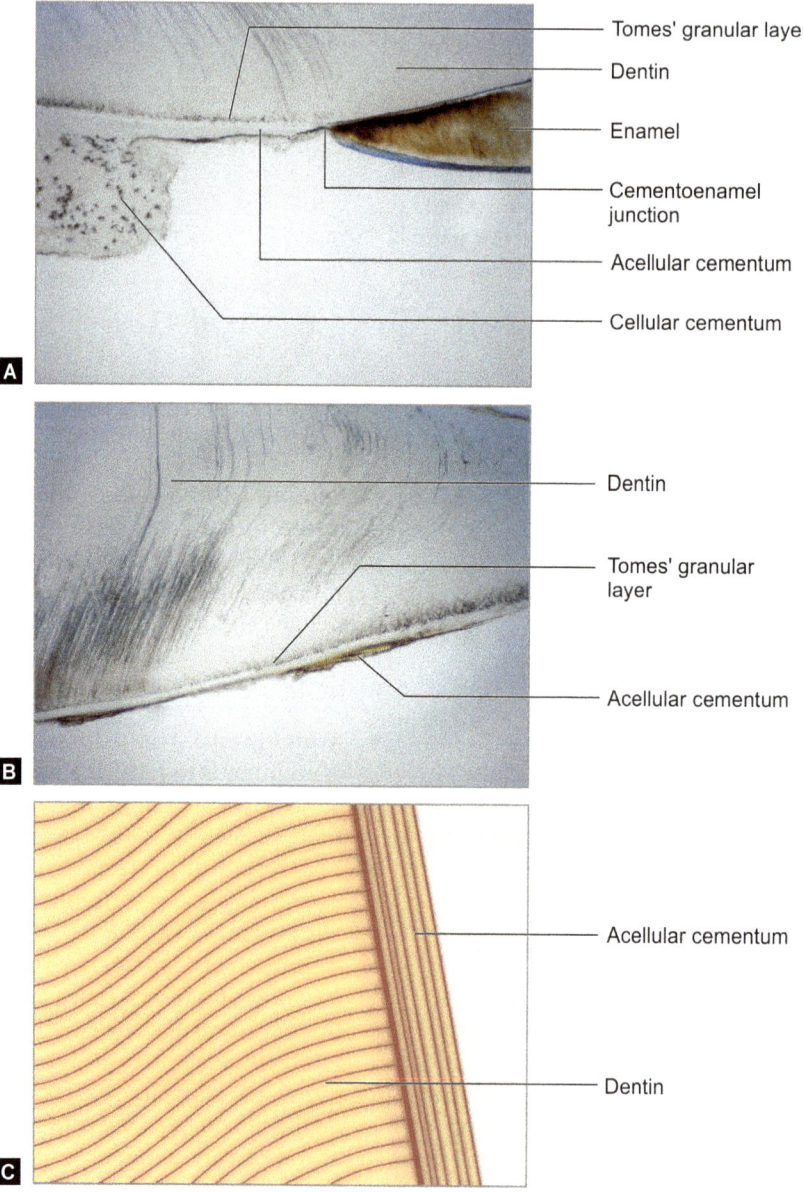

**Figs. 16.2A to C:** Acellular cementum.

# Cementum

but it is often missing in the apical third of the root. It is the thinnest at the cementoenamel junction (20-50 mm) and thicker near the apex or at bifurcation (150-200 mm). The apical foramen is surrounded by cementum. Sometimes cementum extends to the inner wall of dentin for a short distance.

It consists of:
a. Collagen fibrils that make up the bulk of the organic portion of the tissue. The fibrils are arranged in a very complex fashion and usually arranged parallel to the root surface.
b. *Sharpey's fibers*: These are discrete bundles of collagen fibrils, particularly seen in tangential section. They are the fibers of periodontal ligament, incorporated into the matrix of cementum **(Fig. 16.3)**. They run at right angle to the collagen fibers.

In a zone, 10-50 mm wide near the cementodentinal junction, 1-5 mm unmineralized areas are seen. These areas probably represent poorly mineralized cores of Sharpey's fibers. When cementum remains relatively thin, Sharpey's fibers cross the entire thickness of the cementum. With further apposition of cementum, a larger part of the fibers are incorporated in the cementum. The attachment proper is confined to the most superficial or recently formed layer of cementum. This indicates that the thickness of cementum does not enhance functional efficiency by increasing the strength of attachment of the individual fibers.

Scanning electron microscopic features of Sharpey's fiber—in fully mineralized area, the center of Sharpey's fiber is exhibited by low rounded projections. In actively mineralizing front, the sites where individual Sharpey's fibers enter the tooth are exhibited by numerous small openings. They represent the unmineralized core of the fiber.

c. *Ground substance*: Interspersed between the collagen fibrils are electron-dense reticular areas which represent protein polysaccharide materials of the ground substance.

## Cellular Cementum

Cellular cementum is the type of cementum in which cementocytes are incorporated **(Figs. 16.4A to C)**. The rate of development is relatively fast. Cellular cementum is more frequently seen on apical half of root. Acellular cementum can occasionally be found on the surface of cellular cementum **(Fig. 16.5)**. Cellular cementum is frequently formed on the surface of acellular cementum **(Fig. 16.5)**, but it may comprise the entire thickness of apical cementum. It is always thickest around the apex and by its growth, contributes to the length of the root. The cementocytes lie in spaces designated as lacunae **(Fig. 16.6)**. A typical cementocyte has numerous cell processes or canaliculi radiating from its cell body. These processes may branch and they frequently anastomose with those of a neighboring cell. Most of the

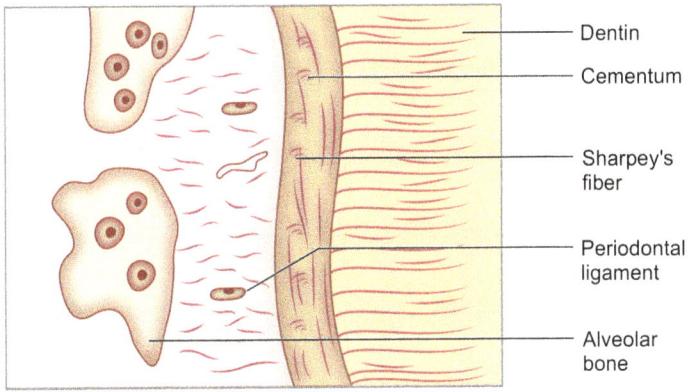

**Fig. 16.3:** Sharpey's fibers.

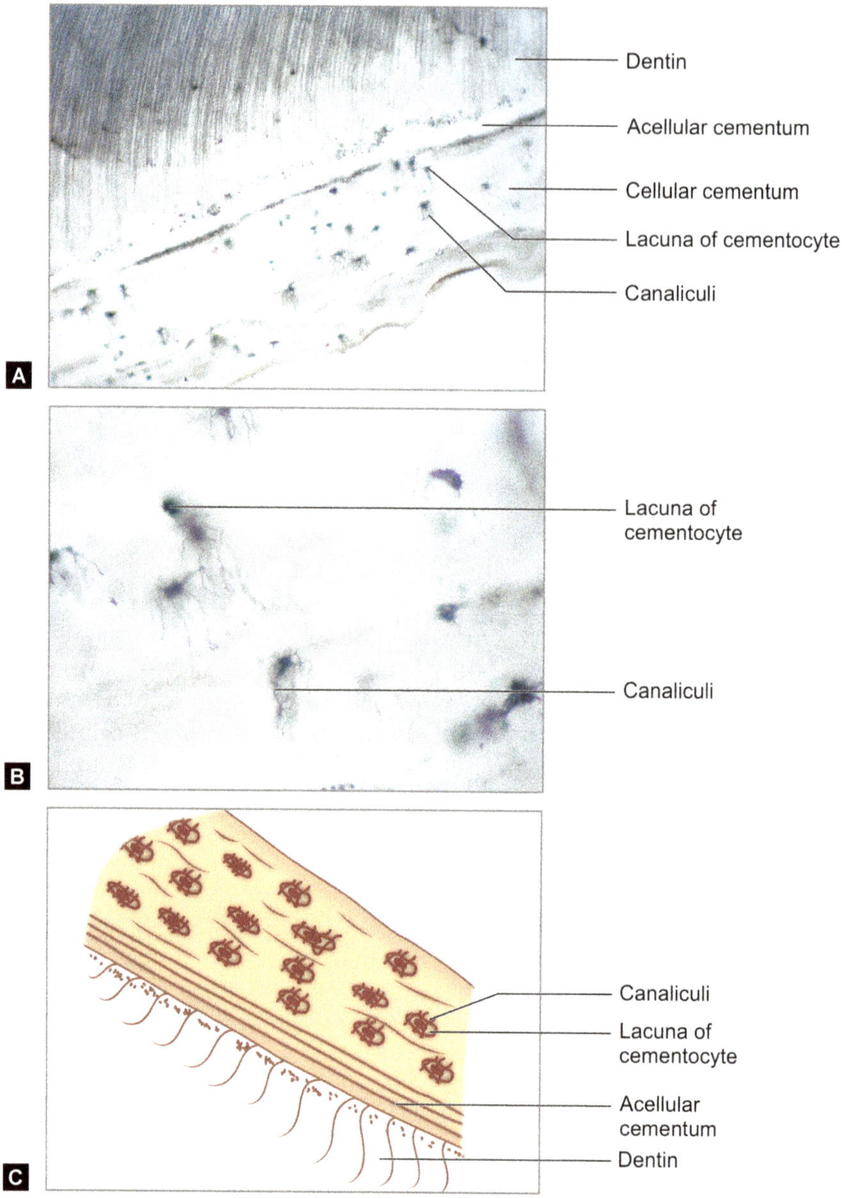

# Cementum

**Figs. 16.4A to C:** Cellular cementum.

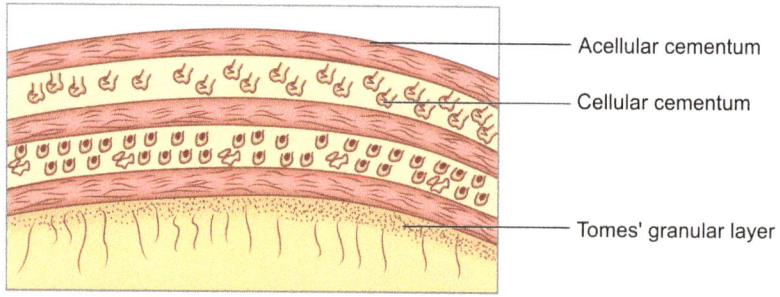

**Fig. 16.5:** Arrangement of cellular and acellular cementum.

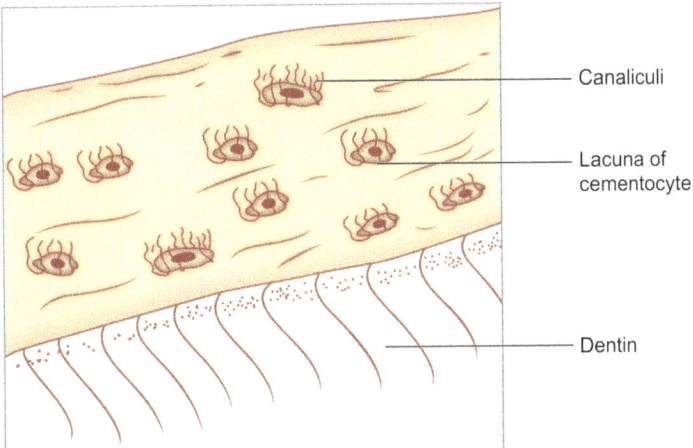

**Fig. 16.6:** Cementocyte.

| TABLE 16.1: Differences between acellular and cellular cementum. | |
|---|---|
| **Acellular** | **Cellular** |
| 1. Absence of cells (cementocytes) in the calcified matrix | 1. Calcified matrix contains lacunae and canaliculi containing cementocytes and their processes |
| 2. Border with dentin is not clearly demarcated | 2. Border with dentin is clearly demarcated |
| 3. Rate of development is relatively slow | 3. Rate of development is relatively fast |
| 4. Incremental lines are relatively close together, thin, and even | 4. Incremental lines are relatively wide apart, thick, and irregular |
| 5. Precementum layer is narrow | 5. Precementum layer is wide |

processes are directed toward the periodontal surface of the cementum. The cytoplasm of the cementocytes contains few organelles. The endoplasmic reticulum appears dilated; mitochondria are sparse.

These features indicate that the cementocytes are in degenerating phase. At a depth of 60 µm, cementocytes show cytoplasmic clumping and vesiculation. Sometimes the lacunae appear to be empty, suggesting complete degeneration of cementocytes **(Table 16.1)**.

## Incremental Lines of Salter

Cementum is deposited in an irregular rhythm, resulting in unevenly spaced incremental lines **(Figs. 16.7A and B)**. Both acellular cementum and cellular cementum are separated by incremental lines into layers, which indicate periodic formation. In acellular cementum, incremental lines tend to be close together and they are thin and even. In the more rapidly formed cellular cementum, the lines are further apart and they are thicker and more irregular. The appearance of incremental lines in cementum is mainly due to differences in the degree of mineralization and also differences in composition of the underlying matrix. Histochemical studies reveal that incremental lines are highly mineralized. They contain collagen and more ground substance.

## SCANNING ELECTRON MICROSCOPY

Extensive variations in the surface topography of cementum can be observed with the scanning electron microscope. Resting cemental surfaces, where mineralization is more or less complete, exhibit low, rounded projections corresponding to the centers of Sharpey fibers. Cemental surfaces with actively mineralizing fronts have numerous small openings that correspond to sites where individual Sharpey's fibers enter the tooth. These openings represent unmineralized cores of the fibers. Numerous resorption bays and irregular ridges of cellular cementum are also observed on root surfaces.

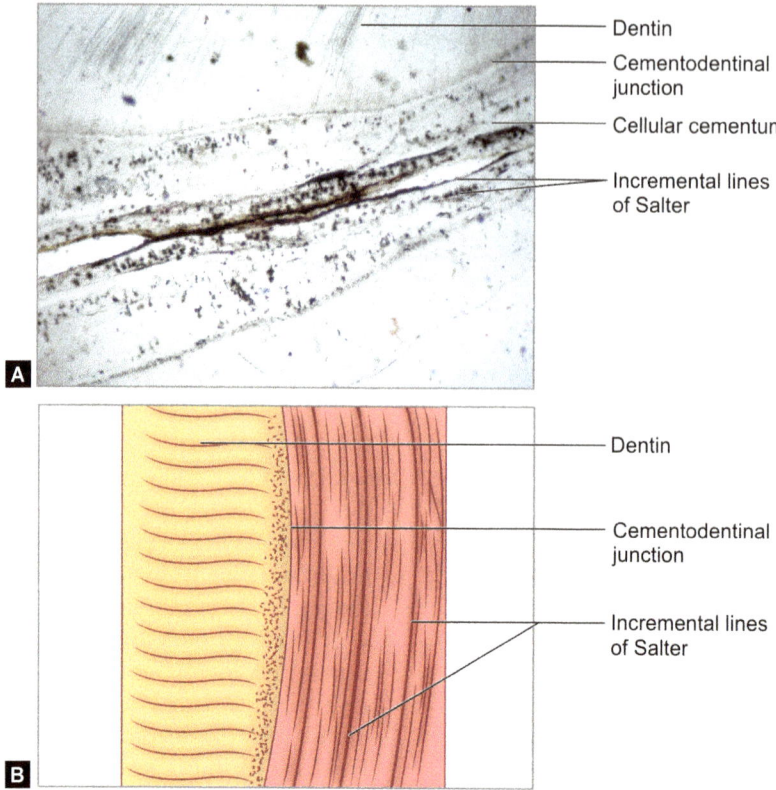

**Figs. 16.7A and B:** Cementodentinal junction and incremental lines of Salter.

## CLASSIFICATION OF CEMENTUM BASED ON THE NATURE AND ORIGIN OF THE ORGANIC MATRIX

Cementum derives its organic matrix from two sources:
1. *From the insertion of Sharpey fibers of the periodontal ligament*: These fibers are referred to as the extrinsic fibers.
2. *From cementoblasts*: These fibers are referred to as intrinsic fibers.

According to the nature and origin of the fibrous matrix, the cementum is classified into:
1. **Extrinsic fiber cementum:** For this type of cementum, all the collagen is derived as Sharpey fibers from the periodontal ligament (ground substance is produced by cementoblast). These fibers continue into the cementum in the same direction as the principal fibers of the ligament (perpendicular or oblique to the root surface). This type of cementum corresponds with primary acellular cementum. It is, therefore, formed slowly and the root surface is smooth. The fibers are well-mineralized.
2. **Mixed fiber cementum:** For this type of cementum, the collagen fibers of the organic matrix are derived from both extrinsic fibers and intrinsic fibers. The intrinsic fibers run between the extrinsic fibers with a different orientation. Indeed, the greater the number of intrinsic fibers in mixed fiber cementum, the greater the separation of the extrinsic fibers. The extrinsic fibers are ovoid or round bundles about 5–7 mm in diameter. The intrinsic fibers are 1–2 mm in diameter. If the formation rate is slow, the mixed fiber cementum may be acellular and well-mineralized. If the formation rate is fast, mixed fiber cementum may be cellular and less mineralized.

3. **Intrinsic fiber cementum:** This type of cementum is comprised only of intrinsic fibers running parallel to the root surface.

## CEMENTODENTINAL JUNCTION

This is a thin smooth boundary line between dentin and cementum in permanent tooth and scalloped in deciduous tooth. The attachment is firm in both sets of dentitions. It is peripheral to Tomes' granular layer. It is debatable whether this layer is a form of dentin or a distinct tissue forming part of the tooth's attachment apparatus and cementing cementum to dentin **(Figs. 16.7A and B)**.

The interface between cementum and dentin is clearly visible in decalcified and stained histologic sections under light microscope. In such preparations, cementum usually stains more intensely than does dentin.

Electron microscopically the cementodentinal junction is not very distinct. A narrow interface zone between the two tissues can be detected where cementum is more electron dense than dentin and some of its collagen fibrils are arranged in relatively distinct bundles while those of dentin are arranged somewhat haphazardly. Since collagen fibrils of cementum and dentin intertwine at their interface in a very complex fashion, it is not possible to determine whether fibrils are of dentinal or cemental origin.

### Intermediate Cementum

Sometimes dentin is separated from cementum by a zone known as the intermediate cementum layer, which does not exhibit the characteristic features of either cementum or dentin. This layer is predominantly seen in apical two-thirds of roots of molars and premolars and rarely observed in deciduous teeth and incisors. This layer represents the entrapped cells of Hertwig's epithelial root sheath in rapidly deposited dentin or cemental matrix. It may be found in continuous layer or in isolated areas.

## CEMENTOENAMEL JUNCTION

It is the region of the tooth where enamel meets the cementum at the cervical line **(Fig. 16.2A)**.

Three possible variations may exist at the cementoenamel junction.
1. The cervical enamel is covered by cementum for a short distance. It occurs in 60% of the teeth. This occurs when the enamel epithelium degenerates at its cervical termination, permitting connective tissue to come in direct contact with enamel surface.
2. In approximately 30% of all teeth, cementum meets the cervical end of enamel in a relatively sharp line.
3. In about 10% of the teeth, enamel and cementum do not meet. This occurs when enamel epithelium in the cervical portion of the root is delayed in its separation from dentin. In such case, there is no cementoenamel junction. Instead, a zone of the root is devoid of cementum and for the time being covered by reduced enamel epithelium.

### Afibrillar Cementum

It is a type of cementum which contains no collagen fiber with a 64 nm periodicity. It is sparsely distributed and consists of a well-mineralized ground substance which may be of epithelial origin. It is thin, acellular layer which covers cervical enamel or intervenes between fibrillar cementum and dentin.

Electron microscope evidence indicates that when connective tissue cells, probably cementoblasts, come in contact with enamel, they produce a laminated, electron-dense, reticular material termed afibrillar cementum. If such afibrillar cementum remains in contact with connective tissue cells for a long time, fibrillar cementum with characteristic collagen fibrils may subsequently be deposited on its surface.

### Cementoblast

These are cementum-forming cells, developed from undifferentiated mesenchymal cells of dental sac which come in contact with dentin after breakage of Hertwig's root sheath. Cementoblasts synthesize collagen and protein polysaccharides (proteoglycans), which form the organic matrix of cementum. These cells have numerous mitochondria, a well-formed Golgi apparatus, and large amount of granular endoplasmic reticulum.

### Cementoid Tissue

The uncalcified matrix of cementum is called cementoid. Under normal conditions, growth of cementum is a rhythmic process and as a new layer of cementoid is formed, the old one calcifies. A thin layer of cementoid can usually be observed on the cemental surface. This cementoid tissue is lined by cementoblast.

### Hypercementosis

Hypercementosis is an abnormal thickening of cementum, may be diffused or circumscribed. It may affect all teeth of the dentition, be confined to a single tooth or even affect only parts of one tooth **(Fig. 16.8)**.

Localized hypercementosis may be observed on enamel pearl (small protuberance of enamel). Occasionally, it is irregular and sometimes contains round bodies that may be calcified epithelial rests. Such knob-like projections are designated as excementoses.

### Cementum Hypertrophy

If the overgrowth improves the functional qualities of the cementum, it is termed as cementum hypertrophy. In localized hypertrophy, a spur or prong-like extensions of cementum may be formed. This condition is frequently found in teeth that are exposed to great stress. The prong-like extensions of cementum provide a layer of surface area for the attaching fibers and thus a firmer anchorage of the tooth to the surrounding alveolar bone is assured.

### Cementum Hyperplasia

If the overgrowth occurs in nonfunctional teeth, it is termed cementum hyperplasia. Extensive hyperplasia of cementum is usually associated with periapical inflammation. The hyperplasia may extend around the entire root of the nonfunctioning teeth or may be localized in small areas. There is reduction in number of Sharpey fibers. In some cases, an irregular overgrowth of cementum can be found as spike-like extensions and calcification of Sharpey fibers and accompanied by cementicles. These are usually associated with injuries of cementum.

### CLINICAL CONSIDERATIONS

1. Cementum is a part of periodontium and gives attachment to periodontal ligament. Formation of cementum continues throughout life and therefore the periodontal ligament must alter or shift according to functional need. During continuous eruption, the width of the periodontal space widens. Deposition of cementum keeps this width constant. The root apex and the bifurcation of the

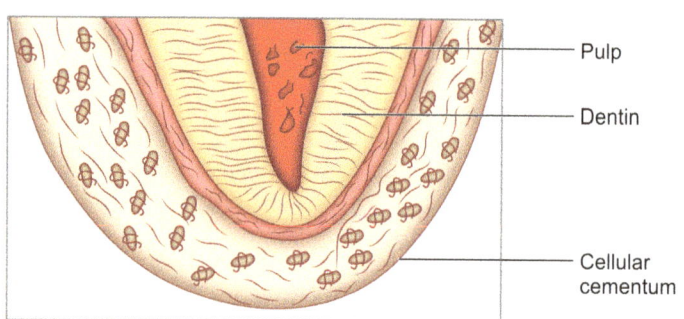

**Fig. 16.8:** Hypercementosis.

roots are the places where this widening is greatest and therefore the thickness of cementum is also greatest in these areas.
2. The continuous formation of cementum is a compensatory reaction against shortening of the crown due to wearing of enamel.
3. Continuous eruption coupled with passive eruption diminishes the length of the clinical root. Deposition of cementum compensates for the deleterious effects of increased leverage due to shortened roots.
4. Cementum is more resistant to resorption than is bone. In careful orthodontic treatment, cementum resorption is minimal or absent but bone resorption leads to tooth migration.
5. Cementum being avascular is not easily damaged by a pressure equal to that exerted on bone.
6. Cementum resorption by trauma can be repaired by cellular or acellular cementum.
*Anatomic repair:* In these cases, repair of cementum is done to re-establish the former outline of the root surface.
*Functional repair:* In these cases, repair after resorption is done both by cementum and bone to restore the periodontal width and to maintain the functional relationship.
7. In case of hypercementosis, normal extraction of teeth is not possible. These cases require surgical removal of tooth.

## QUESTIONNAIRE

1. What is cementum? Discuss physical characteristics, chemical composition, and functions of cementum.
2. What are the different types of cementum? Describe the microscopic features of acellular cementum with diagrams.
3. Describe the microscopic features of cellular cementum. Differentiate between the structures of cellular and acellular cementum.
4. Classify the cementum based on nature and origin of the organic matrix.
5. Write notes on:
    a. Cementodentinal junction.
    b. Cementoenamel junction.
    c. Afibrillar cementum.
    d. Hypercementosis.
    e. Sharpey's fibers.

## BIBLIOGRAPHY

1. Antonio N. Ten Cate's Oral Histology Development, Structure, and Function, 7th edition. Mosby; 2008.
2. Berkovitz BKB, Holland GR, Moxham BJ. A Colour Atlas and Textbook of Oral Anatomy, Histology and Embryology, 4th edition. Mosby: Elsevier; 2009.
3. Das AK. Dental Anatomy and Oral Histology, 1st edition. Current Publishers; 1972.
4. Gaunt WA, Osborn JW, Ten Cate AR. Advances in Dental Histology. Bristol: John Wright and Sons Ltd.; 1967.
5. Kumar GS. Orban's Oral Histology and Embryology, 12th edition. Mosby; 2009.
6. Osborn JW, Ten Cate AR. Advanced Dental Histology, 3rd edition. Bristol: John Wright and Sons Ltd.; 1976.

# CHAPTER 17

# Periodontium

The tissues which surround and support the tooth are collectively called the periodontium. They include the following:
a. Cementum
b. Periodontal ligament
c. Alveolar bone
d. Gingiva, facing the tooth.

The supporting tissues of the tooth form a specialized fibrous joint known as gomphosis and develop from the dental follicle.

## PERIODONTAL LIGAMENT

The periodontal ligament is the dense fibrous connective tissue which occupies the periodontal space between the root of the tooth and the alveolus. It surrounds the tooth root and anchors it to the bony socket. The tooth is attached to the alveolus by bundles of collagenous tissue, vessels, and nerves. These fibers, known as the principal fibers, invest and surround the tooth and are called periodontal ligament. Above the alveolar crest, the ligament is continuous with connective tissues of the gingiva and at the apical foramen, it is continuous with the dental pulp and also communicates with marrow spaces of alveolar bone.

### Functions

#### Physical

a. Attaches the tooth to the bone.
b. Transmits masticatory forces to the bone.
c. Acts as a shock absorber against external forces.
d. Maintains the relation between the tooth and the gingiva.
e. Gives protection to blood vessels and nerves by cushioning.

#### Formative

Cementoblasts are present in periodontal tissues which help in formation of cementum through its cells.

#### Nutritive

The ligament transmits blood vessels which provide anabolites and other substances required by the cells of the ligament, such as cementoblasts, cementocytes, and superficial osteocytes of alveolar bone. The blood vessels are also concerned with the catabolites.

#### Sensory

The nerves supply the blood vessels and also carry pain and proprioceptive sense of localization and pressure. Its mechanoreceptors are involved in the neurological control of mastication.

#### Homeostatic

The cells of the periodontal ligament have the capacity to resorb and synthesize the extracellular substance of the connective tissue of ligament, alveolar bone, and cementum.

### Structure

*The periodontal ligament consists of the following:*
- **Fibers**
    a. *Collagen:* Over 90% of periodontal ligament fibers.
    b. *Oxytalan:* Small amount.
    c. *Reticulin:* Small amount.
- **Ground substance**
- **Cellular elements**
    I. *Connective tissue cells*
        A. Synthetic cells
            a. Fibroblast

b. Osteoblast
c. Cementoblast
B. Resorptive cells
a. Fibroblast
b. Osteoclast
c. Cementoclast
C. Progenitor cells
D. Defense cells
a. Mast cells
b. Macrophages
II. Epithelial rests of Malassez
- **Vessels—arteries, veins, and lymphatics**
- **Nerves.**

## FIBERS OF THE PERIODONTAL LIGAMENT

### Collagen Fibers

The periodontal collagen is mostly Type-I collagen. It is low in hydroxylysine and glycosylated hydroxylysine. The periodontal ligament also contains 20% of Type-III collagen. It is high in hydroxyproline, low in hydroxylysine, and contains cystine. Much of the collagen is gathered together to form bundles which are approximately 5 mm in diameter. They are organized into functional groups and are termed the principal fibers of the periodontal ligament. They follow a wavy course which straightens out under load. They are more numerous at alveolar bone. Collagen fibrils are the banded subunits of the collagen fiber. They are formed by the packing together of individual tropocollagen molecules.

The fibers are arranged in three sets:
1. *The outer set*: Attached to bone and run toward cementum.
2. *The inner set*: Attached to cementum and run toward bone.
3. *Intermediate set*: Joins the outer and inner sets. This group is less matured.

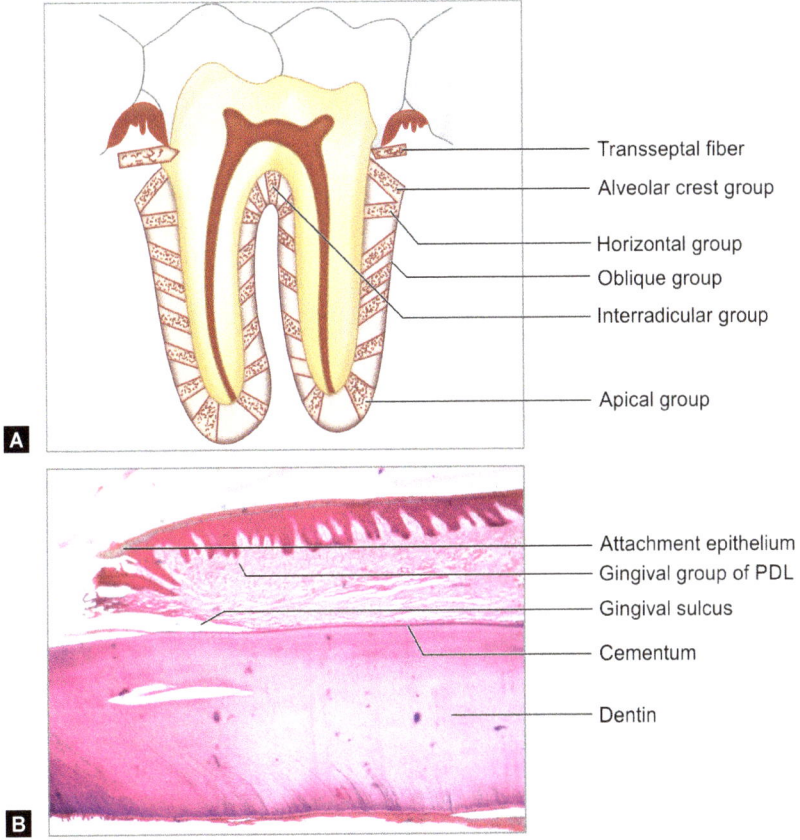

Figs. 17.1A and B

# Periodontium

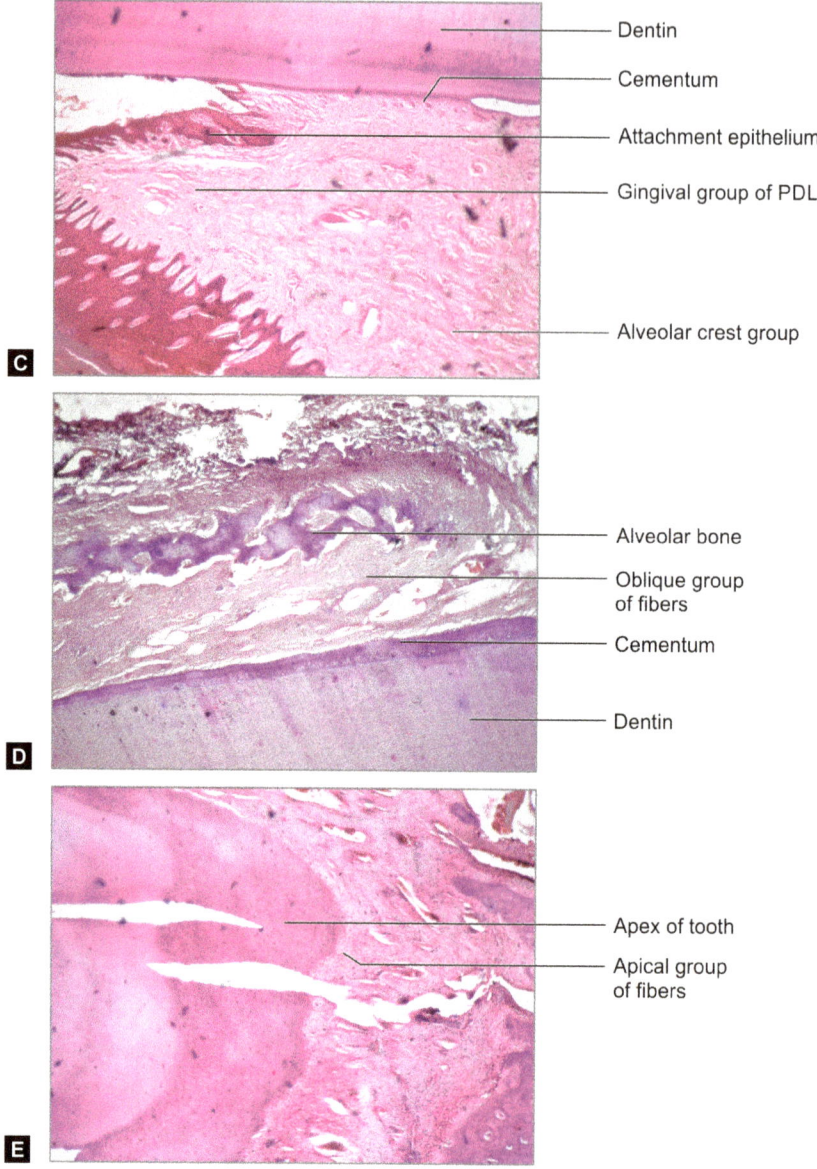

Figs. 17.1C to E
Figs. 17.1A to E: Principal fibers of periodontal ligament.

The principal fibers are classified as follows (Figs. 17.1A to E):
1. Gingival group
2. Transseptal group
3. Alveolar group
   a. Alveolar crest group
   b. Horizontal group
   c. Oblique group
   d. Apical group
   e. Interradicular group.

## Gingival Group

These fibers extend from cervical cementum to free and attached gingiva. The part embedded in cementum is called Sharpey fibers (**Fig. 17.2**).

### Functions
1. To support the gingiva, keeping it closely adapted to the tooth surface.
2. To sustain the gingiva against the forces of mastication.

3. To inhibit apical migration of the epithelial attachment.

*Gingival fibers run in groups, from coronal to apical direction and they are:*

- **Group 1:** This group leaves cementum near epithelial attachment at right angle, runs a short course, bends occlusally, and ends in papillary gingiva.
- **Group 2:** This group runs from cementum straight across to attached gingiva.
- **Group 3:** This group arises from cementum at right angle, crosses over the alveolar crest, and inclines apically between the outer periosteum of alveolar process and epithelium of attached gingiva.
  These groups keep the gingiva firmly against the tooth and keep the attached gingiva closely adapted to the underlying bone and tooth.
- **Group 4:** Circular group—These fibers are circular bands around the teeth. They run over the transseptal fibers crisscrossing gingival fibers.

### Transseptal Group

This is a dense group of fibers seen in proximal areas of teeth, extending from cementum of one tooth to the cementum of adjacent tooth. It forms a strong ligament connecting the neeks of the adjacent teeth on their mesial and distal surfaces above the level of the interdental septum of the alveolar bone. These transseptal fibers link the individual units of the dentition together **(Fig. 17.3)**.

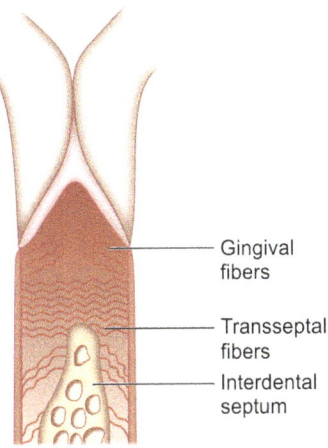

Fig. 17.3: Transseptal fibers.

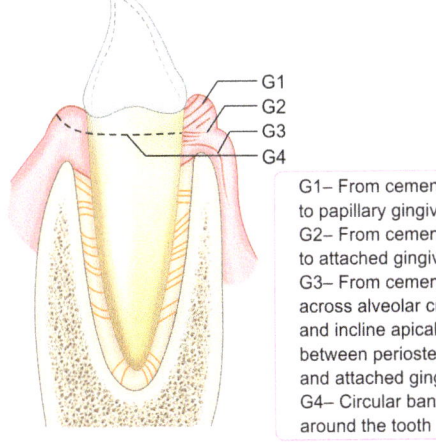

G1– From cementum to papillary gingiva
G2– From cementum to attached gingiva
G3– From cementum across alveolar crest and incline apically between periosteum and attached gingiva
G4– Circular bands around the tooth

**Fig. 17.2:** Gingival fibers.

### Functions

a. They support interproximal gingiva and secure adjacent teeth.
b. After removal of a single tooth and the repair of its socket, the transseptal fibers are reconstructed so as to connect the teeth on either side of the gap. The repair of these fibers, with the subsequent contraction of the fibrous tissue, is one of the factors responsible for the tilting of the teeth on either side of the space left by the last tooth. The transseptal fibers have been shown to be important in the production of physiological mesial drift of the tooth.
c. The transseptal fiber system is capable of turnover and remodeling under normal physiologic condition. Therefore, a sufficiently prolonged retention period following orthodontic tooth movement would allow reorganization of the transseptal fiber system to ensure the clinical stability of the tooth position.

### Alveolar group

This group of fibers extends from cementum to alveolus. They run in five groups **(Fig. 17.4)**:
1. **Alveolar crest group:** This group of fibers is attached at one end to the cervical part of

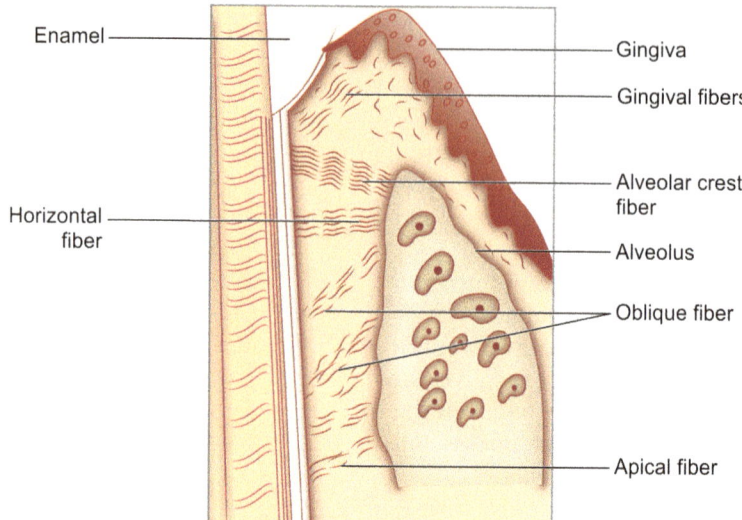

Fig. 17.4: Alveolar group of fibers.

the cementum in relation to the buccal and lingual sides of the teeth. The fibers pass to the alveolar bone and are attached to the rim of the socket (alveolar crest).

*Function*: They anchor the tooth to the alveolus and oppose lateral stress. These fibers limit tilting and extrusion movements of the tooth.

2. **Horizontal group:** These fiber bundles extend from cementum at right angles to the long axis of the tooth to the bone.
*Function*: They resist tooth displacement against lateral pressure.
3. **Oblique group:** These fiber bundles run obliquely from cementum to bone with cemental side apically and alveolar side coronally. These fiber bundles are most numerous and constitute the main attachment of tooth.
*Function*: They sustain occlusal stress and suspend the tooth in a socket.
4. **Apical group:** The bundles of fiber extend from cementum in apical region to surrounding bone.
*Function*: They prevent vestibulooral tipping of tooth.
5. **Interradicular group (Fig. 17.5):** These fiber bundles extend from crest of the interradicular septum to the cementum at furcation of multirooted teeth.
*Function*: They resist tipping and torquing.

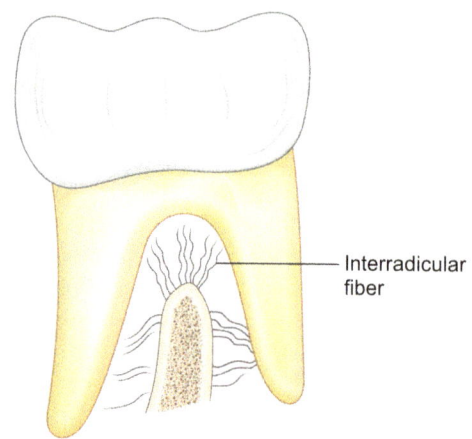

Fig. 17.5: Interradicular fiber.

*Intermediate Plexus*

Under the light microscope, the principal fibers of the periodontal ligament arising from cementum and bone appear to be joined in the midregion of the periodontal space, giving rise to a zone of distinct appearance, the so called intermediate plexus **(Fig. 17.6)**.

Electron microscopic and autoradiographic studies reveal that the intermediate plexus is an artifact arising out of the plane of section. The recent evidence suggests that the collagen fibers do not course only in one bundle but may move from one bundle to the other and join neighboring fibers to form a complex three-dimensional network.

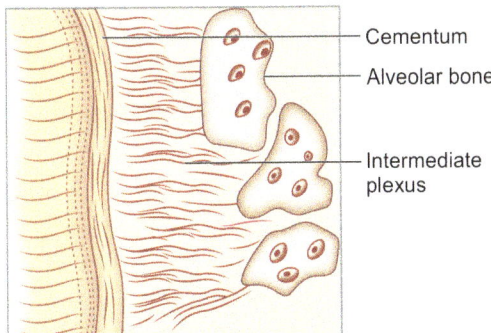

Fig. 17.6: Intermediate plexus.

Though existence of intermediate plexus is controversial, there is a "Zone-of-Shear" a site of remodeling in the periodontal ligament, which allows a tooth to move during eruption. It is either located in the center of periodontal ligament or close to the root surface.

## Oxytalan Fibers

Two immature forms of elastic fibers named oxytalan and elaunin are present in periodontal ligament. The oxytalan fibers run parallel to the root surface in a vertical direction. It bends to attach to the cementum or possibly to the bone and the other end often in the wall of a blood vessel.

In the vicinity of the apex, the oxytalan and the elaunin fibers form a complex network.

### Functions

1. They may play a part in supporting the blood vessels of the periodontal ligament.
2. They are also thought to regulate vascular flow.

## Reticulin Fibers

These fibers are related to the basement membranes within the periodontal ligament (i.e. associated with blood vessels and epithelial cell rests).

## GROUND SUBSTANCE OF THE PERIODONTAL LIGAMENT

The ground substance of the periodontal ligament consists mainly of hyaluronate, glycosaminoglycans, proteoglycans, and glycoproteins. All the components of the periodontal ligament ground substance are presumed to be secreted by the fibroblasts.

### Functions

1. Binding of ion and water.
2. Exchange of ion and water.
3. Control of fibrillogenesis and fiber orientation.
4. The tissue of fluid pressure has been found to be high in periodontal ligament (10 mm Hg above atmospheric pressure). Tissue fluid has been implicated in the tooth support and eruptive mechanisms.
5. A complex glycoprotein called fibronectin present in periodontal ligament promotes attachment of cells to collagen fibrils. As it is attached to cells, it is also involved in cell migration and orientation.
6. Another glycoprotein termed tenascin is present adjacent to alveolar bone and cementum. The role of this glycoprotein in the functions of the periodontal ligament is yet to be known.

## CELLS OF THE PERIODONTAL LIGAMENT (FIG. 17.7)

### Synthetic Cells

#### Fibroblast

The fibroblasts are the most common cells in periodontal ligament and appear as ovoid, elongated, or fusiform in shape, oriented along the principal fibers, and exhibit pseudopodia-like processes.

##### Functions

1. Synthesis of collagen.
2. *In vitro* studies suggest that the periodontal fibroblasts are motile and contractile cells and they are capable of generating a force responsible for tooth eruption.

#### Osteoblast

The osteoblasts are present covering the periodontal surface of the alveolar bone.

##### Function

Synthesis of protein to constitute bony matrix.

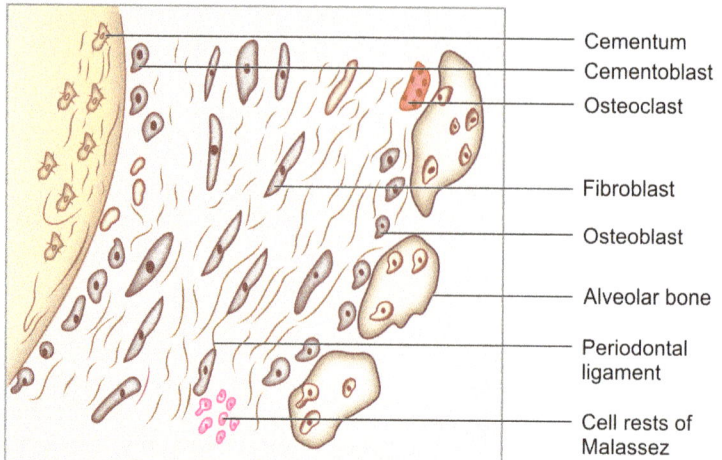

**Fig. 17.7:** Cells of the periodontal ligament.

## Cementoblast

The cementoblasts in various stages of differentiation are seen on the cemental surface of periodontal ligament.

These three synthetically active cells when viewed under electron microscope reveal:
1. Increased transcription of RNA.
2. Production of ribosome.
3. Development of large quantities of rough endoplasmic reticulum (RER).
4. Presence of profuse Golgi saccules and vesicles.
5. Presence of large number of mitochondria.

Under the light microscope, the cells exhibit a large, open-faced or vesicular nucleus with prominent nucleoli and have abundant cytoplasm which is hematoxyphilic due to interaction of the RNA with the acid hematin in the stain.

## Resorptive Cells

### Fibroblast

The periodontal fibroblasts possess the capacity to phagocytose old collagen fibers and degrade them by the activity of proteolytic enzyme collagenase. Thus, collagen turnover appears to be regulated by fibroblasts.

### Osteoclast

These are the cells that resorb bone. Light microscopically the osteoclasts are large, multinucleated or small, mononuclear cells, formed from circulating monocytes. They contain eosinophilic cytoplasm and occupy bays in bone known as Howship's lacunae (**Fig. 17.8**). Electron microscope reveals numerous mitochondria, lysosomes, Golgi saccules, ribosomes, and little RER. The plasma membrane toward resorbing bone is raised in folds and is known as ruffled border. Osteoclasts are rich in acid phosphatase. Resorption of bone is accomplished by demineralization and disintegration of organic matrix.

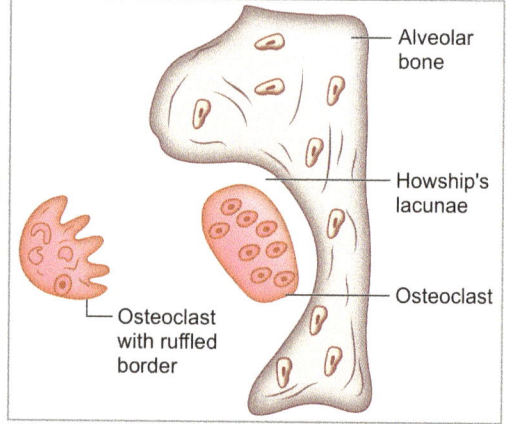

**Fig. 17.8:** Howship's lacunae.

### Cementoclasts

They resemble osteoclasts and are located in Howship's lacunae on the surface of the cementum.

## Periodontium

### Progenitor cells

The progenitor cells in the periodontal ligament replace the differentiated cells dying at the end of their lifespan or as a result of trauma. They are small, close-faced nucleus with little cytoplasm. They have the capacity to undergo mitotic division. The cells that divide in response to normal biologic requirements are located predominantly in the vicinity of blood vessels.

### Defense Cells (Fig. 17.9)

#### Mast cells

These are small, round, or oval cells having 12–15 mm diameter. They have numerous cytoplasmic granule containing heparin and histamine. Mast cell histamine plays a role in the inflammatory reaction.

### Macrophages

These are derived from blood monocytes and are capable of phagocytosis. It contains horseshoe or kidney-shaped nucleus which exhibits a dense uneven layer of peripheral chromatin. The surface of the cell is raised into microvilli and cytoplasm contains numerous free ribosomes and lysosomes in which phagocytosed material may be seen.

### Epithelial Rests of Malassez

These are the remnants of Hertwig's epithelial root sheath, described by Malassez in 1884. These are found close to the cementum in periodontal ligament. They persist as a network, strands, islands, or tubule-like structures near and parallel to the surface of the roots **(Fig. 17.10)**.

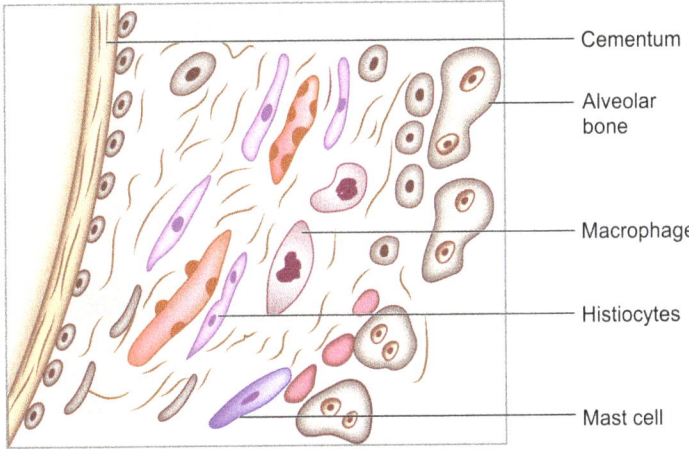

**Fig. 17.9:** Defense cells.

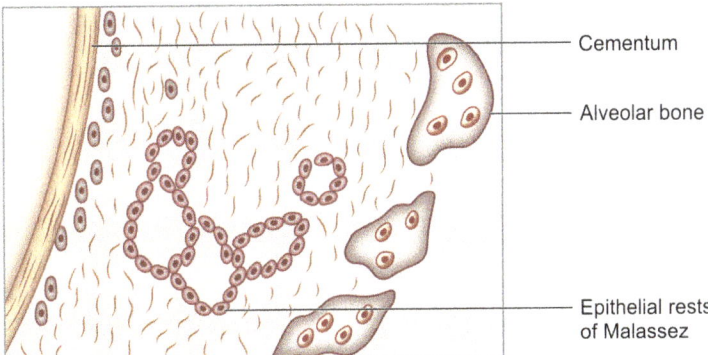

**Fig. 17.10:** Epithelial rests of Malassez.

Electron microscopic observations show that the epithelial cell rests exhibit tonofilaments and they are attached to one another by desmosomes. They are surrounded by a periodic acid Schiff (PAS) positive, argyrophilic fibrillar material, sometimes by hyaline capsule from which they are separated by basal lamina. They diminish in number with age. Either they undergo degeneration or calcification to form cementicles. Their physiologic role in the functioning periodontal ligament is unknown. Under certain pathologic conditions, the cells of the epithelial rests undergo rapid proliferation and can produce a variety of cysts and tumors that are unique to the jaws.

## BLOOD VESSELS AND NERVES OF THE PERIODONTAL LIGAMENT

### Blood Vessels

The arterial vessels of the periodontal ligament are derived from three sources:
1. From apical vessels that supply the dental pulp.
2. From intra-alveolar vessels. These branches run horizontally, penetrating the alveolar bone to enter the periodontal ligament.
3. From gingival vessels. These enter the periodontal ligament from coronal direction.

The arterioles and capillaries form a rich network in the periodontal space adjacent to the bone. There is a rich vascular plexus at the apex and in the cervical part of the ligament. The venous vessels tend to run axially to drain to the apex. There are numerous arteriovenous anastomoses and glomerulus-like structures.

### Lymphatics

A network of lymphatic vessels follows the path of the blood vessels and flow from the ligament toward and into the adjacent alveolar bone.

### Nerves

The periodontal ligament is well innervated. The nerve fibers entering the periodontal ligament are derived from two sources:

a. The nerve bundles enter near the root apex and pass up through the periodontal ligament.
b. The finer branches of the nerve enter the middle and cervical portions of the ligament through openings in the alveolar bone.

The nerves of the periodontal ligament are of two types:
1. **Nonmyelinated:** They are autonomic nerves having a diameter of about 0.5 mm and supply the blood vessels.
2. **Myelinated:** The average diameter of myelinated nerve fibers is about 5 mm (some are having 15 mm diameter). They are sensory nerve fibers. The sensations felt by the nerves of the periodontal ligament are that of pain, pressure, and touch through finer myelinated nerves and proprioception (sense of localization, chewing forces, movement, food texture, etc.) through larger myelinated nerves.

### Cementicles (Fig. 17.11)

These are calcified bodies located at any level of the periodontal ligament. They are more frequently encountered near the tip of the root. As isolated calcified bodies, fused to or incorporated in the cementum, they are known as free, adherent, and interstitial cementicles, respectively. They do not grow larger than 0.2 mm. They are composed of calcified layers surrounding degenerating cell remnants of Hertwig's epithelial root sheath or phleboliths (vein stones).

## CLINICAL CONSIDERATIONS

1. Orthodontic tooth movement depends on resorption and formation of both bone and periodontal ligament. These activities can be stimulated by properly regulated pressure and tension. The stimuli are transmitted through the medium of the periodontal ligament. If the movement of the teeth is within physiologic limits, the initial compression of the periodontal ligament on the pressure side is compensated for by bone resorption,

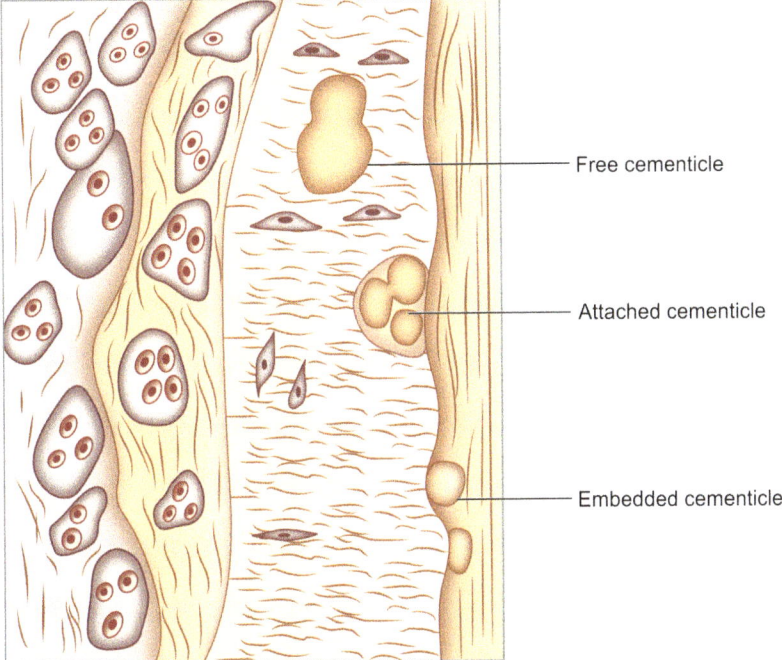

Fig. 17.11: Cementicles.

whereas on the tension side, bone apposition is seen.
2. Inflammatory diseases of the pulp progress to the apical periodontal ligament with the formation of granuloma.
3. Epithelial cell rests in periodontal ligament form cyst or neoplasm on stimulation.
4. Gingivitis or inflammation of the gingiva is the most common dental disease of humans. If not controlled or treated, it extends to the periodontal ligament and bone, and produces their slow but progressive destruction.

## QUESTIONNAIRE

1. What is periodontium? Enumerate the functions of periodontal ligament.
2. What are the component structures of periodontal ligament? Enumerate the principal fibers of periodontal ligament. Discuss the course and functions of each group with neat diagram.
3. Discuss about the composition and function of ground substance of periodontal ligament.
4. Describe the cellular components of periodontal ligaments along with their functions.
5. Discuss about the resorptive cells and defense cells of periodontal ligament.
6. Write notes on:
    a. Epithelial rests of Malassez.
    b. Intermediate plexus.
    c. Cementicles.

## BIBLIOGRAPHY

1. Antonio N. Ten Cate's Oral Histology Development, Structure, and Function, 7th edition. Amsterdam: Mosby; 2008.
2. Berkovitz BKB, Holland GR, Moxham BJ. A Colour Atlas and Textbook of Oral Anatomy, Histology and Embryology, 4th edition. Amsterdam: Mosby Elsevier; 2009.
3. Das AK. Dental Anatomy and Oral Histology, 1st edition. Kolkata: Current Books International; 1972.
4. Gaunt WA, Osborn JW, Ten Cate AR. Advances in Dental Histology. Bristol: John Wright and Sons Ltd.; 1967.
5. Kumar GS. Orban's Oral Histology and Embryology, 12th edition. Amsterdam: Mosby; 2009.

6. Newman MG, Takei HH, Klokkevold PR. Carranza's Clinical Periodontology, 10th edition. St. Louis: Saunders; 2007.
7. Osborn JW, Ten Cate AR. Advanced Dental Histology, 3rd edition. Bristol: John Wright and Sons Ltd.; 1976.
8. Provenza DV. Fundamentals of Oral Histology and Embryology. Philadelphia: JB Lippincott Company; 1972.

# CHAPTER 18
# Alveolar Bone

The part of maxilla or mandible which supports and protects the teeth is known as alveolar bone (process) **(Figs. 18.1A and B)**. It is dependent on the presence of teeth for its development and maintenance. It is developed along with eruption of teeth and gradually atrophies after extraction or exfoliation of teeth.

Anatomically, no distinct boundary exists between the body of the maxilla or the mandible and their respective alveolar processes. An arbitrary boundary at the level of the apices of the teeth separates the alveolar processes from the body of the mandible and maxilla.

## FUNCTION

1. Alveolar bone forms the bony socket to hold the root of tooth as well as attaches it through the periodontal ligament.
2. It gives attachment to the muscle.
3. It provides a framework for bone marrow.
4. It acts as a reservoir for ion (especially calcium).
5. The most important biologic property of bone is its plasticity, allowing it to remodel according to the functional demands placed upon it. This property is essential for orthodontic tooth movement.

## STRUCTURE OF BONE

Bone is a mineralized connective tissue. It is composed of:
a. Intercellular calcified material known as bone matrix.
b. Bone cells.
c. Periosteum and endosteum.

### Bone Matrix

It has inorganic component, organic component, and water.

|  | By weight | By volume |
|---|---|---|
| Inorganic material | 60% | 36% |
| Organic material | 25% | 36% |
| Water | 15% | 28% |

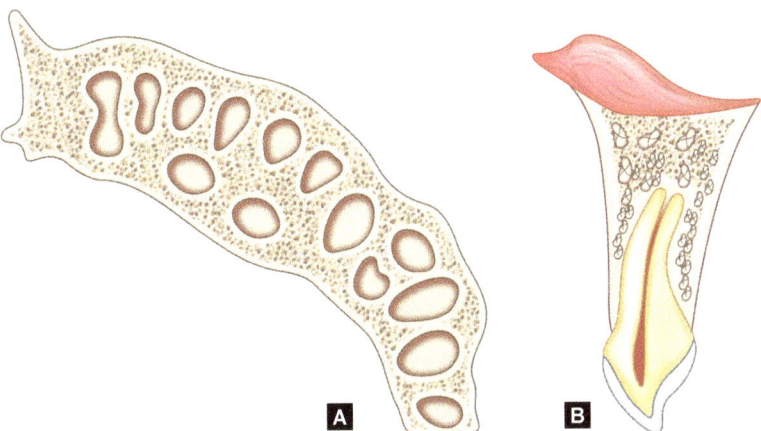

**Figs. 18.1A and B:** Alveolar bone: (A) Horizontal section; (B) Labiolingual section.

- **Inorganic:** Calcium and phosphorus are abundant but bicarbonate, citrate, magnesium, potassium, and sodium are also found. The mineral phase is hydroxyapatite $[Ca_{10}(PO_4)_6(OH)_2]$ in the form of needle-like crystallites or thin plates about 8 nm thick and of variable length.
- **Organic:** About 90% of the organic material is present as Type-I collagen. Ground substance contains proteoglycans and small amounts of other proteins like osteocalcin, osteonectin, and osteopontin.

## Bone Cells

- Osteoblast
- Osteocytes
- Osteoclast
- Osteoprogenitor cells
- Bone-lining cells.

### Osteoblast

Osteoblasts are specialized fibroblast like cells of mesenchymal origin. They differentiate from progenitor cells of connective tissue. These are bone-forming cells and are found on the surface in the area of active bone formation **(Fig. 18.2)**.

They are cuboidal with basophilic cytoplasm, prominent round nucleus toward the basal end of the cell, extensive endoplasmic reticulum, Golgi material, numerous mitochondria, and vesicle. They are active in the formation of collagen fibrils and ground substance that constitute organic matrix. They produce homogeneous intercellular substance called osteoid tissue. They also take part in calcification. Alkaline phosphatase is a useful marker for identification of cells at bony surfaces.

### Osteocytes

Some osteoblasts are entrapped in osteoid tissue during its formation and are termed osteocytes **(Fig. 18.3)**. They occupy a space called lacuna and anastomose with each other by means of processes contained in canaliculi. The processes of osteocytes communicate with each other and with the central canal of a haversian system.

In ground section, osteocytes are lost and lacunae appear black in transmitted light. Osteocytes show few organelles revealing little sign of cellular activity. Osteocytes are thought to play a role in calcium homeostasis.

### Osteoclast

The osteoclasts are large multinucleated cells responsible for resorption of bone. They arise as a result of fusion of blood cells of the myelomonocyte cell line. Osteoclasts are found in bay-like depressions in the bone called Howship lacunae **(Fig. 18.4)**.

The part of the cell in contact with the bone shows a convoluted surface, the ruffled border,

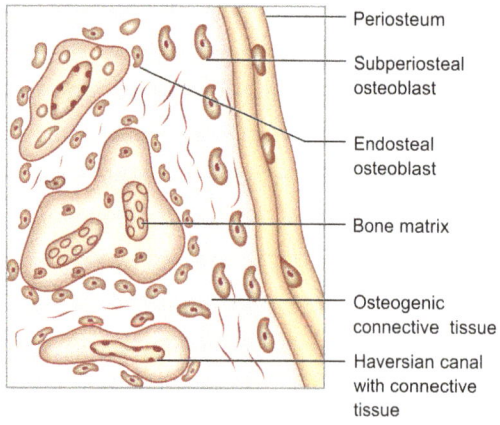

**Fig. 18.2:** Osteoblasts.

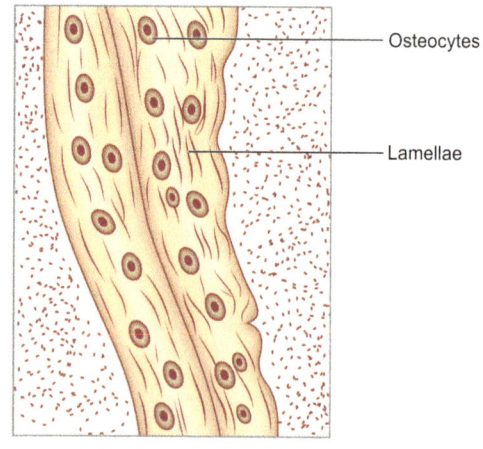

**Fig. 18.3:** Osteocytes.

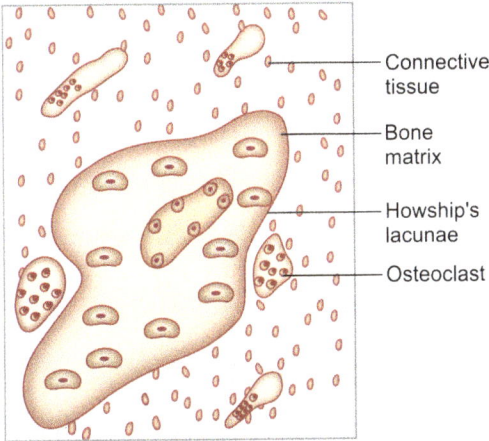

Fig. 18.4: Osteoclasts.

which is surrounded by a clear zone that has no organelles but only fine granular cytoplasm with microfilaments. Acid phosphatase is used as a marker to identify the cells.

## Osteoprogenitor Cells

These are mesenchymal, fibroblast-like cells, regarded as forming a stem cell population to generate osteoblasts. They are situated in the vicinity of the blood vessels of the periodontal ligament.

## Bone-lining Cells

When alveolar bone is not being deposited or resorbed, the surface is lined by relatively undifferentiated, flattened cells termed bone-lining cells. They may be related to ion exchange and the process of osteoblasis (bone deposition) and osteoclasis (bone resorption).

## Periosteum and Endosteum

External and internal surfaces of bone are covered by layers of bone-forming cells and connective tissue called periosteum and endosteum. The periosteum consists of an outer layer of collagen fibers and fibroblast and inner layer of osteoprogenitor cell (which differentiate into osteoblast).

The endosteum lines all internal cavities within the bone and is composed of a single layer of osteoprogenitor cells and a very small amount of connective tissue.

## Functions

1. Periosteum and endosteum provide nutrition to osseous tissue.
2. They supply new osteoblasts for repair and growth of bone.

## TYPES OF BONE TISSUES

There are three types of bone tissues. They are mature bone, immature bone, and bundle bone.

## Mature Bone

The mature bone shows incremental lines or lamellae and is called lamellated bone. Each lamella is 4–12 mm thick. They are demarcated from each other by bands of intercellular cement approximately 0.1 mm thick. The collagen fibers within each lamella are parallel with each other, but have different orientation to those in adjacent lamellae. The osteocytes are evenly distributed. It can be compact or spongy bone.

## Compact Bone

The compact bone is thick and solid. The lamellae are arranged in the form of concentric cylinders surrounding a narrow canal. Each canal is surrounded by 5–20 lamellae, which are known as circumferential lamellae. The central vascular (haversian) canal together with concentric lamellae is known as haversian system or osteon (**Figs. 18.5A and B**). A cement line of mineralized matrix (about 1 μm thick) delineates the haversian system.

The longitudinally running haversian canals are connected by transversely running Volkmann's canals (**Fig. 18.6**). Osteocytes through their canaliculi are in communication with the haversian canals.

Haversian canals are connected by transversely running Volkmann's canals (**Fig. 18.6**). Osteocytes through their canaliculi are in communication with the haversian canals. As a result of remodeling, fragments of previous haversian systems may be present and are known as interstitial lamellae.

## Alveolar Bone

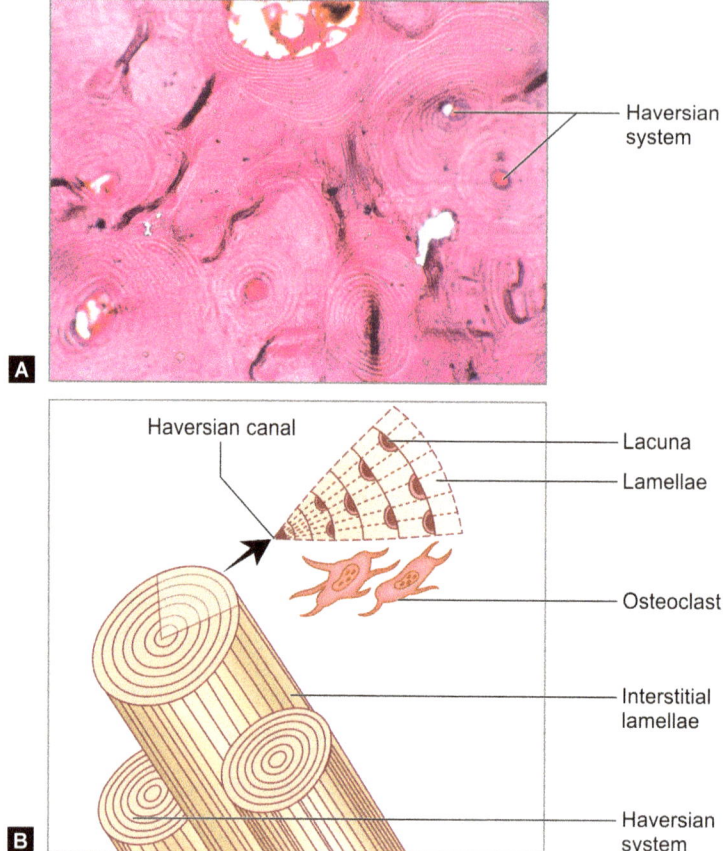

Figs. 18.5A and B: Haversian system.

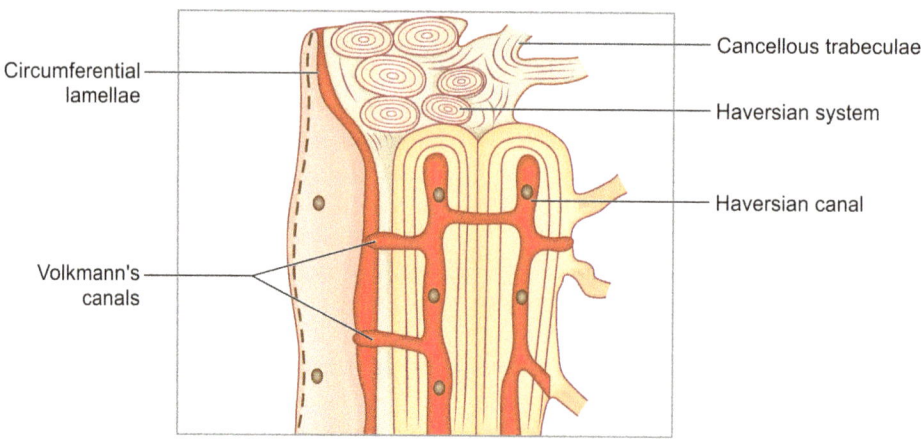

Fig. 18.6: Volkmann's canals.

### Spongy Bone (Cancellous Bone)

In spongy bone, the lamellae are apposed to each other to form trabeculae about 50 mm thick. The marrow cavity is interrupted by a network of bony trabeculae which are not arranged randomly but aligned along lines of stress. These internal trabeculae support the outer cortical crust of compact bone.

### Immature Bone

There are more osteocytes than lamellated bone. The cells and collagen fibrils are arranged haphazardly. The fibrils are coarser and more in number. It contains less ground substance and it is less calcified.

### Bundle Bone

Collagen fibers of periodontal ligaments (Sharpey's fibers) are embedded in it. It is more calcified. This type of bone is restricted to alveolar bone proper. Parts of jaw bones are given in **Flowchart 18.1**.

Alveolar bone or alveolar process (**Fig. 18.7**) consists of two parts:

- **Alveolar bone proper:** It forms the socket wall and gives attachment to the periodontal ligament. The alveolar bone proper, which forms the inner wall of the socket, is perforated by many openings that carry branches of interalveolar nerves and blood vessels into the periodontal ligament. Therefore, the alveolar bone proper is also known as cribriform (sieve like) plate.

The alveolar bone proper consists partly of lamellated bone and partly of bundle bone (**Fig. 18.8**). Some lamellae of lamellated bone are arranged roughly parallel to the surface of the adjacent

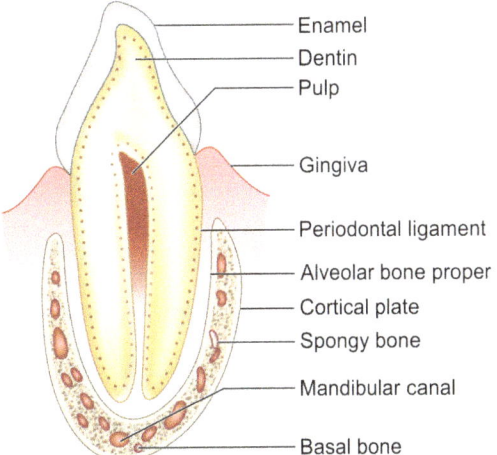

**Fig. 18.7:** Parts of alveolar bone.

marrow spaces, whereas others form haversian system.

Bundle bone is that bone in which the principal fibers of the periodontal ligament are anchored. It is termed as bundle bone as the bundles of the principal fibers continue into the bone as Sharpey's fibers. The bundle bone is characterized by the scarcity of the fibrils which are arranged at the right angles to the Sharpey's fibers. As fibrils are less in bundle bone, it appears darker in hematoxylin- and eosin-stained section and much lighter in preparations stained with silver compared

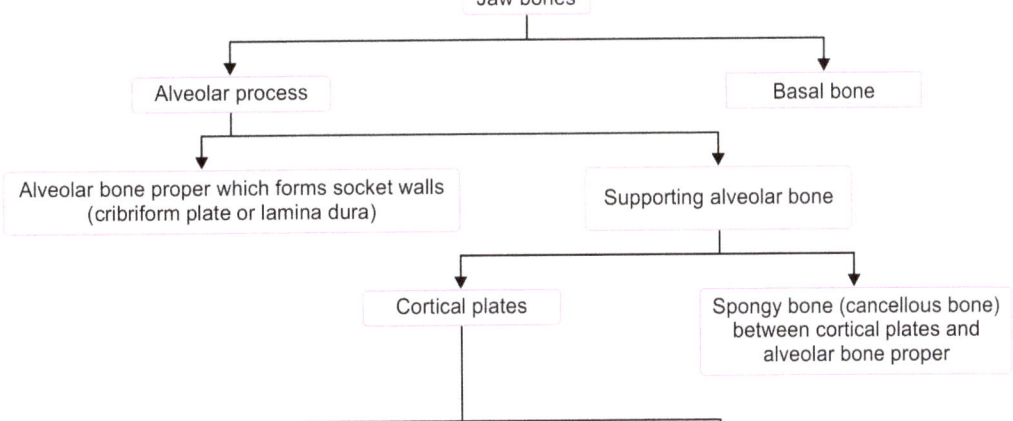

**Flowchart 18.1:** Parts of jaw bones.

# Alveolar Bone

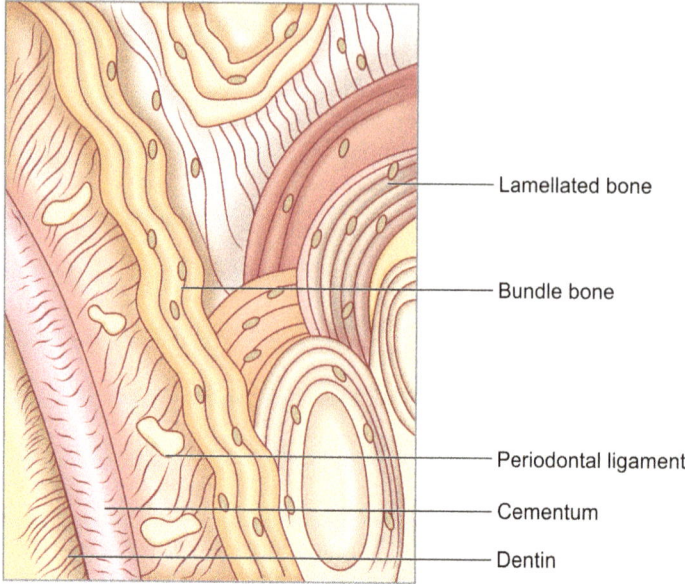

Fig. 18.8: Lamellated and bundle bone.

to lamellated bone. Bundle bone contains more calcium, salts per unit area than other types of bone tissue. Therefore, in roentgenograms, bundle bones are seen as dense radiopacities and are known as lamina dura.

- **Supporting alveolar bone:** It consists of two parts:
  a. *Cortical plates*: It is compact bone forming the outer and inner plates of alveolar processes **(Fig. 18.9)**. It is continuous with the compact layers of the maxillary and mandibular body.

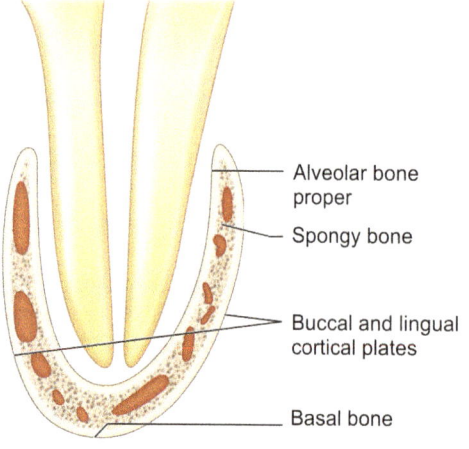

Fig. 18.9: Cortical plates.

It is much thinner in the maxilla than in the mandible. In the maxilla, the outer cortical plate is perforated by many small openings through which blood and lymph vessels pass. In the anterior region, supporting bone is very thin. No spongy bone is found in this region and the cortical plate is fused with the alveolar bone proper.

In the middle, the cortical bone of the alveolar process is dense. They are thickest in the premolar and molar regions, especially on the buccal side. In the anterior region, cortical plate is thin and is fused with the alveolar bone proper.

In a healthy mouth, the distance between the cementoenamel junction and the free border of alveolar bone proper is fairly constant **(Fig. 18.10A)** and the shape of the outline of the crest of the alveolar septa is dependent on the position of the adjacent teeth. If the neighboring teeth are inclined, the alveolar crest is oblique **(Fig. 18.10B)** which is most pronounced in the premolar and molar region. The interdental septa contain perforating canals of Zuckerkandl

# Alveolar Bone

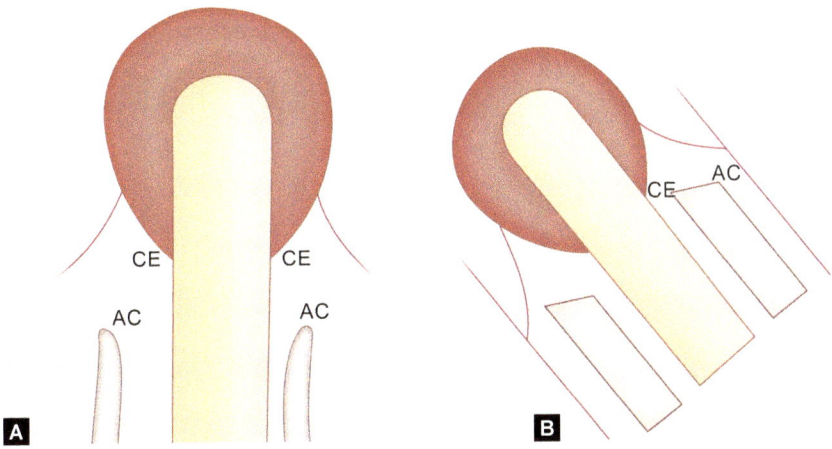

**Figs. 18.10A and B:** Relation between cementoenamel (CE) junction of adjacent teeth and shape of alveolar crest (AC).

and the interradicular septa contain canals of Hirschfeld which house the interdental and interradicular arteries, veins, lymph vessels, and nerves.

Histologically, the cortical plates consist of longitudinal lamellae and haversian systems.

b. *Spongy bones:* It is the cancellous bone between cortical plates and alveolar bone proper **(Figs. 18.11A and B)**. Radiologically, the spongy bone is of two types.
- *Type I*: Interdental and interradicular trabeculae are regular

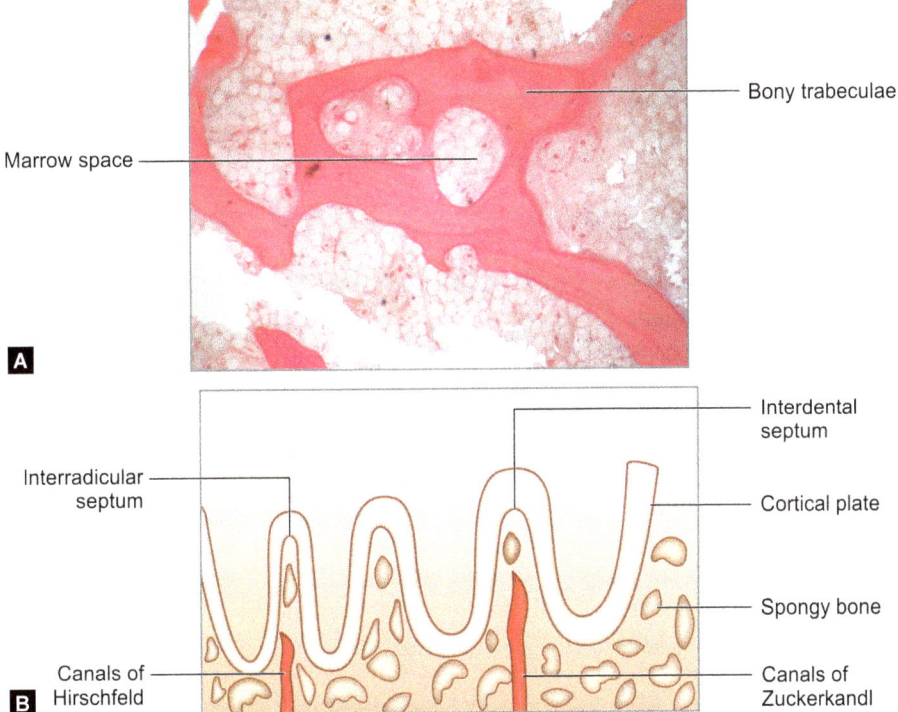

**Figs. 18.11A and B:** Spongy bone.

Regular ladder-like arrangement of interdental and interradicular trabeculae (as shown in radiograph)

Irregularly arranged interdental and interradicular trabeculae (as shown in radiograph)

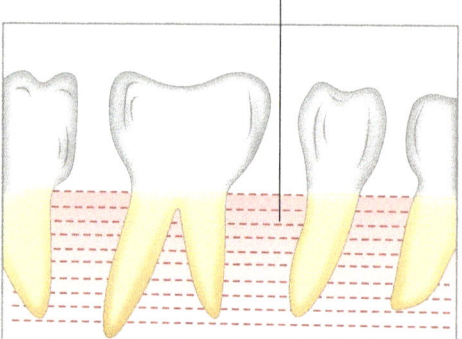

Fig. 18.12: Type-I alveolar spongiosa.

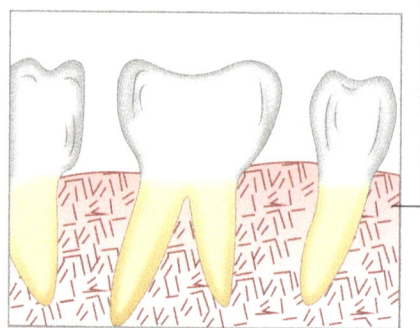

Fig. 18.13: Type-II alveolar spongiosa (diagram of radiological feature).

and horizontal in a ladder-like arrangement (**Fig. 18.12**). It is mostly seen in mandible and shows the trajectory pattern of spongy bone.
- *Type II*: It shows irregularly arranged, numerous, delicate interdental and interradicular trabeculae (**Fig. 18.13**). It lacks a distinct trajectory pattern. This arrangement is more common in maxilla.

The marrow spaces in the process usually contain fatty marrow. In the condylar process, angle of the mandible, maxillary tuberosity region, and hematopoietic cellular marrow is found.

## PHYSIOLOGIC CHANGES IN ALVEOLAR PROCESS

In the jaws, structural changes are correlated to the growth, eruption, movements, wear, and loss of teeth. All these processes are made possible only by a coordination of destructive and formative activities.

Osteoblasts secrete the Type-I collagen and noncollagenous organic matrix. The unmineralized matrix is osteoid tissue. Hydroxyapatite crystals are deposited on and in between the molecules of collagen and noncollagenous organic matrix. A superficial layer of osteoid tissue is present as mineralization always lags behind the production of bone matrix. Some osteoblasts are embedded in the matrix and are known as osteocytes. Enzymes responsible for synthesis of bone are (1) ATPase, (2) alkaline phosphatase, and (3) pyrophosphatase. Osteoclasts are responsible for resorption of bone. During bone resorption, three processes occur in more or less rapid succession. They are:
1. Decalcification
2. Degradation of matrix
3. Transport of soluble products to extracellular fluid or blood vascular system.

Bone decalcification is achieved at the ruffled border of the osteoclast by secretion of citric acid and lactic acid. After decalcification, pieces of matrix are released by the activity of cathepsin B-1 (lysosomal acid protease) and collagenase enzymes. After degradation of the matrix, the breakdown products of bone are transported to the extracellular fluids and to blood vascular system.

## INTERNAL RECONSTRUCTION OF BONE

Remodeling is a natural process occurring in most bones throughout life. This activity is especially important to the alveolar process during:
a. Physiologic eruptive movements of the teeth.
b. Physiologic mesial drift.
c. Orthodontic mesial or distal movements of teeth.

## Resting Lines

Bone is laid down rhythmically and results in formation of regular parallel lines **(Fig. 18.14)** which, because they are formed in periods of relative quiescence, are termed as resting lines. These lines are prominent in bundle bone during drift of teeth.

## Resorption Tunnel

When the bone undergoes osteoclastic activity, the resorbed bone is replaced by proliferating loose connective tissue. This area of resorption is called the *resorption tunnel* or cutting cone.

## Reversal Lines

These are intensely hematoxyphilic scalloped line seen at the junction of resorbed bone and the new bone formed after cessation of resorption. They are irregular scalloped line, being composed of series of concavities, which were once the sites of the resorptive Howship's lacunae **(Fig. 18.15)**.

During remodeling, the compact bone may be replaced by spongy bone or spongy

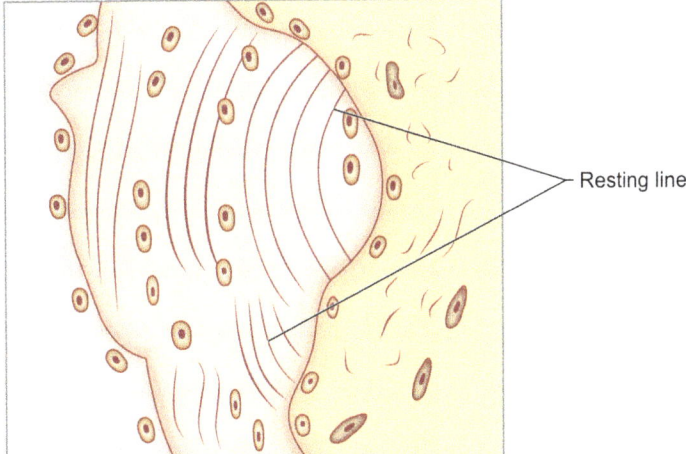

**Fig. 18.14:** Resting lines of bone.

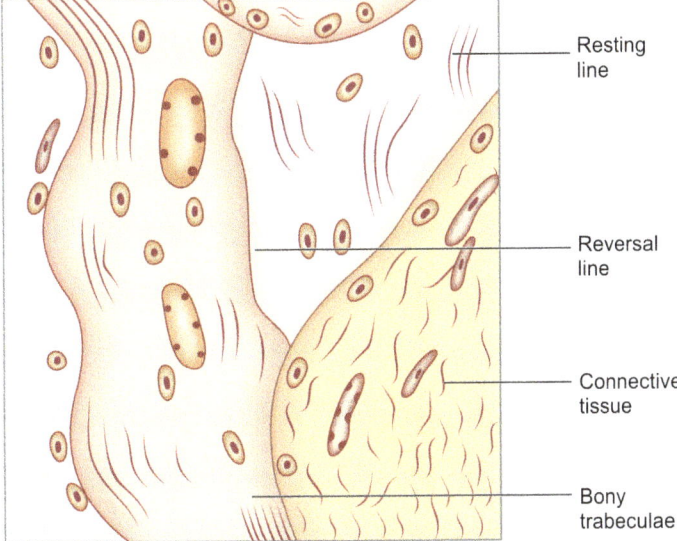

**Fig. 18.15:** Reversal lines of bone.

bone may change into compact bone. This is known as internal reconstruction of bone.

## CLINICAL CONSIDERATIONS

1. Bone being highly plastic enables the orthodontic movement of teeth. Bone is resorbed on the side of pressure with the help of cyclic adenosine monophosphate (cAMP) and apposed on the side of tension.
2. During healing of fractures or extraction wounds, an embryonic type of bone is formed which is later replaced by mature bone.
3. Periodontal disease leads to resorption of alveolar bone.
4. Synthetic inorganic products are currently used for the augmentation of the alveolar ridges and for filling bone defects produced by periodontal disease.
5. After exfoliation of tooth, alveolar bone undergoes gradual atrophy. Sometimes resorption is so severe that the fabrication of a functional prosthesis may become difficult.

## QUESTIONNAIRE

1. What is alveolar bone? Enumerate the functions of alveolar bone.
2. Discuss composition and basic microscopic structure of bone.
3. What are periosteum and endosteum?
4. What are the different types of bones?
5. Discuss different parts of alveolar bone with diagram.
6. What are the physiological changes in alveolar process?
7. Discuss resting lines and reversal lines.
8. Write notes on:
   a. Cribriform plate.
   b. Lamina dura.
   c. Bundle bone.
   d. Haversian system.

## BIBLIOGRAPHY

1. Antonio N. Ten Cate's Oral Histology Development, Structure, and Function, 7th edition. Amsterdam: Mosby; 2008.
2. Berkovitz BKB, Holland GR, Moxham BJ. A Colour Atlas and Textbook of Oral Anatomy, Histology and Embryology, 4th edition. Amsterdam: Mosby Elsevier; 2009.
3. Das AK. Dental Anatomy and Oral Histology, 1st edition. Kolkata: Current Books International; 1972.
4. Gaunt WA, Osborn JW, Ten Cate AR. Advances in Dental Histology. Bristol: John Wright and Sons Ltd.; 1967.
5. Junqueira LC, Jose C. Basic Histology, Text and Atlas, 10th edition. New York: Lange Medical Books McGraw-Hill; 1998.
6. Kumar GS. Orban's Oral Histology and Embryology, 12th edition. Amsterdam: Mosby; 2009.
7. Newman MG, Takei HH, Klokkevold PR. Carranza's Clinical Periodontology, 10th edition. St. Louis: Saunders; 2007.
8. Osborn JW, Ten Cate AR. Advanced Dental Histology, 3rd edition. Bristol: John Wright and Sons Ltd.; 1976.
9. Provenza DV. Fundamentals of Oral Histology and Embryology. Philadelphia: JB Lippincott Company; 1972.
10. Scott JH, Symons NBB. Introduction to Dental Anatomy, 9th edition. London: Churchill Livingstone; 1982.

# CHAPTER 19

# Oral Mucous Membrane

The moist lining of oral cavity is known as oral mucous membrane or oral mucosa. At the lips, the oral mucosa is continuous with the skin and at the pharynx, it is continuous with the moist mucosa lining the rest of the intestine. It has a superficial epithelial lining and a deeper connective tissue layer. The epithelium of oral mucosa anterior to buccopharyngeal membrane is ectodermal in origin.

The oral mucous membrane is very similar to skin but there are differences in certain aspects **(Table 19.1)**.

## FUNCTIONS OF THE ORAL MUCOSA

### 1. Protection

The oral mucosa separates and protects deeper tissues and organs in the oral region from mechanical forces like compression, stretching, and shearing at the time of biting and chewing food. The epithelium of oral mucosa provides a barrier to microorganisms, toxins, and various antigens.

### 2. Sensation

In the oral cavity, there are receptors that respond to temperature, touch, and pain. There are also taste buds, which are not found anywhere else in the body. Certain receptors in the oral mucosa respond to the taste of water and signal the satisfaction of thirst. Reflexes such as swallowing, gagging, retching, and salivating are also initiated by receptors in the oral mucosa.

### 3. Immunological Defense

It has a role in immunological defense, both humoral and cell mediated.

### 4. Lubrication and Buffering

Minor salivary glands within the oral mucosa provide lubrication and buffering as well as secretion of some antibodies.

### 5. Digestive Function

Food is tasted and masticated and the saliva secreted into oral cavity lubricates the food to facilitate swallowing. Enzymes in saliva initiate digestion in oral cavity.

### 6. Thermal Regulation

In some animals (dog), the mucosa plays a major role in regulation of body temperature as considerable body heat is dissipated through the oral mucosa by panting.

**TABLE 19.1:** Differentiating features between skin and oral mucosa.

| Skin | Oral mucosa |
|---|---|
| 1. Skin provides covering for the external surface of the body | 1. Oral mucosa covers the oral cavity from vermilion zone to pharynx |
| 2. It is pale brown in color | 2. It is coral pink in color |
| 3. It has dry surface with folds and wrinkles | 3. It has moist, smooth surface (except dorsum of tongue and palatine rugae) |
| 4. It is composed of two different layers known as epidermis and dermis or corium | 4. It is composed of two different layers known as epithelium and lamina propria |
| 5. Skin contains numerous hair follicles, sebaceous glands, and sweat glands | 5. The glandular component of oral mucosa is represented by minor salivary gland |

## ORGANIZATION OF THE ORAL MUCOSA

The oral cavity consists of two parts:
1. Vestibule—bounded by the lips and cheeks.
2. Oral cavity proper.

*Anteriorly*: Separated from the vestibule by the alveolus, bearing the teeth and gingiva.

*Superiorly:* Hard and soft palate.

*Inferiorly*: Floor of the mouth, base of the tongue.

*Posteriorly*: Pillars of the fauces and the tonsils.

## CLASSIFICATION OF ORAL MUCOSA (ACCORDING TO FUNCTION)

### 1. Masticatory Mucosa

This is a type of mucosa which is subjected to friction due to mastication. The masticatory mucosa tends to be bound to bone and does not stretch. It bears forces generated when food is chewed, e.g. mucosa of gingiva and hard palate **(Figs. 19.1 and 19.2)**.

### 2. Lining Mucosa

This is a type of mucosa which is subjected to less friction due to mastication. It covers musculature and is distensible, adopting itself to the contraction and relaxation of cheeks, lips, and tongue and to the movement of mandible produced by muscles of mastication, e.g. lips, cheeks, vestibule, inferior surface of tongue, floor of the mouth, and soft palate **(Figs. 19.1 and 19.2)**.

### 3. Specialized Mucosa

The specialized mucosa is so called because it bears the taste buds, which have a sensory function, e.g. dorsum of tongue.

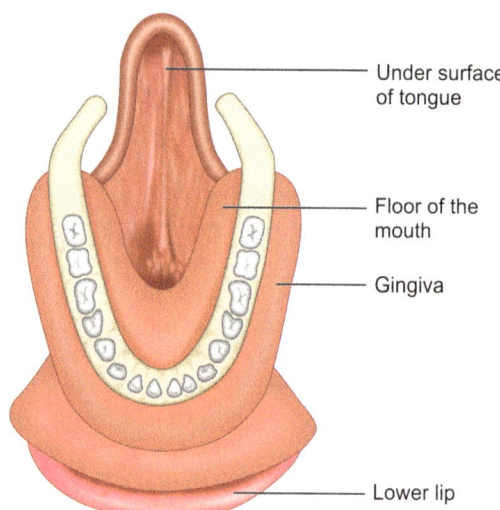

**Fig. 19.2:** Anatomic location of different types of mucosa in oral cavity—Part B.

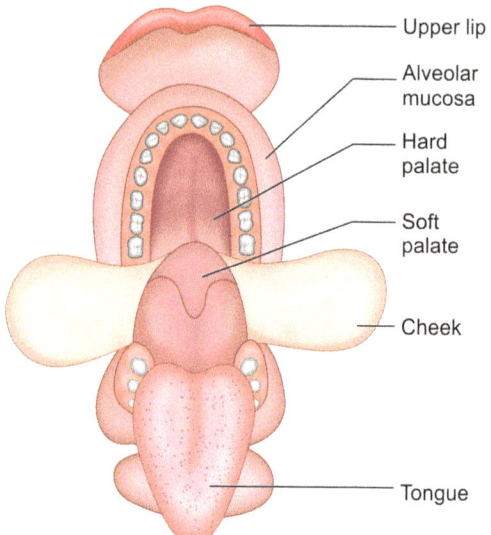

**Fig. 19.1:** Anatomic location of different types of mucosa in oral cavity—Part A.

## CLINICAL APPEARANCE

1. *Color:* The usual color of oral cavity is coral pink. The color depends upon:
   a. Thickness of epithelium.
   b. Degree of keratinization.
   c. State of dilatation of small blood vessels in the underlying connective tissue.
   d. Amount of melanin in epithelium.
2. It is moist as salivary glands pour their secretion into it.
3. Sometimes sebaceous glands of skin are present in oral mucosa and are manifested as pale yellow spots known as Fordyce's spots.
4. In general, the oral mucosa is smooth except dorsum of tongue (due to the presence of papillae/rugae).

5. The healthy gingiva shows a pattern of fine surface stippling, consisting of small indentations of the mucosal.
6. *Linea alba*: It is a whitish keratinized ridge along buccal mucosa in the occlusal plane of the teeth and represents the effect of abrasion from the surface of tooth.
7. The oral mucosa varies considerably in its firmness and texture. The lining mucosa of the lips, cheeks is soft and pliable whereas gingiva and hard palate are covered by a firm and immobile layer.

## COMPONENT TISSUES OF ORAL MUCOSA

The main tissue components of oral mucosa are:
a. Oral epithelium
b. Lamina propria
c. Submucosa
d. Mucoperiosteum.

### Oral Epithelium

The epithelium of the oral mucous membrane is of the stratified squamous variety. It may be keratinized and nonkeratinized, depending on location. Masticatory mucosa (gingiva and hard palate) and specialized mucosa (dorsum of tongue) are keratinized. Lining mucosa (cheek, lip, floor of the mouth, under surface of tongue, alveolar mucosa, vestibule, soft palate) are nonkeratinized. The cells of the epithelium consist of two functional populations:
1. *A progenitor population:* Its function is to divide and provide new cells.
2. *A maturing population:* The cells in this group continually undergo a process of differentiation or maturation to form a protective surface layer.

After cell division, each daughter cell makes the decision either to recycle in the progenitor population or to enter the maturing compartment. The decision-making period is known as the dicophase. Turnover time of epithelium is the time taken by a cell to divide, pass through the entire epithelium, and to desquamate from the surface. It is 41–51 days in gingiva and 25 days in the cheek mucosa. Cell division, growth, and differentiation of oral epithelium are regulated by a soluble glycoprotein, cytokine.

### *Keratinized Oral Epithelium*

The different layers **(Figs. 19.3A to D)** are:
a. The basal cell layer (stratum basale).
b. The prickle cell layer (stratum spinosum).
c. The granular cell layer (stratum granulosum).
d. The keratinized layer (stratum corneum).

### *The basal cell layer (stratum basale)*

The basal cell layer is a layer of cuboidal or columnar cells adjacent to the basement membrane. The basal cells and some

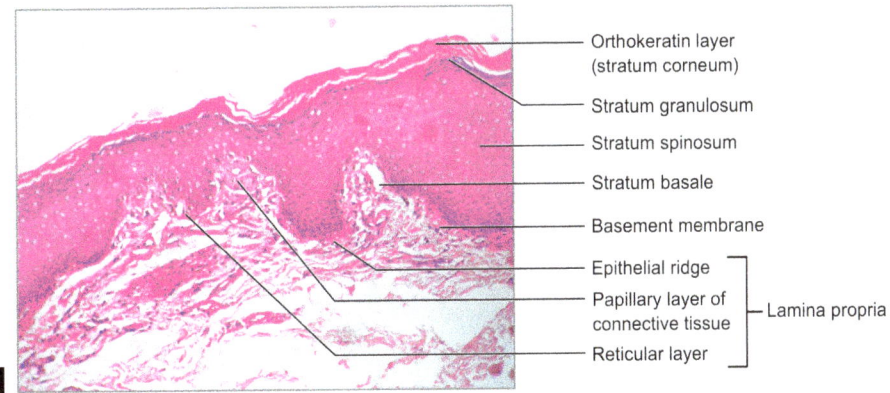

Fig. 19.3A

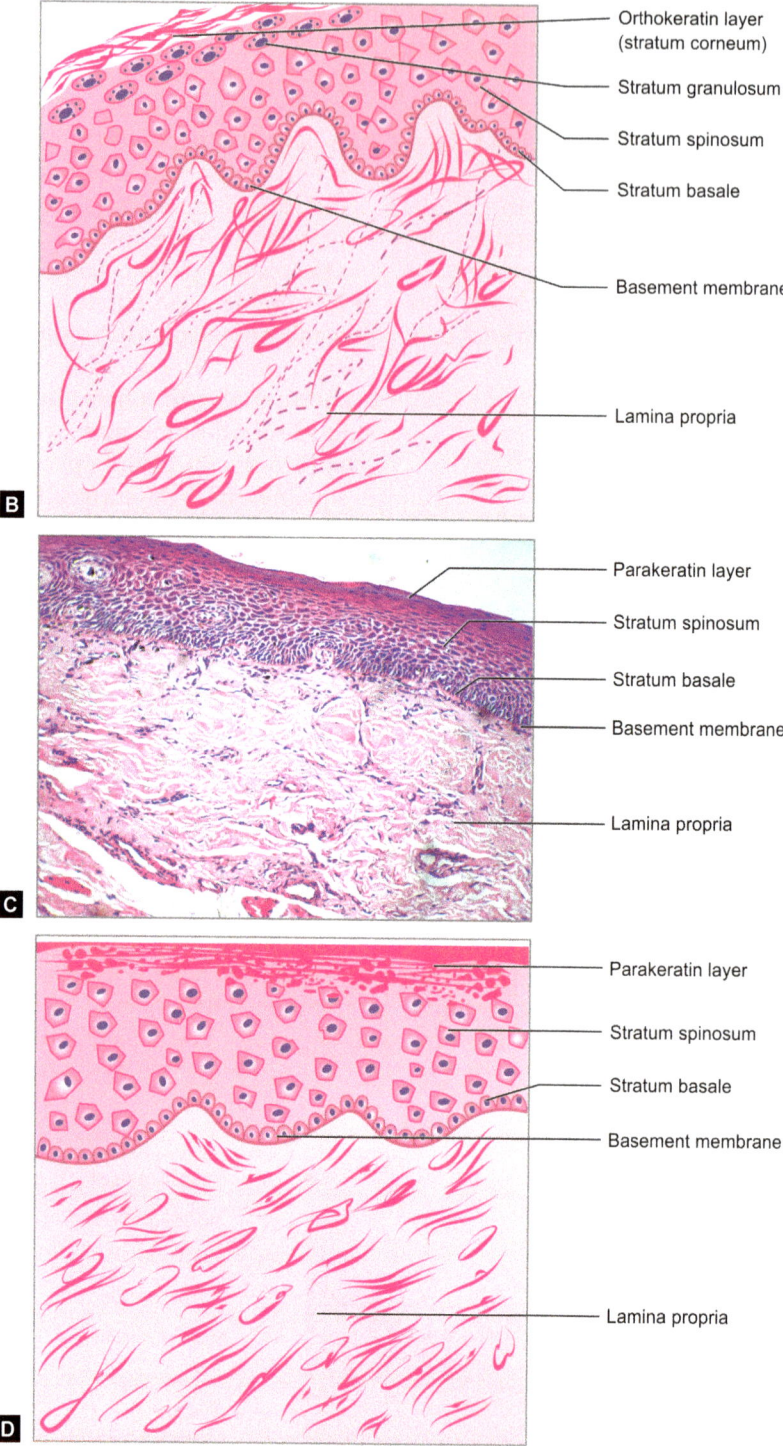

**Figs. 19.3B to D**

**Figs. 19.3A to D:** (A and B) Histology of orthokeratinized oral epithelium; (C and D) Histology of parakeratinized oral epithelium.

# Oral Mucous Membrane

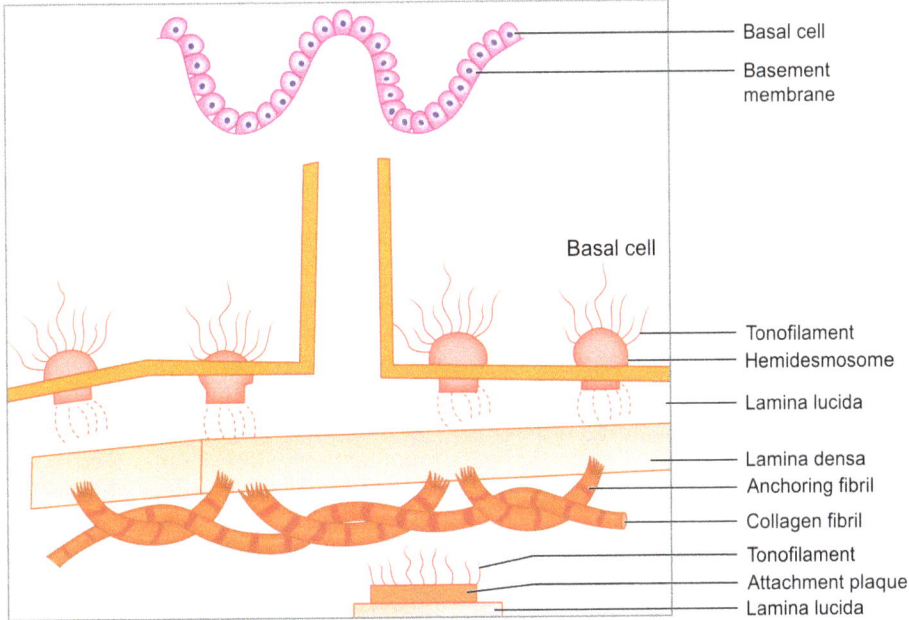

Fig. 19.4: Hemidesmosome.

superficial parabasal cells are capable of cell division. So they are also known as *stratum germinativum*. The basal cells are attached to underlying basement membrane and connective tissue by hemidesmosomes (**Fig. 19.4**). The lateral borders of adjacent basal cells are closely apposed and connected by desmosomes (**Fig. 19.5**). The basal cells contain tonofilament in relation to desmosome and hemidesmosomes. Tight and gap junctions are also present at basal cells. Ribosomes and rough endoplasmic reticulum are indicative of protein synthesizing activity. Nucleolus, mitochondria, and Golgi material are also present.

Desmosomes are circular or oval areas of adjacent cell membranes, adhering by specialized intracellular thickenings known as attachment plaque (formed by a protein known as desmoplakin) into which bundles of tonofilaments insert. These filaments loop around within the plaques and pass out again without crossing the adjacent cells. During histologic processing, the desmosomes usually remain intact, which appear as intercellular bridges light microscopically. Adhesion between basal cells and connective tissue is provided by hemidesmosomes which are present on basement membrane of basal cells. They possess single attachment plaque with tonofilaments inserted. The desmosomes, hemidesmosomes, and tonofilaments form a mechanical linkage that distributes and dissipates localized forces applied to the epithelial surface over a wide area.

The gap junction is the region where membranes of adjacent cells run closely together, separated by only a small gap. There appear to be small interconnections between the membranes across these gaps. Such junctions may allow electrical or chemical communication between the cells.

The tight junctions are so tightly apposed that there is no intercellular space. These junctions may serve to seal off and compartmentalize the intercellular area.

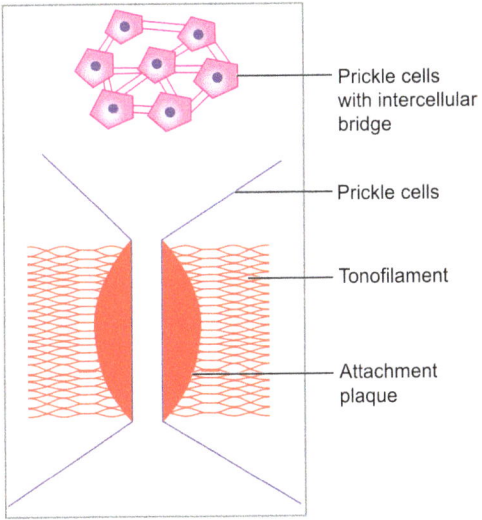

Fig. 19.5: Desmosome.

### The prickle cell layer (stratum spinosum)

Above the basal cells, there are several rows of irregularly polyhedral cells, longer than basal cells. They are known as prickle cell layer or stratum spinosum. Light microscopically, it appears that the cells are joined by intercellular bridges. Electronmicroscopically the *intercellular bridges* are desmosomes and tonofilaments. These spinous cells are most active in protein synthesis.

> The term prickle arises from prickly appearance of the cells. During histological preparations, the cells shrink and are attached to one another at the site of desmosomes which give a spiny or prickle-like profile. Greek word for prickle is acanthi. So the increased thickness of prickle cells is known as acanthosis and separation of the prickle cells by degeneration of intercellular bridges is termed as acantholysis.

### The granular cell layer (stratum granulosum)

Superficial to the prickle cell layer, there are larger flattened cells containing small granules that stain intensely with acid dyes such as hematoxylin (i.e. they are basophilic). This layer is the granular layer, or stratum granulosum, and the granules are called keratohyaline granules. In gingiva, these granules are difficult to see under light microscope as they are masked by the superficial nucleated keratin layer.

Though this layer still synthesizes protein, the nuclei show signs of degeneration and pyknosis.

Tonofilaments are more dense in quantity and are associated with keratohyaline granule. The membrane-coating granules known as keratinosome or Odland body are found in upper spinous and granular cell layer. They discharge their contents into intercellular space forming an intercellular lamellar material, which contributes to the permeability barrier.

### The keratinized layer (stratum corneum)

The surface layer or stratum corneum is composed of flat cells, stained bright pink with eosin, and do not contain nuclei, ribosome, mitochondria, and keratohyaline granule. The pattern of maturation of the cells to form anucleated squames is known as orthokeratinization **(Figs. 19.3A and B)**.

The masticatory mucosa (e.g. parts of the hard palate and much of the gingiva) reveals a variation of keratinization where the surface layer shows pyknotic nuclei and partially lysed cell organelles. This process is known as parakeratinization **(Figs. 19.3C and D)**.

The keratinized cell becomes compact and dehydrated and covers a greater surface area than basal cells and prickle cells but smaller than granular cells. Ultrastructurally the cells of the cornified layer are composed of densely packed filaments developed from the tonofilaments, altered and coated by the basic protein of the keratohyaline granule, filaggrin. There is also a sulfur-rich component called loricrin. The dehydrated squames of keratin are shed in few hours and are replaced by cells from underlying layers.

The epithelial cells that ultimately keratinize are called keratinocytes. All epithelial cells have intermediate filaments made of keratin.

### Nonkeratinized Oral Epithelium

It does not produce cornified surface layers.

The different layers **(Fig. 19.6)** are:
a. The basal cell layer (stratum basale)
b. The intermediate cell layer (stratum intermedium)
c. The superficial cell layer (stratum superficial).

*a. The basal cell layer*
The cells are similar to the basal cells of keratinized oral epithelium.

*b. The intermediate cell layer*
The cells are larger than prickle cells and there is accumulation of glycogen. Morphologically, they are not spinous and biochemically they do not keratinize. Rarely, they contain keratohyaline granule and sparsely distributed intermediate keratin filament. The cells are attached by desmosomes and the cell surfaces are more closely apposed.

*c. The superficial cell layer*
The nonkeratinized epithelium is devoid of stratum granulosum and stratum corneum. The superficial cells are large, flattened.

# Oral Mucous Membrane

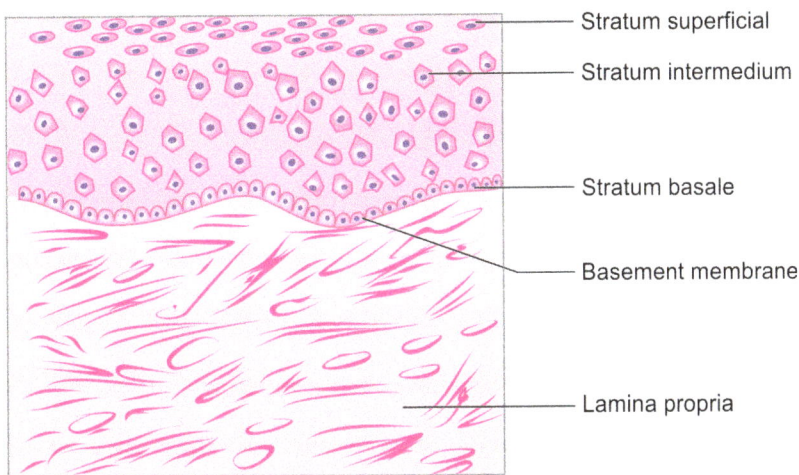

Fig. 19.6: Histology of nonkeratinized oral epithelium.

TABLE 19.2: Differences between masticatory and lining mucosa.

| | Masticatory mucosa | Lining mucosa |
|---|---|---|
| Site | Gingiva, hard palate, dorsum of tongue | Lips, cheeks, soft palate, floor of the mouth, ventral surface of tongue, and vestibule |
| Color | Light pink, modified by melanin pigment | Red, modified by melanin pigment |
| Surface | Stippled | Smooth |
| Elasticity | Tightly bound | Elastic |
| Stratum corneum or Stratum superficial | Extremely flattened, dehydrated cells, in which cell organelles and nuclei are lost. Cells filled only with packed fibrillar material; when pyknotic nuclei are retained, it is parakeratinization | Slightly flattened nucleated cells with fewer organelles, dispersed tonofilaments, and glycogen |
| Stratum granulosum or Stratum intermedium | Flattened cells with keratohyaline granule, tonofibril, Odland bodies | Slightly flattened cells with dispersed tonofilaments and glycogen |
| Stratum spinosum | Large ovoid cells with prominent tonofibril bundles, Odland bodies in upper layers | Large ovoid cells with dispersed tonofilament |
| Stratum basale | Cuboidal or columnar cells containing bundles of tonofibrils and other cell organelles | Cuboidal or columnar cells with sparse tonofibrils |

They contain loosely arranged tonofilament, nuclei, and few cell organelles. They are not dehydrated. So the surface is flexible and tolerant of both compression and distention **(Table 19.2)**.

## Nonkeratinocytes in the Oral Epithelium

Nonkeratinocyte cells in the oral epithelium do not contain large numbers of tonofilaments and desmosomes seen in epithelial keratinocytes and none participates in the process of maturation.

They constitute 10% of the cell population in the oral epithelium. They lack desmosomal attachment to adjacent cells and during histological processing, the cytoplasm shrinks around the nucleus to produce the clear halo. So they are also termed as clear cells. They are named as **(Table 19.3)**:
1. Melanocyte
2. Langerhans cell
3. Merkel cells
4. Lymphocyte.

## Oral Mucous Membrane

**TABLE 19.3:** Characteristics of nonkeratinocytes in oral epithelium.

| Cell type | Origin | Level in epithelium | Specific staining | Ultrastructure | Function |
|---|---|---|---|---|---|
| Melanocytes | Neural crest cells | Basal | Dopa oxidase tyrosinase, silver stain | Dendritic, no desmosomes or tonofilaments, premelanosomes and melanosomes are present | Synthesis of melanin pigment granules (melanosome and transfer to surrounding keratinocytes) |
| Langerhans cells | Bone marrow | Predominantly suprabasal | Hematoxylin and eosin stain, ATPase, cell surface antigen markers | Dendritic, no desmosomes or tonofilament, Langerhans granule present | Act as part of the immune system as antigen presenting cells |
| Merkel's cells | Neural crest cell | Basal | PAS stain | Nondendritic, sparse desmosome and tonofilament, electron dense vesicles and associated nerve axon | Tactile sensory cell |
| Lymphocyte | Bone marrow, lymph node, spleen | Variable | Cell surface antigen marker (OKT-3) | Large circular nucleus, scant cytoplasm. No desmosome, tonofilament | Associated with inflammatory response in oral mucosa |

### Junction of the Epithelium and Lamina Propria

The interface between the epithelium and connective tissue is usually corrugated.

The upward projection of connective tissue is called connective tissue papillae (**Figs. 19.7A and B**) which interdigitate with epithelial ridges or pegs, sometimes called rete ridges. The epithelium does not contain blood vessels and connective tissue papillae carry blood vessels and nerves. The interlocking arrangement of the connective tissue papillae and the epithelial ridges increases the area of contact between the lamina propria and epithelium. This additional area facilitates exchange of material between the epithelium and the blood vessels in the connective tissue and also serves to strengthen the attachment to the connective tissue.

Light microscopically, in a hematoxylin and eosin stained section, the interface

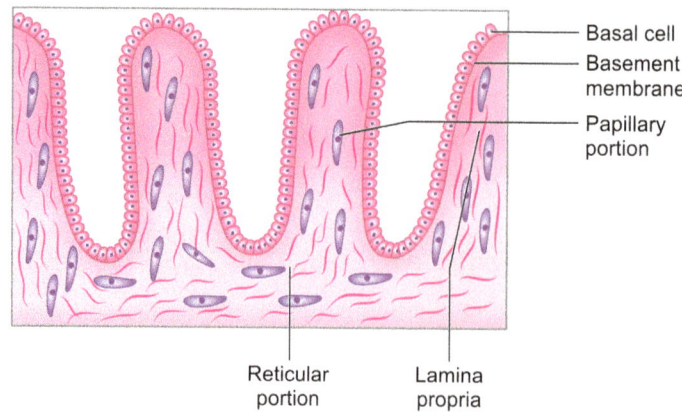

**Fig. 19.7A:** Junction of epithelium and lamina propria.

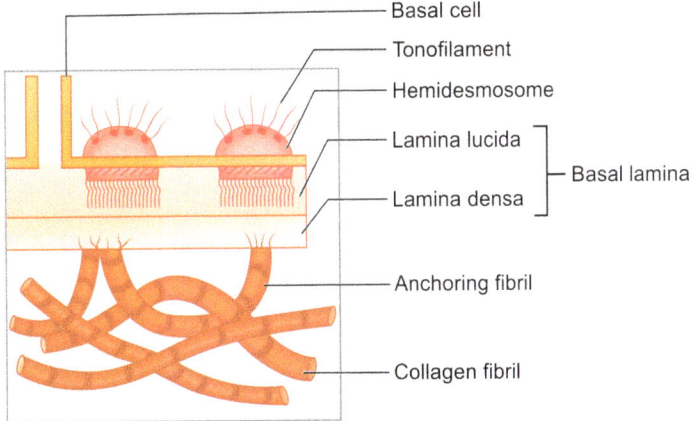

**Fig. 19.7B:** Junction of epithelium and lamina propria.

between epithelium and connective tissue appears as a structureless layer about 1–2 mm thick and it is known as basement membrane. This zone stains positively with periodic acid Schiff as it contains neutral mucopolysaccharide.

It also contains fine argyrophilic reticular fiber. Electron microscopically the basement membrane is known as basal lamina. It has two parts:

### *Lamina Lucida*

It is clear zone adjacent to epithelium and epithelial in origin. It is 45 nm wide. Basal cells are attached to lamina lucida by hemidesmosomes. Fine filaments termed anchoring filaments traverse lamina lucida opposite to hemidesmosome. Lamina lucida contains glycoprotein.

### *Lamina Densa*

It is a finely granular or filamentous material about 50 nm thick and placed below lamina lucida and it is connective tissue in origin. Inserted into lamina densa are small loops of finely banded fibrils called anchoring fibrils. Collagen fibrils run through these loops and are thus interlocked with the lamina densa to form a flexible attachment. It contains laminin and Type-IV collagen. Anchoring fibrils consist of Type-VII collagen and collagen that runs through the loops of anchoring fibrils is Type-I and Type-III collagen.

## Lamina Propria

The connective tissue supporting the oral epithelium is termed lamina propria. It comprises:

a. Superficial papillary layer (associated with the epithelial ridges).
b. Deeper reticular layer (which lies between the papillary layer and the underlying structure).

The lamina propria consists of the cells, blood vessels, neural elements, and fibers (collagen and elastic) embedded in an amorphous ground substance (containing proteoglycans and glycoproteins) **(Table 19.4)**.

> The term reticular means net-like and refers to the arrangement of the collagen fibers. The lamina propria consists of the cells, blood vessels, neural elements, and fibers (collagen and elastic) embedded in an amorphous ground substance (containing proteoglycans and glycoproteins).

## Submucosa

In many regions (e.g. cheeks, lips, parts of the hard palate), a layer of loose fatty or glandular connective tissue containing the major blood vessels and nerves separates the oral mucosa from underlying bone or muscle. This region is known as submucosa of oral cavity. Its composition determines the flexibility of the attachment of oral mucosa to the underlying structures.

## TABLE 19.4: Cell types in lamina propria of oral mucosa.

| Cell type | Morphology | Function | Distribution |
|---|---|---|---|
| Fibroblast | Stellate or elongated with abundant rough endoplasmic reticulum | Secretion of collagen fiber and ground substance | Throughout lamina propria |
| Histiocyte | Spindle-shaped or stellate, often dark-staining nucleus, many lysosomal vesicle | Precursor of functional macrophage | Throughout lamina propria |
| Macrophage | Round with pale staining nucleus, contains lysosomes and phagocytic vesicles | Phagocytosis, including antigen processing | Areas of chronic inflammation |
| Monocyte | Round with dark-staining kidney-shaped nucleus | Phagocytic cell | Areas of inflammation |
| Mast cell | Round or oval with basophilic granules, staining metachromatically | Secretion of histamine, heparin, serotonin | Throughout lamina propria, often subepithelial |
| Polymorphonuclear leukocyte | Round with lobulated nucleus | Phagocytosis | Site of acute inflammation |
| Lymphocyte | Round with dark-staining nucleus | Participate in humoral or cell mediated immune response | Site of inflammation |
| Plasma cell | Cartwheel nucleus, profuse rough endoplasmic reticulum | Synthesis of immunoglobulin | Areas of chronic inflammation |
| Endothelial cell | Associated with basal lamina | Lining of blood and lymphatic | Lining vascular channels of lamina propria |

### Mucoperiosteum

In the regions of gingiva and parts of hard palate, oral mucosa is attached directly to the periosteum of underlying bone, with no intervening submucosa. This is called mucoperiosteum which provides a firm inelastic attachment.

> A common feature of all epithelial cells is that they contain keratin intermediate filaments which resemble tonofilaments and are 7–11 nm in width. Similarly, connective tissue contains vimentin, muscle tissue contains desmin, and nerve cells contain neural filaments.

## STRUCTURE OF MUCOSA IN DIFFERENT REGIONS OF THE ORAL CAVITY

In different parts of the mouth, the mucosa has different roles and experiences different degrees and types of stress during mastication, speech, and facial expression. As a consequence, the structure of oral mucosa varies in terms of the thickness of the epithelium, the degree of keratinization, the complexity of the connective tissue, epithelium interface, the composition of lamina propria, and the presence or absence of submucosa.

### Keratinized Area

A. Masticatory mucosa: (1) Hard palate and (2) Gingiva.
B. Vermilion zone of lip.

### Masticatory Mucosa

The masticatory mucosa is keratinized, e.g. hard palate and gingiva.

The common features:
a. The pedicles (serrations in cells to strengthen the attachment to the connective tissue).
b. The increase in number and length of the desmosomes.
c. The density of the tonofilaments.
d. Complimentary grooves and ridges all appear to be adaptations of keratinizing epithelium to resist forces and to bind the epithelium to the connective tissue.

# Oral Mucous Membrane

Hard palate and gingiva have similarities in thickness, keratinization, and lamina propria but they have differences in submucosa.

## Hard palate (Fig. 19.8)

The following zones in the hard palate can be distinguished **(Fig. 19.8)**:
a. Gingival region—adjacent to teeth.
b. Midpalatine raphe—from incisive or palatine papilla posteriorly.
c. Anterolateral fatty zone between the raphe and gingiva.
d. Posterolateral glandular area between raphe and gingiva.

The mucosa of the hard palate is thick, orthokeratinized or parakeratinized, stratified squamous epithelium, long connective tissue papillae, thick dense collagenous tissue, and moderate vascular supply with short capillary loops. There is no submucosa in the region of midpalatine raphe and attached gingiva and the lamina propria binds down directly to bone (mucoperiosteum). Between the raphe and gingiva, the palate contains submucosa with neurovascular bundles, adipose tissue (predominantly anteriorly), and minor mucous glands (predominantly posteriorly) **(Fig. 19.9)**.

The nasal surface of hard palate is lined by a respiratory mucosa of ciliated columnar epithelium.

- **Incisive papilla:** The oral incisive (palatine) papilla is formed of dense connective tissue covered by keratinized epithelium. It contains the oral parts of the vestigial nasopalatine ducts. They are blind ducts of varying length lined

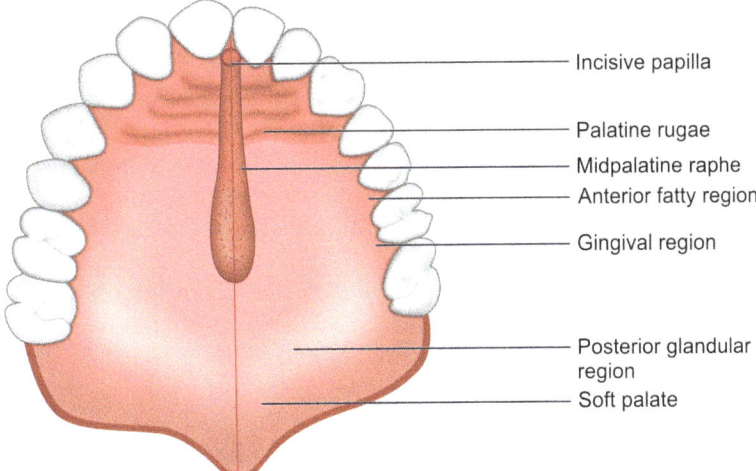

**Fig. 19.8:** Hard palate.

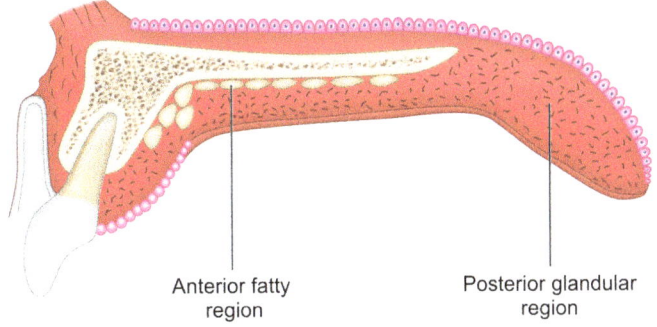

**Fig. 19.9:** Diagram of sagittal section through palate.

by simple or pseudostratified columnar epithelium, rich in goblet cell.
- **Palatine rugae:** They are irregular, asymmetric, ridges of mucosa extending laterally from the incisive papilla and the anterior part of the raphe. Their core is made of a dense connective tissue layer with fine interwoven fibers.
- **Epithelial pearls:** In the midline, especially in the region of the incisive papilla, concentrically arranged keratinized epithelial cells are found in the lamina propria. They are remnants of the epithelium formed in the line of fusion between the palatine processes.

*Gingiva (Fig. 19.10)*

Gingiva is that part of oral mucosa which surrounds the tooth and covers the alveolus. It can be divided into (Fig. 19.10):
- **Free gingiva:** About 1–1.5 mm of coronal part of gingiva is loosely attached to the tooth and is called free gingiva. The potential space between tooth and free gingiva is called gingival sulcus or gingival crevice. The region apical to this, where the gingiva is bound to the underlying tooth, is the junctional epithelium. From facial or lingual aspects, the margins of free gingiva appear as a wavy line and it is known as *marginal gingiva*. The free gingiva in the interproximal area is known as papillary *gingiva* or *interproximal gingiva*.
- **Attached gingiva:** The gingiva apical to the free gingiva is firmly attached to the underlying structures by gingival fibers of periodontal ligament and is called attached gingiva. The surface of attached gingiva has a stippled or pitted appearance. This is due to high connective tissue papillae elevating the epithelium.

The junction of free and attached gingiva produces a scalloped depressed line known as *free gingival groove*, which runs parallel to the margin of gingiva. The attached gingiva is continuous with alveolar mucosa. This border is scalloped and is called mucogingival junction. On the palatal surface of the maxillary teeth, there is no alveolar mucosa. Here, the attached gingiva merges with the palatal mucosa, with no clearly demarcated boundary. The attached gingiva may be slightly depressed between adjacent teeth corresponding to the depression on the alveolar process between the eminences of the sockets. These depressions on the gingiva are called *interdental folds*.

The interdental papilla is that part of the gingiva that fills the space between two adjacent teeth. When viewed from oral or vestibular aspect, the surface of the interdental papilla is triangular. In a three-dimensional view, the interdental papilla of the posterior teeth is tent-shaped, whereas it is pyramidal between anterior teeth.
- **Col:** It is the concave area of interdental papilla between the higher oral and vestibular corners and it fits below the contact point. The col is covered by thin

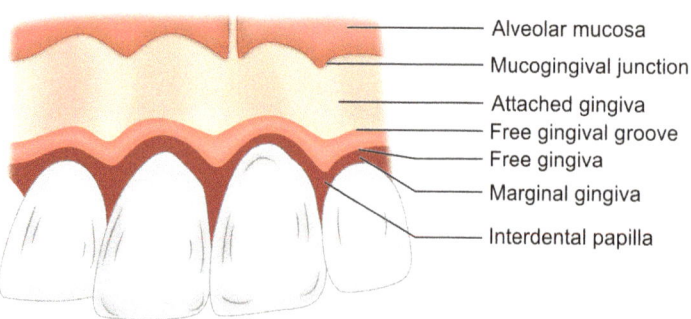

**Fig. 19.10:** Diagram of surface characteristics of gingiva.

nonkeratinized epithelium and is more vulnerable to periodontal disease.

The gingiva is covered by stratified squamous epithelium, which may be nonkeratinized or orthokeratinized but predominantly parakeratinized. The epithelium covers a dense lamina propria with long, slender papillae, dense collagenous connective tissue which is not highly vascular but contains long capillary loops with numerous anastomoses. There is no distinct layer of submucosa and mucosa is firmly attached by collagen fibers to cementum and periosteum of alveolar process.

## Vermilion Zone of Lip

The transitional zone between the skin of the lip and the mucous membrane of the lip is the red zone, or the vermilion border. It is found only in humans. It is covered by a moderately thick, keratinized epithelium, numerous densely arranged long papillae of the lamina propria, reaching deep into the epithelium and carrying large capillary loops close to the surface. As the blood vessels are visible through the thin, translucent epithelium, the zone appears red. Some sebaceous glands are present in submucosa and it is firmly attached to the underlying muscle.

## Nonkeratinized Areas

a. Lining mucosa
b. Specialized mucosa.

## Lining Mucosa

### Labial mucosa and buccal mucosa (lip and cheek)

These are covered by thick, nonkeratinized stratified squamous epithelium. The lamina propria shows short and comparatively broad papillae; the basement membrane zone is wavy. There is dense fibrous connective tissue containing collagen and some elastic fibers, rich vascular supply giving off anastomosing capillary loops into papillae. Mucosa is firmly attached to the underlying muscle by collagen and elastin (buccal mucosa to buccinator muscle and labial mucosa to orbicularis oris). There are adipose tissue, minor salivary glands, and sometimes ectopic sebaceous gland (Fordyce's spot).

### Vestibular fornix and alveolar mucosa

The labial and buccal mucosae are reflected from vestibular fornix to the alveolar mucosa covering bone. They are covered by thin, nonkeratinized stratified squamous epithelium. Connective tissue papillae are short and absent. Connective tissue contains many elastic fibers, capillary loops close to surface and salivary gland. In the fornix (vestibule), the mucosa is loosely connected to underlying structures, allowing the necessary movements of the lips and cheeks. The alveolar mucosa is also loosely attached to underlying periosteum.

### Ventral surface of the tongue, floor of the mouth

**Epithelium:** These areas are covered by thin, nonkeratinized stratified squamous epithelium.

- *Lamina propria:*
  a. **Ventral surface of tongue:** Lamina propria contains thin, numerous short papillae, some elastic fibers, few minor salivary glands, and capillary network in subpapillary layer; reticular layer is relatively avascular.
  b. **Floor of the mouth:** Lamina propria contains short papillae, elastic fiber, and extensive vascular supply with short anastomosing capillary loops.
- *Submucosa*
  a. **Ventral surface of tongue:** Submucosa binds the mucous membrane tightly to the connective tissue surrounding the bundles of the muscles of the tongue.
  b. **Floor of the mouth:** Submucosa contains adipose tissue and it is loosely attached to the underlying structures to allow the free movement of tongue.

### Soft palate

The covering epithelium is nonkeratinized stratified squamous epithelium. The papillae of connective tissue are few and short, and show a distinct layer of elastic fibers separating from submucosa. It is highly vascular with a well-developed capillary network. The submucosa is loose, diffuse, containing numerous salivary gland and taste buds.

## Specialized Mucosa

### Dorsal surface of tongue

The dorsum of tongue **(Fig. 19.11)** is divided grossly into an anterior two-thirds (body of tongue) and a posterior one-third (base of tongue) by a V-shaped indistinct groove, the sulcus terminalis. The angle of the V shows a depression called *foramen cecum*. The anterior part is covered by a keratinized stratified squamous epithelium with four types of papillae. They are filiform, fungiform, foliate, and circumvallate papillae. The posterior one-third of tongue is nonkeratinized and studded with small lymphatic nodule (or follicles).

- **Filiform papillae (Figs. 19.12A and B):** They are about 2.5 mm long, conical in shape (flame-shaped), and arranged in rows parallel to the sulcus terminalis. The epithelial covering of these papillae is thick. Each papilla consists of a loose connective tissue core covered by a keratinized stratified squamous epithelium with many secondary papillae. They do not contain taste buds.
- **Fungiform papillae (Figs. 19.13A and B):** They are isolated, short, flat topped, elevated, reddish, dome-shaped (mushroom shaped), 2 mm long, and 1 mm wide. They are disposed among the filiform papillae but are much less in number compared to filiform papillae. They are covered by a relatively thin, nonkeratinized epithelium. The color is derived from a rich capillary network visible through the relatively thin epithelium. They bear few taste buds.
- **Foliate papillae:** They are seen as four to eight parallel mucosal folds at the bilateral lateral borders near the posterior part of the body of the tongue. They are well-developed at birth but become rudimentary during adult life. They bear taste buds and excretory ducts from von Ebner glands.
- **Circumvallate papillae (Figs. 19.14A and B):** These are largest of the papillae, 10–12 in number, and are situated in front of sulcus terminalis. They are mushroom-shaped (resemble inverted truncated cone) submerged circular structures, 1 mm high and 2.5 mm wide, surrounded on all sides by a trench or crypt. These papillae have a connective tissue core that is covered on the superior surface by a keratinized epithelium. The epithelium covering the lateral walls is nonkeratinized and contains multiple taste buds. Small serous glands (of von Ebner) empty into the base of the trench.
- **Taste buds (Fig. 19.15):** These are chemoreceptive organs responsible for taste, located particularly within the epithelium around the walls of the circumvallate papillae, on the upper surface of fungiform papillae in the lateral wall of foliate papillae, and in the mucosa of the soft palate. Histologically, taste buds are small ovoid or barrel-shaped intraepithelial organs about 80 mm high and 40 mm thick. They extend from the basal lamina to the surface of the epithelium and are separated from underlying connective tissue by basal lamina. Their outer surface is almost covered by flat epithelial cells, which surround a small opening, the taste pore. They consist of two types of cells:
  a. *Supporting cells (sustentacular cells)*: The cells are wide with round, faintly stained nucleus. They are without hair and are found in the peripheral part of the organ.
  b. *Taste cells*: They are long, fusiform with dark-staining centrally located oval nuclei. The cells occupy the core of the taste organ. The ends of the cells facing the taste pore bear hairs which are modified microvilli. The hairs project

# Oral Mucous Membrane

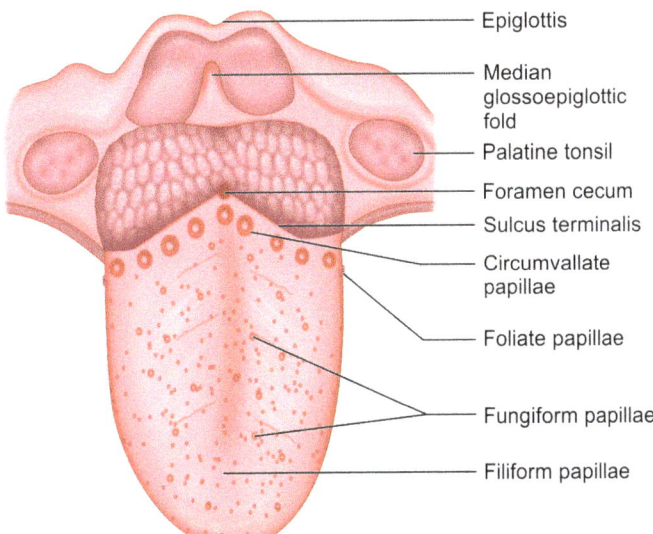

**Fig. 19.11:** Diagram of tongue.

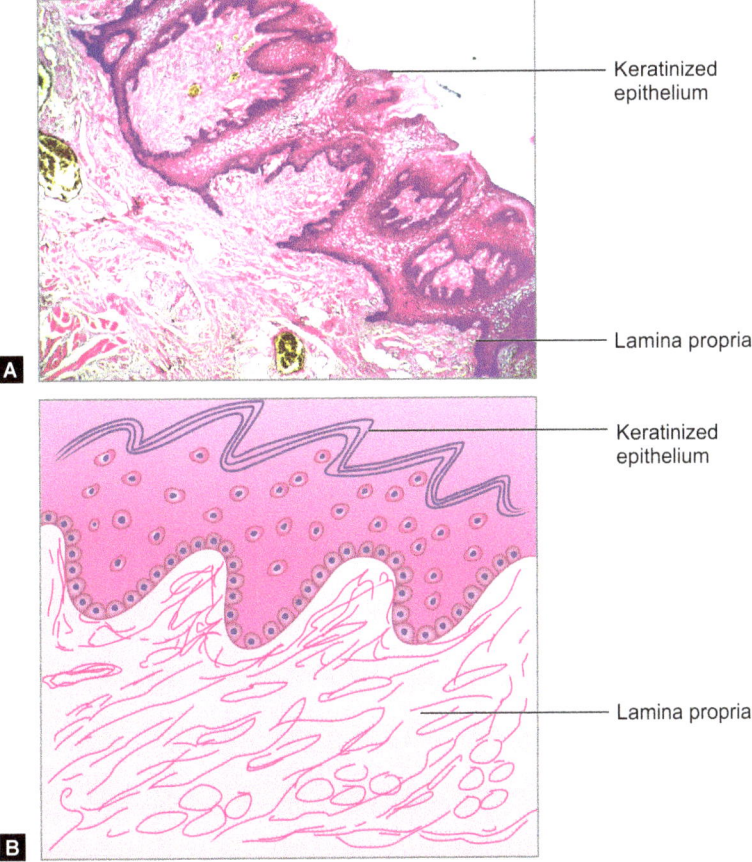

**Figs. 19.12A and B:** Filiform papillae.

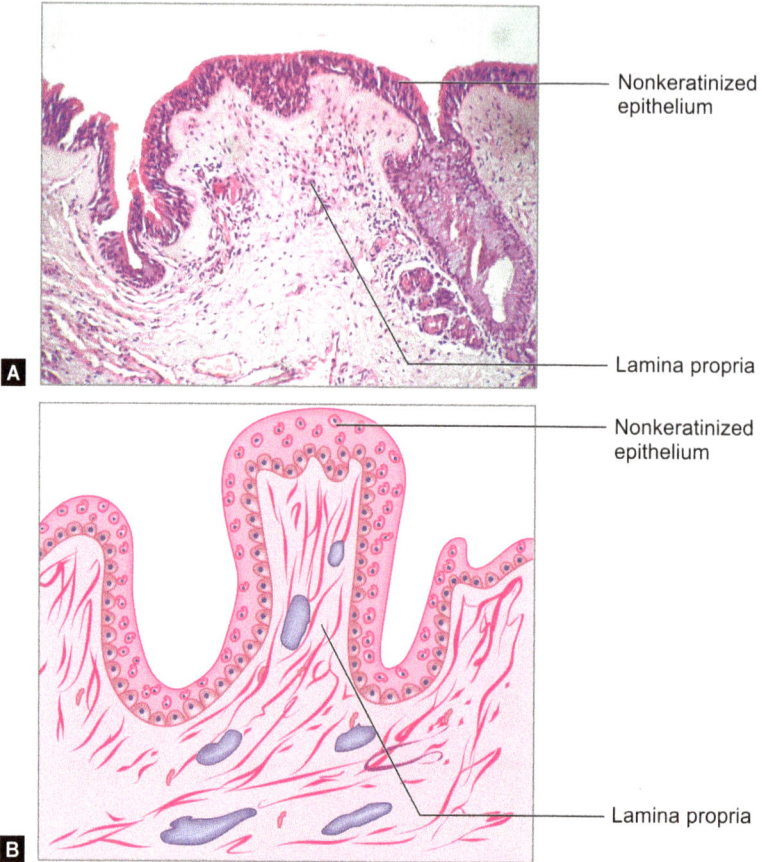

**Figs. 19.13A and B:** Fungiform papillae.

**TABLE 19.5:** Distribution of primary taste sensations.

| Taste | Site | Name of papillae | Nerve |
| --- | --- | --- | --- |
| Sweet | Tip of tongue | Fungiform papillae | Chorda tympani |
| Salty | Lateral border of tongue | Fungiform papillae | Chorda tympani |
| Bitter | Posterior part of tongue | Circumvallate papillae | Glossopharyngeal nerve |
| Sour | Lateral border and posterior part of tongue | Foliate papillae | Glossopharyngeal nerve |

into the lumen of the pore. The top of the taste canal is open to allow the entrance of fluids **(Table 19.5)**.

Taste stimuli are probably generated by the adsorption of molecules onto membrane receptors on the surface of the taste bud cells, which activates a signaling cascade mediated by membrane associated proteins such as transducin and gustducin. The change in membrane polarization that follows stimulates release of transmitter substances, which, in turn, stimulate unmyelinated afferent fibers of the glossopharyngeal nerve, which surround the lower half of the taste cells.

## Gingival Sulcus and Dentogingival Junction

### Gingival Sulcus

The gingival sulcus **(Fig. 19.16)** is the shallow crevice or space around the tooth bounded by the surface of the tooth on one side and sulcular epithelium on the other. The inferior boundary of the gingival sulcus is the attachment of the junctional epithelium and the coronal extent is the epithelium lining the free margin of the gingiva on the other. In

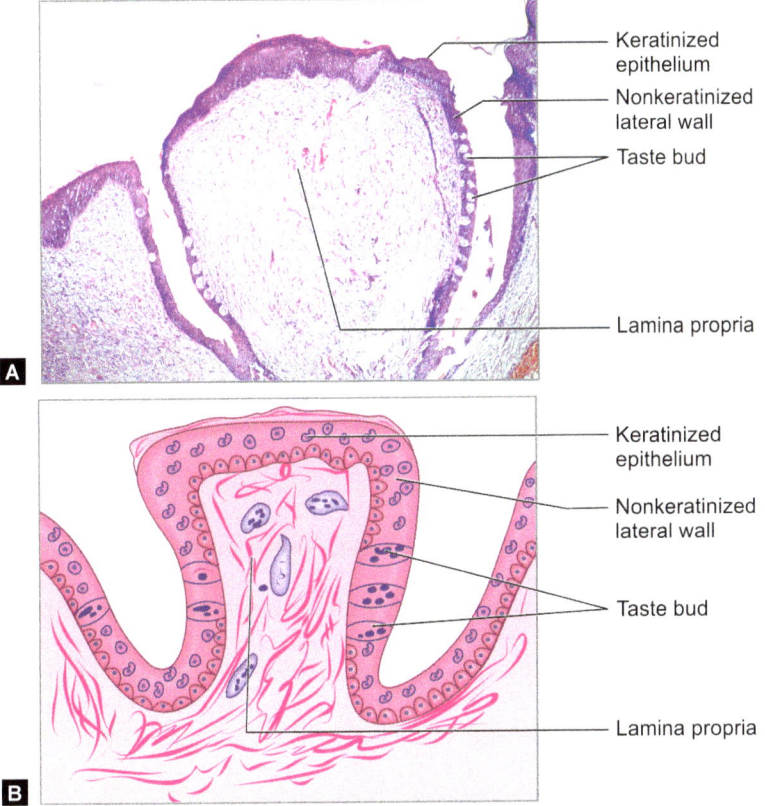

**Figs. 19.14A and B:** Circumvallate papillae.

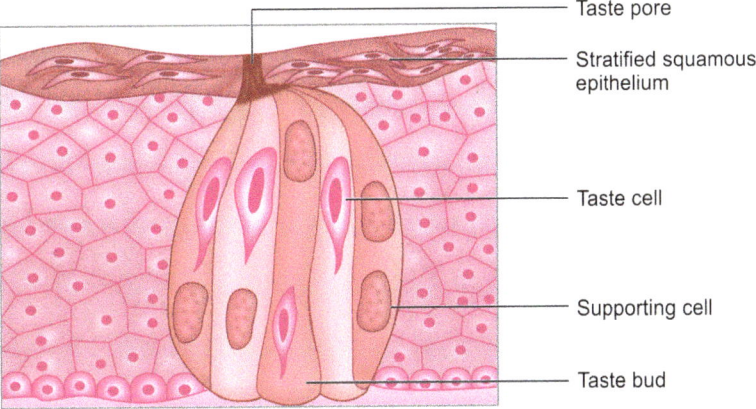

**Fig. 19.15:** Taste bud.

clinically healthy gingiva in human, the depth of the sulcus varies from 0 to 6 mm.

The sulcular epithelium lines the gingival sulcus. It is a thin, nonkeratinized, stratified squamous epithelium without rete pegs and extends from the coronal limit of the junctional epithelium to the crest of gingival margin. It acts as a semipermeable membrane through which injurious bacterial products pass into gingiva and through which tissue fluid from gingiva seeps into sulcus.

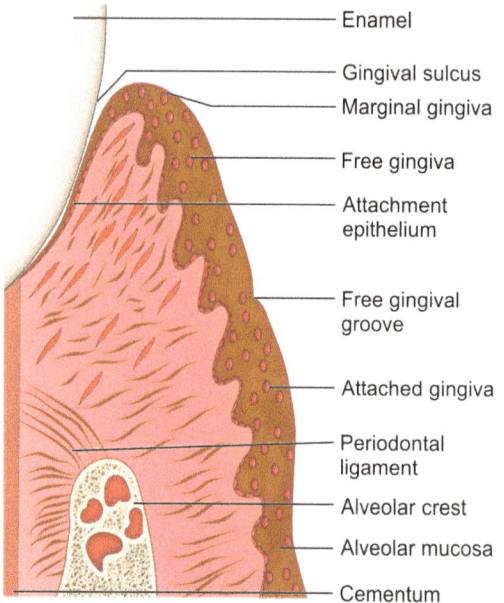

Fig. 19.16: Gingival sulcus and junctional epithelium.

## Sulcular Fluid

The gingival sulcus contains a fluid that seeps into it from the gingival connective tissue through the thin sulcular epithelium. The gingival fluid is believed to:
- Cleanse material from sulcus.
- Contain plasma protein that may improve adhesion of the epithelium to the tooth.
- Possess antimicrobial properties.
- Exert antibody activity in the defense of the gingiva.

## Dentogingival Junction (Junctional Epithelium)

The junctional epithelium consists of a collar-like band of nonkeratinizing stratified squamous epithelium. It is three to four layers thick in early life, but the number of layers increases with age to 10 or even 20. These cells can be grouped in two strata, basal and suprabasal.

## Development of Gingival Sulcus and Junctional Epithelium (Figs. 19.17A and B)

After completion of enamel formation, the ameloblasts leave a thin membrane on the surface of the enamel, the primary enamel cuticle. It is connected to interprismatic enamel. Then four layers of enamel organ are reduced to few layers of flat cuboidal cells known as reduced enamel epithelium. It covers entire enamel up to cementoenamel junction and is attached to the primary enamel cuticle.

At the time of eruption of tooth, the reduced enamel epithelium fuses with the oral epithelium. The epithelium surrounding the tip of the crown degenerates and the crown emerges through the perforation into the oral cavity. The reduced enamel epithelium

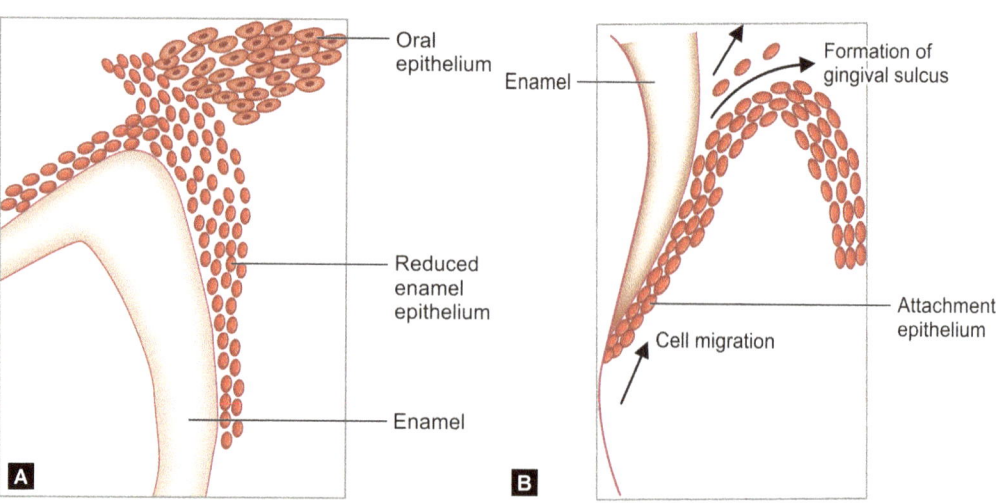

Figs. 19.17A and B: Development of gingival sulcus and junctional epithelium.

attached to enamel is known as primary attachment epithelium which is continuous with oral epithelium. The remnant of the primary enamel cuticle is known as *Nasmyth membrane.*

The shallow groove between gingiva and tooth surface is gingival sulcus. It is bounded by the attachment epithelium at its base and by the gingival margin laterally. Gradually, the tooth emerges into plane of occlusion and the reduced enamel epithelium (primary attachment epithelium) is totally replaced by oral epithelium. It is now known as *secondary attachment epithelium.* The attachment epithelium is attached to tooth by a basal lamina and hemidesmosomes. It is submicroscopic, 40 nm wide, and is known as *epithelial attachment.*

### Migration of Attachment Epithelium

The site and extent of attachment epithelium is not static but is changing. With advancing age, there is an apical migration of the attachment and consequently an increase in the height of the clinical crown by passive eruption. The migration can be described in four stages:
1. The lower end of the attachment epithelium is at the cementoenamel junction and the bottom of the crevice is on the enamel **(Fig. 19.18A)**.
2. The attachment epithelium is partly on the enamel and partly on the cementum **(Fig. 19.18B)**. The bottom of the crevice is on enamel.
3. The attachment epithelium lies entirely on cementum and the bottom of the crevice at the cementoenamel junction **(Fig. 19.18C)**.
4. The attachment epithelium and the bottom of the crevice are on the cementum **(Fig. 19.18D)**.

### Deepening of Sulcus (Pocket Formation)

The gingival sulcus deepens as a result of separation of junctional epithelium from actively erupting tooth. The more shallow a sulcus, the more likely that the gingival margin is not inflamed. Lymphocytes and plasma cells in the connective tissue at the bottom of the gingival sulcus constitute a barrier against the invasion of bacteria and the penetration of toxins.

## AGE CHANGES

1. In elderly person, the oral mucosa becomes smooth, dry (due to atrophy of salivary gland), thin (atrophic), and friable. These features lead to the symptoms of burning sensations and abnormal taste.

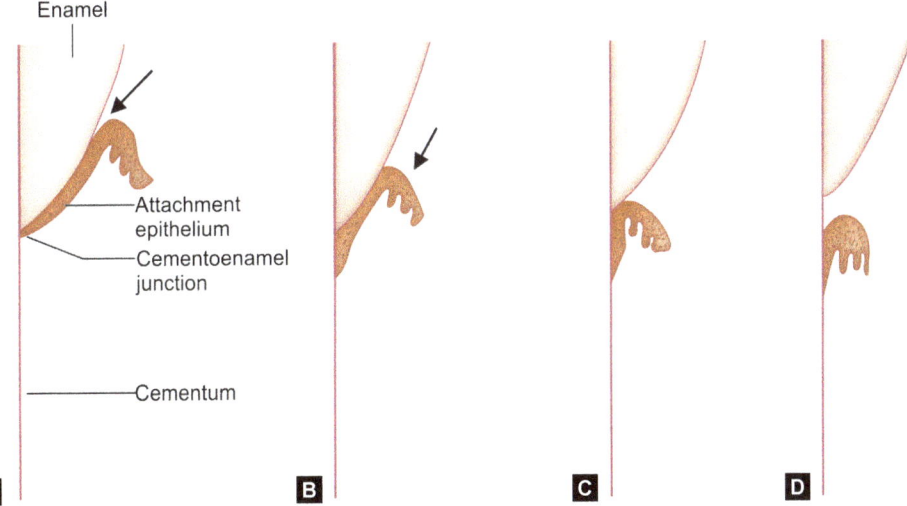

**Figs. 19.18A to D:** Migration of attachment epithelium.

2. Development of nodular varicose veins on the under surface of tongue.
3. Reduction in number of filiform papillae.
4. Histologically, the epithelium becomes thin, epithelium connective tissue interface becomes flattened, and Langerhans cells become fewer (decline in cell mediated immunity). Lamina propria shows decreased cellularity, increased collagen, and marked atrophy of salivary glands.

## CLINICAL CONSIDERATIONS

1. Oral mucous membrane is clinically very important. It reflects signs of a large volume of systemic diseases. Nutrition deficiencies, skin diseases, infectious diseases, and blood disorders are manifested orally.
2. Deepening of gingival sulcus leads to periodontal diseases.
3. Use of pan, betel nut, and tobacco may cause precancer (leukoplakia, submucous fibrosis, or cancerous change of oral mucosa).
4. In denture bearing areas, mucosa must be firm and moist.
5. In old age, thin and dry oral mucosa leads to severe burning sensation.

## QUESTIONNAIRE

1. Define oral mucosa. What are the functions of oral mucosa?
2. Classify oral mucosa.
3. Describe the microscopic features of oral mucosa with diagram.
4. Differentiate between keratinized and nonkeratinized epithelium.
5. Discuss the characteristic features of nonkeratinocytes.
6. Discuss the structural variations of mucosa in different regions of oral cavity.
7. What is specialized mucosa? Enumerate different tongue papillae. Discuss the macroscopic and microscopic features of tongue papillae.
8. Describe the structure and function of taste bud.
9. Discuss the dentogingival junction with diagram.
10. What are the age changes in oral mucosa?

## BIBLIOGRAPHY

1. Antonio N. Ten Cate's Oral Histology Development, Structure, and Function, 7th edition. Amsterdam: Mosby; 2008.
2. Berkovitz BKB, Holland GR, Moxham BJ. A Colour Atlas and Textbook of Oral Anatomy, Histology and Embryology, 4th edition. Amsterdam: Mosby Elsevier; 2009.
3. Das AK. Dental Anatomy and Oral Histology, 1st edition. Kolkata: Current Books International; 1972.
4. Gaunt WA, Osborn JW, Ten Cate AR. Advances in Dental Histology. Bristol: John Wright and Sons Ltd.; 1967.
5. Kumar GS. Orban's Oral Histology and Embryology, 12th edition. Amsterdam: Mosby; 2009.
6. Newman MG, Takei HH, Klokkevold PR. Carranza's Clinical Periodontology, 10th edition. St. Louis: Saunders; 2007.
7. Osborn JW, Ten Cate AR. Advanced Dental Histology, 3rd edition. Bristol: John Wright and Sons Ltd.; 1976.
8. Provenza DV. Fundamentals of Oral Histology and Embryology, Philadelphia: JB Lippincott Company; 1972.

# CHAPTER 20

# Salivary Glands

## DEFINITION OF GLAND

A gland is a unit of structure and function, involved in the manufacture and discharge of a secretion.

## CLASSIFICATION OF GLANDS

### According to Number of Cells Involved
a. Unicellular, e.g. goblet cells
b. Multicellular, e.g. salivary gland.

### According to Size
a. Major, e.g. parotid
b. Minor, e.g. mucous glands of lip.

### According to Morphology
a. Alveolar (acinar)
b. Tubular
c. Tubuloacinar.

### According to Branching of the Duct
a. Simple (nonbranching)
b. Compound (branching).

### According to the Presence of Ducts
a. Exocrine (ducts are present), e.g. salivary gland.
b. Endocrine (ducts are absent), e.g. pituitary.

### According to Type of Secretion
a. Serous, e.g. parotid
b. Mucus, e.g. minor salivary gland of cheek
c. Mixed (seromucus), e.g. submandibular.

### According to Damage of Secretory Cells at Discharge
a. Merocrine (no damage), e.g. salivary glands
b. Apocrine (cells contribute part of their protoplasmic substance to their secretion), e.g. some sweat glands.
   Holocrine (there is extreme damage of the cell; secretion consists of altered cells of the gland itself), e.g. sebaceous gland.

## CLASSIFICATION OF SALIVARY GLANDS

Salivary glands are multicellular, merocrine, exocrine glands. They may be classified according to size, location or type of secretion (Table 20.1).

**TABLE 20.1: Classification of salivary glands.**

| Name | Size | Location | Type of secretion |
|---|---|---|---|
| Parotid | Major | Cheek | Pure serous |
| Submandibular | Major | Floor of the mouth | Mixed (predominantly serous) |
| Sublingual | Major | Floor of the mouth | Mixed (predominantly mucus) |
| Superior labial and inferior labial | Minor | Lip | Mixed (predominantly mucus) |
| Buccal and retromolar | Minor | Cheek | Mixed (predominantly mucus) |
| Posterolateral palatine | Minor | Hard palate | Pure mucus |
| Palatine | Minor | Soft palate | Pure mucus |
| Glossopalatine | Minor | Glossopalatine fold | Pure mucus |
| Anterior lingual (Blandin-Nuhn) | Minor | Body of tongue | Mixed (predominantly mucus) |
| Posterior lingual (von Ebner) | Minor | Base of tongue | Pure serous |
| Posterior lingual (tonsil, lingual) | Minor | Base of tongue | Pure mucus |

# Salivary Glands

## STRUCTURAL PATTERN OF THE SALIVARY GLAND (FIG. 20.1)

Salivary glands consist of two main elements:
a. The parenchyma—the glandular secretory tissue.
b. The stroma—the supporting connective tissue.

## Capsule

The gland is surrounded by capsule that consists mostly of collagenous tissue with few elastic and reticular fibers.

## Trabeculae

From the capsule, connective tissue septae or strands traverse the glands and divide them into lobules. These septae carry blood vessels, nerves, and excretory ducts. The septal connective tissue consists of mesenchymal cells, fibroblasts, plasma cells, lymphocytes, and fat cells. The connective tissue of the septae spreads into the lobules forming stroma for the secretory units.

## Secretory Cells

Each lobule contains numerous secretory units and each unit consists of a cluster of grape-like structure (the acini) positioned around a lumen **(Fig. 20.2)**.

A secretory acinus may be serous, mucous, or mixed. It is responsible for the production of primary secretion. It empties into an intercalated duct lined by cuboidal

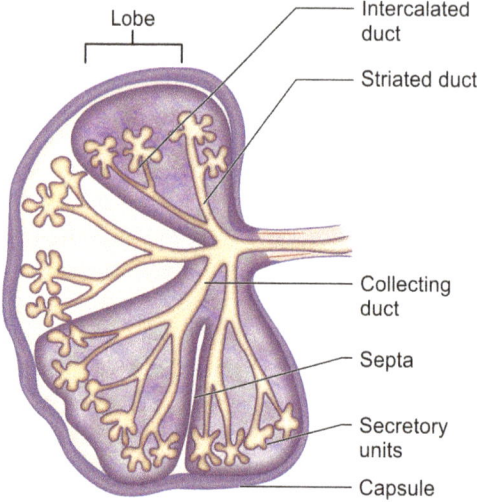

**Fig. 20.1:** General organization of a salivary gland.

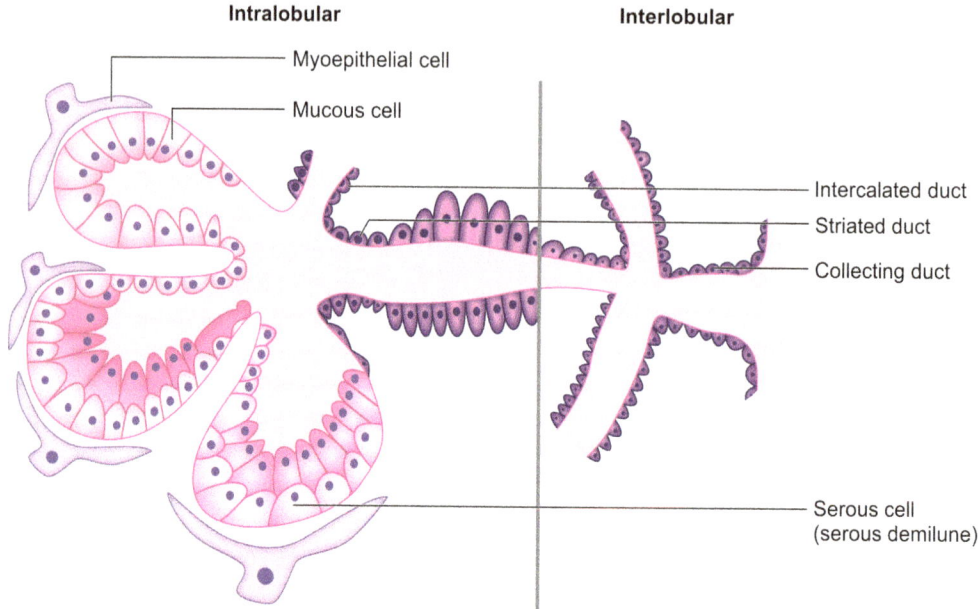

**Fig. 20.2:** Secretory elements of salivary gland.

# Salivary Glands

epithelium, which in turn joins a larger striated duct formed of columnar cells. Both the intercalated and striated ducts are intralobular and affect the composition of the secretion passing through them. Plasma cells (secrete the immunoglobulins) are found around the intralobular ducts. The striated ducts empty into the relatively inert excretory ducts, which carry the saliva to the mucosal surface and which may be lined near their termination by a layer of stratified squamous epithelial cells. The excretory ducts are interlobular.

## Mucous Acinus (Mucous Cell)

Mucous cells are large pyramidal cells with broad-base resting on the basement membrane and narrow apex directed toward lumen **(Figs. 20.3A and B)**. The nucleus is round or oval and is placed near the base. The cells form alveoli or tubules. In H and E stain, they take pale blue color and with periodic acid Schiff stain, the mucous acini appear purplish.

Ultrastructurally, the mucous cell contains prominent Golgi complexes (which reflect the

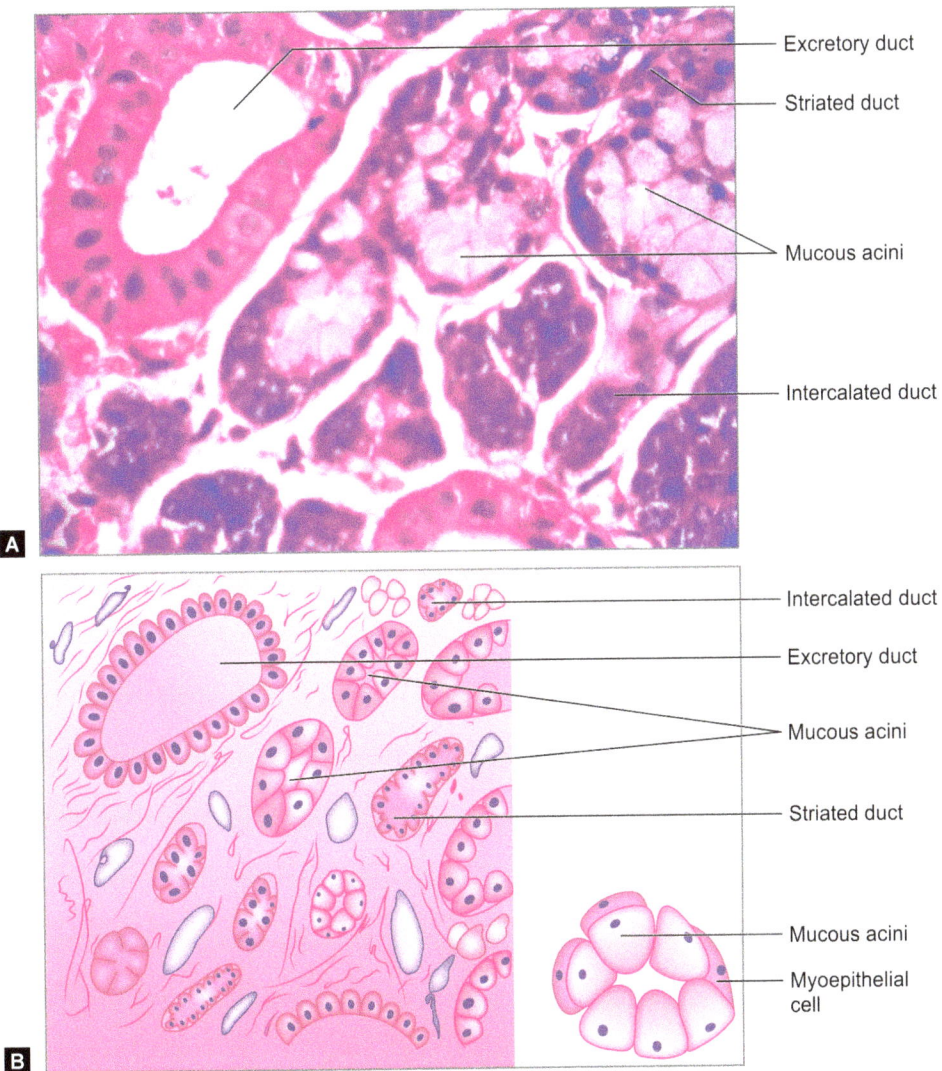

**Figs. 20.3A and B:** Mucous acini.

cell's increased carbohydrate metabolism) and pale, electron lucent secretory droplets containing scattered flocculent material. In early stages of synthesis of secretory products, large amount of rough endoplasmic reticulum is present. In resting phase, all cellular organelles are less conspicuous. Intercellular canaliculi are found leading to demilunes and also occur between mucous cells.

The secretory products (mucigen) are emptied into secretory capillaries which drain into intercalated duct and then out of the gland. After mucigen is emptied into the lumen, it acquires water by virtue of its hydrophilic property and results in mucin. Mucin contains large amount of carbohydrate, sialic acid and occasionally sulphated sugar. It changes to mucus, which is a heavy, viscous, opalescent fluid. It functions for lubrication and protection of the oral tissues.

### Serous Acinus (Serous Cells) (Figs. 20.4A and B)

The serous cells are smaller. They are pyramidal in shape, with its broad-base resting on a thin basement membrane and

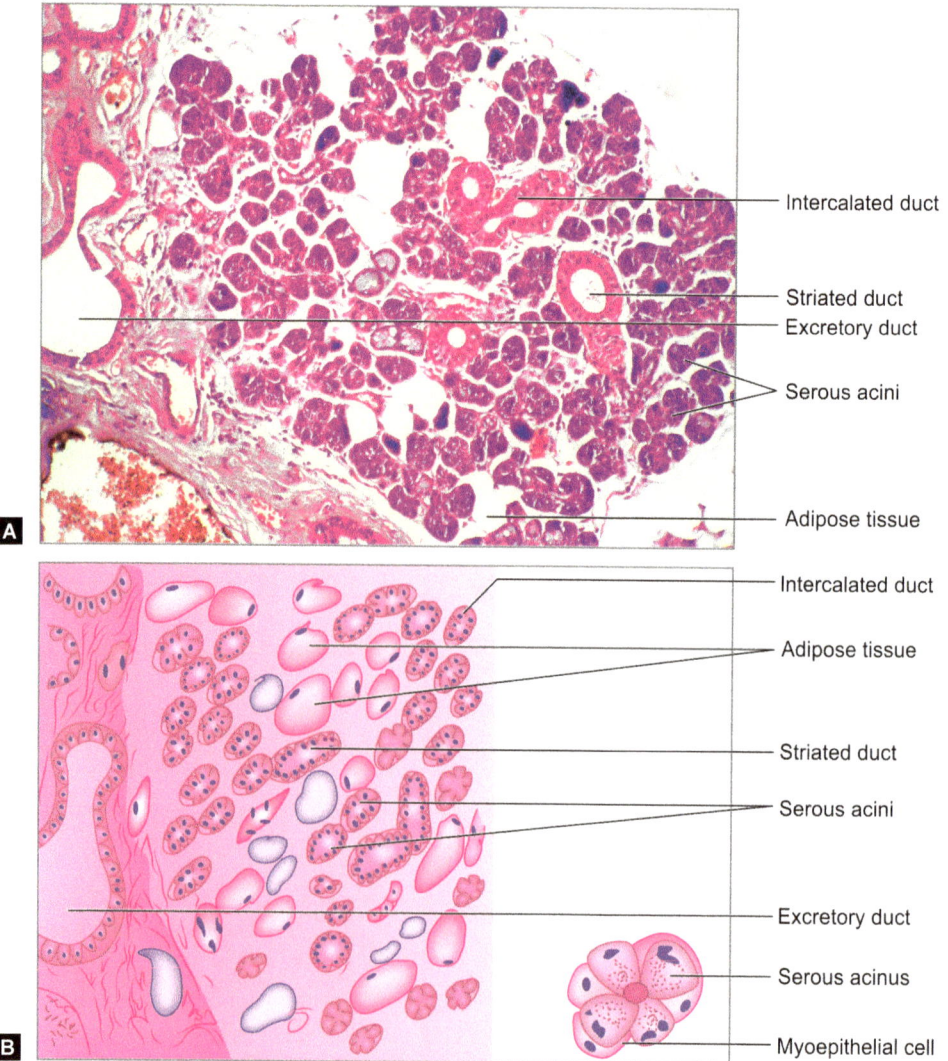

**Figs. 20.4A and B:** Serous acini.

# Salivary Glands

**TABLE 20.2: Difference between serous and mucous cells.**

| Serous cells | Mucous cells |
|---|---|
| 1. The cells of the serous acini are smaller and pyramidal in shape; the apex is situated toward the central narrow lumen | 1. The cells of the mucous acini are large and pyramidal, a broad-base is resting on a basement membrane, and narrow apex is directed toward wider lumen |
| 2. The nucleus is spherical and is placed in the basal third of the cell | 2. The nucleus is flattened and is placed near the base |
| 3. The cytoplasm is deep basophilic and contains numerous coarse basophilic zymogen granule in H and E stain | 3. In H and E stain, mucus cell appears pale blue, the apical part stains intensely with mucicarmine stain |
| 4. Ultrastructurally the cells contain Golgi complex but less conspicuous than mucous cells | 4. Ultrastructurally the mucus cells contain prominent Golgi cell complex and its secretory material is stored in droplets |
| 5. The serous cells have large amount of rough endoplasmic reticulum packed basally and laterally to the nucleus | 5. In resting cells, the rough endoplasmic reticulum and mitochondria are less conspicuous |
| 6. The interdigitations between adjacent serous cells are more | 6. The interdigitations between adjacent mucus cells are few |
| 7. The secretion is watery and its amylase helps to breakdown starch | 7. The secretion is thick and viscous. It has little or no enzymatic activity and serve mainly for lubrication and protection of oral tissues |
| 8. The secretion of the granule content occurs by exocytosis. The granule membrane fuses with the plasma membrane at the lumen. The opening of fused portion causes exteriorization of granule content without loss of cytoplasm | 8. The secretion of mucous droplets occurs by different mechanisms. The membrane of mucous droplet fuses with the apical plasma membrane. The fused membrane ruptures and the mucous droplet is discharged along with the membrane |

its narrow apex bordering on the lumen. The spherical nucleus is located in the basal region of the cell. The distal part of the cell adjacent to the lumen contains numerous, coarse, basophilic granules, called zymogen granules (1 mm in diameter), which are the precursors of ptyalin.

Ultrastructurally, the basal part of the cytoplasm is filled with ribosome, rough endoplasmic reticulum (RER), a closed system of membranous sacs or cisternae. Golgi apparatus is located apical or lateral to the nucleus. Mitochondria are found throughout the cell. Many narrow canaliculi run between the cells and join the lumen. Both the canaliculi and lumen are lined by short microvilli. The secretory proteins are synthesized by membrane-bound ribosomes, transferred to the cisternal space of RER, and migrate to the Golgi apparatus, where carbohydrate addition and other post-translational modifications are completed, and they are packaged into secretory granules which are discharged by exocytosis at the secretory surface of the cell **(Table 20.2)**.

## Serous Crescent (Figs. 20.5A and B)

In a mixed salivary gland, the mucous cells are situated more near the duct, while serous cells occupy the blind end of the acinus. In certain glands, the terminals of the acini are partially surrounded by serous cells. This appears like a crescent and is called serous crescent of Giannuzzi or demilunes of Heidenhain.

## Myoepithelial Cells (Basket Cell)

The myoepithelial cells **(Fig. 20.6)** are flattened cells found interposed between the basement membrane and the basal plasma membrane of the secretory epithelial cells and intercalated duct cells. There is usually one myoepithelial cell per secretory end piece (two or three myoepithelial cells are also found). The body of the cell is small, filled mostly with a flattened nucleus, and four to eight cytoplasmic processes radiate from cell body to embrace the long axis of the secretory unit. In ordinary H and E stained section under light microscope, only their nuclei are visible. The typical stellate-shaped cells with

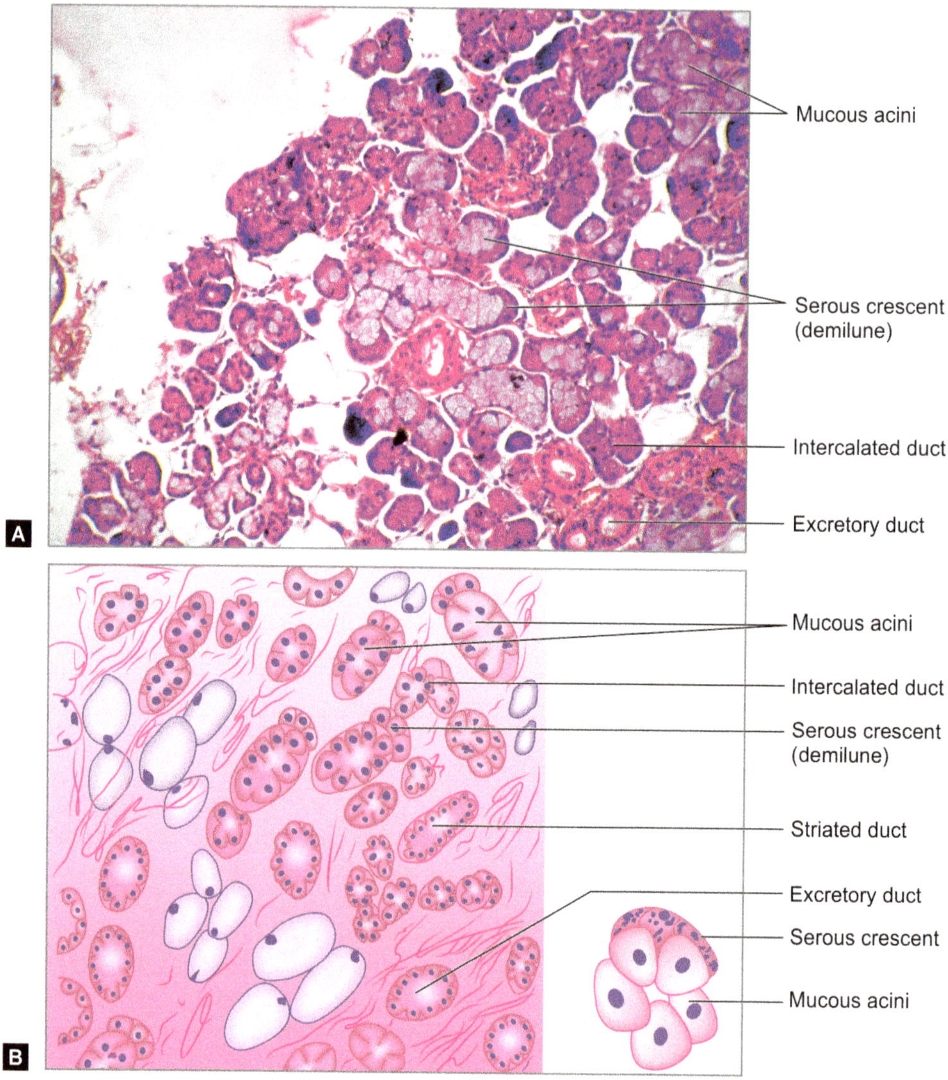

# Salivary Glands

**Figs. 20.5A and B:** Mixed acini showing serous crescent.

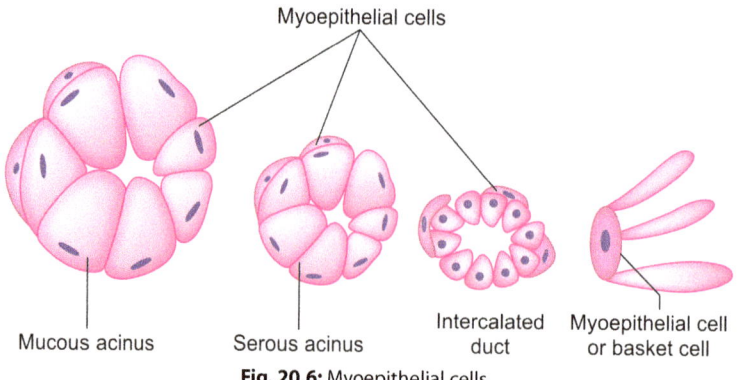

**Fig. 20.6:** Myoepithelial cells.

processes are observed by immunofluorescent techniques. Their appearance is reminiscent of a basket cradling the secretory unit, hence the name "basket cell".

The ultrastructural features reveal:
a. Desmosomal attachments between the myoepithelial cells and the secretory cells to provide structural stability, to prevent the processes from sliding over the acinar or duct cells during contraction.
b. Processes filled with longitudinally oriented microfilaments, about 6 nm thick.
c. Small, dense, dark bodies frequently present between the thin filaments.
d. Other cytoplasmic organelles, located in the perinuclear region of the cell.
e. Numerous micropinocytic vesicles located on the plasma membrane of the myoepithelial cells.

***Functions***
1. Myoepithelial cells are considered to have a contractile function helping to expel secretions from the lumina of the secretory units and ducts.
2. They act as a support for the secretory cells, preventing overdistension as secretory products accumulate within the cytoplasm.
3. They contract and widen the diameter of the intercalated ducts, thus lowering or raising their resistance to outflow.
4. They may aid to rupture the acinar cells packed with mucus secretion.

The myoepithelial cells are considered to be of epithelial origin because they are situated between the parenchymal cell and its basement membrane.

**Oncocytes:** They are large cells with small central pyknotic nucleus and abundant eosinophilic cytoplasm. They are seen frequently in the parotid and submandibular glands of older people.

## DUCTAL SYSTEM

The ductal system of salivary glands is a varied network of ducts characterized by progressively smaller diameter membranes. The network contains three classes of ducts:

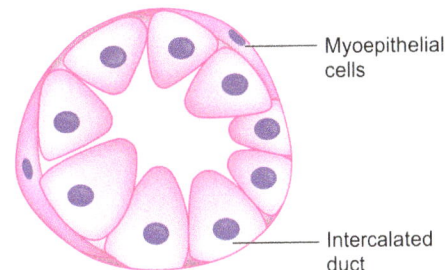

**Fig. 20.7:** Intercalated ducts.

intercalated, striated, and terminal or excretory. The ductal system is not a simple conduit, for it actively participates in the production and modulation of saliva. Within a lobule, the smallest ducts are the intercalated ducts which connect the terminal secretory units to the next larger ducts, the striated ducts. In the interlobular connective tissue, the ducts join to form large excretory duct.

### Intercalated Ducts

The secretion of the terminal end pieces passes first through the intercalated ducts **(Fig. 20.7)**. These small diameter ducts are lined by short, cuboidal cells with centrally placed nuclei and little cytoplasm, containing some rough endoplasmic reticulum situated basally and some Golgi complexes apically. Secretory granules are occasionally found in these cells, especially in cells closest to the secretory end piece. These cuboidal cells have a few microvilli projecting into the lumen of the duct, and their lateral borders interdigitate with each other and are interconnected by means of junctional complexes situated apically, as well as scattered desmosomal attachments below the junctional complexes. Myoepithelial cells, or their processes, are usually present between the basement membrane and the ductal cells. Intercalated ducts are especially prominent in salivary glands with a serous secretion and therefore occur frequently in the parotid gland.

### Striated Ducts

The intercalated duct passes into the striated duct **(Fig. 20.8)**. Striated ducts are lined by columnar cells, which have centrally placed

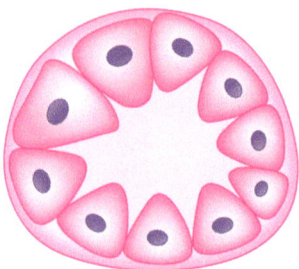

**Fig. 20.8:** Striated ducts.

nuclei and intensely eosinophilic cytoplasm, making the ducts clearly recognizable in H and E stained sections. The most characteristic feature of such cells, however, is their prominent striations at the basal end of the cells, giving the ducts their name. These striations are seen by electron microscopy as particularly deep indentations of the basal plasma membrane into the cell. They also extend beyond the lateral boundaries of the cell as a series of foot processes that, in turn, possess complex secondary extensions. The lateral processes interlock in a highly complex fashion with adjacent cells and at the same time provide a large increase in the surface area of the basal plasma membrane. Many elongated mitochondria following the long axis of the folds occur in the cytoplasm between the folds. Around the nucleus are a few profiles of rough endoplasmic reticulum, along with some Golgi complexes.

The apical cytoplasm often contains a few scattered vesicles, smooth endoplasmic reticulum, free ribosomes, and lysosomes. The luminal surface of the striated cell is characterized by short, stubby microvilli and again adjacent cells are united by junctional complexes and desmosomal attachments. Occasional dark cells containing numerous mitochondria and scattered small basal cells are also present. Striated ducts are also surrounded by a number of longitudinally oriented small blood vessels.

Interspersed between cells of the ductal epithelium of both intercalated and striated ducts are cells described simply as clear cells. They are thought to be of two types, one macrophage like and the other lymphocytic and both are involved in immune surveillance.

The specialized structure of the striated ducts implies a particular function. They modify the secretions passing through them. The fluid is characterized by an isotonic protein content, a high sodium content (hypertonic), and a low potassium content (hypotonic). As it passes along the striated duct, it changes to a generally hypotonic state. The massive infoldings of the basal plasma membrane, associated with the elongated mitochondria, are thought to reflect the sodium pumping capacity of the cell wall in this location. Thus, sodium, extracted from the cell, passes into the tissue fluid and establishes a concentration gradient between the cell and luminal fluid. Sodium therefore diffuses into the cells from the luminal fluid; at the same time, active transport of potassium occurs in the opposite direction. Bicarbonate ions are also actively secreted. Because under normal conditions of flow, the striated duct cells do not absorb water, these ionic changes result in the formation of a hypotonic solution.

## Terminal Excretory Ducts

After passing through the striated ducts, salivary fluid is secreted into the oral cavity through the terminal excretory ducts. The histology of these ducts varies as they pass from the striated ducts to the oral cavity. Near the striated ducts, they are lined by a pseudostratified epithelium, consisting of tall, columnar cells (much like striated cells) admixed with small basal cells and goblet cells **(Fig. 20.9)**. As the terminal excretory ducts approach the oral cavity, their epithelium changes to a stratified epithelium merging with that of the oral cavity at the ductal orifice. The main excretory ducts modify the final saliva by altering its electrolyte concentration, rendering it hypotonic, and perhaps also adding a mucoid component. Special eosinophilic cells, loaded with mitochondria, tend to be found in the ducts, particularly in mucosal glands. These cells are known as oncocytes **(Table 20.3)**.

- **Connective tissue elements:** Fibroblasts, macrophages, mast cells, occasional leukocytes, fat cells, and plasma cells

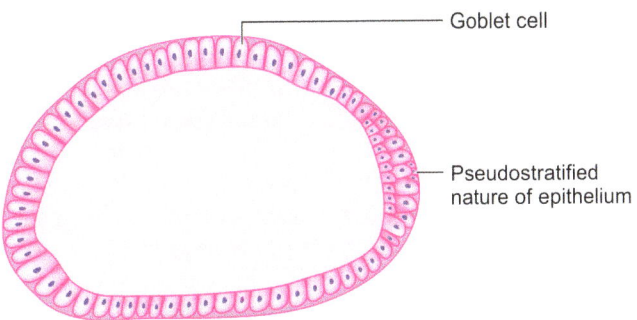

**Fig. 20.9:** Terminal excretory ducts.

**TABLE 20.3: Characteristic features of three major salivary glands.**

| Characteristics | Parotid | Submandibular | Sublingual |
|---|---|---|---|
| Location | Superficial portion is lying in front of the external ear and its deeper part is filling the retromandibular fossa | It is located in the submandibular triangle behind and below the free border of the mylohyoid muscle with a small extension above mylohyoid muscle | It lies between the floor of the mouth and mylohyoid muscle |
| Main excretory duct | Stenson's duct opens into the oral cavity on the buccal mucosa opposite the maxillary second molar. The opening is usually marked by a small papilla | Wharton's duct opens at a small papilla at the side of the lingual frenum on the floor of the mouth | Bartholin's duct opens with or near the submandibular duct |
| Type | It is a compound, branched, alveolar gland, and purely serous | It is compound, branched, alveolotubular gland. It is mixed gland with serous element predominance | It is a compound branched tubuloalveolar gland. It is a mixed gland with mucous predominance |
| Capsule | It is well capsulated | It is well capsulated | There is no capsule |
| Duct system | The intercalated ducts are long and branching. Pale-staining striated ducts are numerous | The intercalated ducts are shorter and striated ducts are longer | The intercalated and striated ducts are poorly developed. Mucous tubules may open directly into ducts lined with cuboidal, columnar cells without basal striations |

along with collagen and reticular fibers are embedded in a ground substance composed of proteoglycans and glycoproteins. The vascular supply to the glands is also embedded within the connective tissue. They enter the glands along the excretory ducts and branch to follow them into the individual lobules. The main branches of the nerves supplying the glands follow the course of the vessels, breaking up into terminal plexuses in connective tissue adjacent to the terminal portions of the parenchyma.

## SALIVA

Saliva is the fluid produced and secreted into oral cavity by salivary glands.

### Quantity of Saliva

Pure glandular secretion is collected by special devices from the ducts. Whole saliva is obtained from the mouth, usually by expectoration. In addition to the components contributed by the glands, whole saliva contains desquamated oral epithelial cells, leukocytes, microorganisms and their products, fluid from the gingival sulcus, and food remnants.

The amount of saliva secreted varies from person to person, depending on type of food taken, age, degree of mechanical stimulation, emotional condition, etc. The total volume of saliva secreted daily by humans is approximately 750 mL of which:
- 60%—from submandibular gland
- 30%—from parotid gland
- 5%—from sublingual gland
- 5%—from minor salivary gland
- pH of saliva—varies from 5.6 to 7.6 (average is 6.8).

## Composition

- Water—99.5%
- Inorganic component—0.2%
- Organic component—0.3%.

Inorganic constituents are bicarbonates, chlorides, phosphates of calcium, magnesium, potassium, bromide, iodide, fluoride, copper, oxygen, and carbon dioxide.

Organic constituents are:
- *Proteins:* Glycoproteins, intrinsic salivary proteins, serum proteins like albumin and globulin, and mucin.
- *Enzymes:* Ptyalin, lysozyme, lipase, and phosphatase.
  Blood group substances, antibodies, blood clotting factors, lipids, amino acids, urea, and cholesterol.
- *Vitamins:* Pantothenic acid, riboflavin, nicotinic acid, and vitamin K.
- *Carbohydrate:* Galactose, mannose, fucose, and glucose.

Desquamated epithelial cells and salivary corpuscles (resemble leukocytes, derived from gingival sulcus).

## Functions of Saliva

### 1. Protection

Saliva is a lubricant. Its glycoprotein content makes it mucinous and protects the lining mucosa by forming a barrier against noxious stimuli, microbial toxins, and minor trauma. Its fluid consistency also provides a mechanical washing action, which flushes away nonadherent bacterial and acellular debris from the mouth.

It prevents accumulation of acidogenic plaque microorganisms and hence prevents cariogenic activity of microbes. The calcium-binding proteins in saliva help to form salivary pellicle, which behaves as a protective membrane.

### 2. Buffering

The buffering capacity of saliva prevents potential pathogens from colonizing the mouth. Plaque microorganisms can produce sugars, which are rapidly buffered and cleared by saliva and thus prevent demineralization of enamel. Much of the buffering capacity of saliva resides in its bicarbonate and phosphate ions. Negatively charged residues on salivary proteins are also thought to serve as buffers; a salivary peptide, stalin, plays a significant role in raising the pH of dental plaque after exposure to fermentable carbohydrate. The ability of saliva to buffer acid is very important because saliva and plaque pH are generally lower in caries active individuals.

### 3. Digestion

Saliva is important for digestion. It provides taste activity, neutralizes esophageal contents, dilutes gastric chime, forms the food bolus, and because of its amylase contents, breaks down starch.

### 4. Taste

Saliva is required to dissolve substances to be tasted and to carry them to the taste buds. It also contains a protein, called gustin, that is thought to be necessary for growth and maturation of the taste buds.

### 5. Antimicrobial Action

Saliva contains a spectrum of proteins with antibacterial properties such as histatin. Lysozyme is an enzyme that can hydrolyze the cell walls of some bacteria. Lactoferrin binds free iron and in so doing deprives bacteria of this essential element. Antibodies are present in saliva. The major salivary immunoglobulin, secretory IgA, has the capacity to clump or agglutinate microorganisms. This ability, along with the cleansing action of saliva, serves to remove clumps of bacteria.

## 6. Maintenance of Tooth Integrity

Saliva is saturated with calcium and phosphate ions. The high concentration of these ions ensures that ionic exchange with the tooth surface is directed to the tooth. This exchange begins as soon as the tooth erupts because although the crown is fully formed morphologically when it erupts, it is crystallographically incomplete. Interaction with saliva results in posteruptive maturation through diffusion of such ions as calcium, phosphorus, magnesium, and chloride into the surface apatite enamel crystals. This maturation increases surface hardness, decreases permeability, and heightens the resistance of enamel to caries.

## 7. Clotting Time

The bleeding time of oral tissues is shorter than that of other tissues. When saliva is experimentally mixed with blood, the clotting time may be greatly accelerated.

## 8. Tissue Repair

Experimental studies in mice have shown that the rate of wound contraction is significantly increased in the presence of saliva, which is thought due to the presence of epidermal growth factor in the saliva produced by the submandibular glands. The occurrence of growth is lower in human saliva.

## 9. Excretion

Saliva excretes body metabolites (electrolytes, water, and protein).

## Control of Secretion

The physiologic control of salivary gland secretion is mediated through the activity of the autonomic nervous system. The release of neurotransmitters from the vesicles in the nerve terminals adjacent to the parenchymal cells stimulates them to discharge their secretory granules and secrete water and electrolytes.

The neurotransmitters interact with specific receptors located on the plasma membrane of the acinar cell.

Norepinephrine, the sympathetic transmitter, interacts with both $\alpha$ and $\beta$-adrenergic receptors. Acetylcholine interacts with the cholinergic receptor.

$\beta$-adrenergic receptors stimulate protein secretion.

$\alpha$-adrenergic and cholinergic receptors stimulate low levels of protein, water, and electrolyte secretions.

Receptors for the peptide transmitter substance P are also present on salivary gland cells. Substance P stimulates secretion similar to that caused by $\alpha$-adrenergic and cholinergic agonists. Vasoactive intestinal polypeptide (VIP) is present in nerve endings in the salivary glands and has been shown to induce secretion by some glands. Receptor stimulation results in increase in the intercellular concentration of "second messengers", which trigger additional events leading to the cellular response. In the case of $\alpha$-adrenergic, cholinergic, and substance P receptors, the membrane permeability to calcium ion is increased and a marked influx of calcium ion into the cell occurs. The increased cytoplasmic calcium ion concentration causes potassium ion efflux, water and electrolyte secretion, and a low level of exocytosis.

Stimulation of the $\beta$-adrenergic receptor activates the plasma membrane enzyme adenylate cyclase, which catalyzes the formation of 3', 5'-cyclic adenosine monophosphate (cyclic AMP) from adenosine triphosphate. The increased intracellular concentration of cyclic AMP activates cyclic AMP-dependent protein kinase, an enzyme that phosphorylates other proteins, which in turn may be involved in the process of exocytosis.

Cyclic AMP may also stimulate release of calcium ion from intracellular stores, thereby increasing its cytoplasmic concentration. Thus, calcium ion may be the common intracellular mediator for all of the receptors;

the different cellular responses may reflect the different sources of calcium ion or differing local concentration or both. Calcium ion may have additional effects, including stimulation of guanylate cyclase activity and an increase in the concentration of 3′, 5′-cyclic guanosine monophosphate (cyclic GMP).

However, the role of cyclic GMP in the secretory process has not yet been determined. Adjacent secretory cells are joined to one another by specialized intercellular junctions called gap junctions. These junctions are permeable to ions and small molecules; thus, changes in the intracellular concentration of these substances in one cell are reflected by parallel changes in the adjacent cells. Therefore, physiologic stimulation probably results in a response by secretory units (acini) rather than individual cells.

The discharge of secretory granules involves translocation to the luminal cell surface and fusion of the granule membrane with the plasma membrane. The microtubules and microfilaments may act as a cytoskeletal framework or contractile mechanism for granule movement.

## CLINICAL CONSIDERATIONS

1. The salivary glands are subject to a number of pathologic conditions.
   These include inflammatory diseases, such as viral, bacterial, or allergic sialadenitis, a variety of benign and malignant tumors, autoimmune diseases, such as Sjögren's syndrome, and genetic diseases, such as cystic fibrosis.
2. One of the most common surface lesions of the oral mucosa is a vesicular elevation called mucocele. This is produced from the severance of the duct of a minor salivary gland and pooling of the saliva in the tissues.
3. A blockage of a salivary gland duct may occur after formation of a mucous or calcified plug within the duct.
4. The major glands, especially the parotid, may become enlarged during starvation, protein deficiency, alcoholism, pregnancy, diabetes mellitus, and liver disease.
5. In conditions associated with the reduction or absence of salivary flow (xerostomia), the incidence of decay increases. Reduction in salivary flow is most often in patients with sicca syndrome or Sjögren's syndrome, after irradiation of the head and neck region, or because of the use of various therapeutic pharmacologic agents.
6. Age changes in the salivary glands, particularly prominent in the parotid, consist of a gradual replacement of parenchyma with fatty tissue. Since the parotid is the major source of serous saliva, with advancing age, patients often complain of dryness and an increase in the viscosity of saliva.

## QUESTIONNAIRE

1. Define and classify glands.
2. Classify salivary glands.
3. Describe serous and mucous acini with diagrams.
4. Differentiate between serous and mucous acini.
5. Discuss the structure and function of myoepithelial cell.
6. Describe ductal system of salivary gland with diagram.
7. Discuss the composition and function of saliva.

## BIBLIOGRAPHY

1. Antonio N. Ten Cate's Oral Histology Development, Structure, and Function, 7th edition. Amsterdam: Mosby; 2008.
2. Berkovitz BKB, Holland GR, Moxham BJ. A Colour Atlas and Textbook of Oral Anatomy, Histology and Embryology, 4th edition. Amsterdam: Mosby Elsevier; 2009.
3. Das AK. Dental Anatomy and Oral Histology, 1st edition. Kolkata: Current Books International; 1972.
4. Gaunt WA, Osborn JW, Ten Cate AR. Advances in Dental Histology. Bristol: John Wright and Sons Ltd.; 1967.
5. Kumar GS. Orban's Oral Histology and Embryology, 12th edition. Amsterdam: Mosby; 2009.
6. Osborn JW, Ten Cate AR. Advanced Dental Histology, 3rd edition. Bristol: John Wright and Sons Ltd.; 1976.

# Index

Page numbers followed by *f* refer to figure, and *t* refer to table.

## A

Accessory canals 168, 169
Acellular cementum 131, 178, 178*f*, 181*t*
 arrangement of 180*f*
 formation of 132*f*
Acid phosphatase activity 140
Adjacent teeth, cementoenamel
  junction of 203*f*
Advanced bell stage 119
Afibrillar cementum 183
Air sinuses, growth of 107
Alveolar bone 197, 197*f*
 parts of 201*f*
 proper 201
 supporting 202
Alveolar crest, shape of 203*f*
Alveolar group 188, 189
Alveolar mucosa 219
Alveolar nerve
 anterior-superior 59*f*
 posterior-superior 59*f*
 superior 59*f*
Alveolar process 204
Alveolar spongiosa 204*f*
Amelin 126
Ameloblastin 126
Ameloblasts 127*f*
 covering maturing enamel 128
 cross-sections of 127*f*
 life cycle of 123
Amelogenesis 123
 prerequisite for 125
Amelogenin 126, 144
Amelotin 126, 127
Amniotic cavity 91
Anodontia 122
Anterior wall 70
Antibodies, production of 173
Antimicrobial action 236
Apical cementum 179
Apical foramen 5, 168
Apical group 190
Arteries 56*f*
Articular capsule 65
 histology of 65*f*
Articular disk 65
 histology of 65*f*
Articular fibrous covering 64
Articular tubercle, histology of 64*f*
Attached denticle 175, 175*f*
Attached gingiva 218
Attachment epithelium, migration
  of 225*f*
Auriculotemporal nerve 63
Autoradiography 85

Axial 5
 root center 5
 surface 5
 wall 5

## B

Balanced occlusion 73
Basal cell layer 209, 212
Basion 80
Basket cell 231
Bifid tongue 108
Bilaminar germ disk 91, 91*f*
Blastocyst 90, 90*f*
Blood vessels 173, 194
Bone 123*t*
 cells 198
 deposition 135, 135*f*
 immature 201
 internal reconstruction of 204
 lining cells 199
 matrix 197
 mature 199
 preparation of ground sections
  of 87
 remodeling 137
 removal of 140
 resting lines of 205*f*
 reversal lines of 205*f*
 structure of 197
 tissues, types of 199
Bonwill triangle 74, 75*f*
Bony component 64
Brain stimulates sutural growth of
  skull cap, growth of 106*f*
Branchial arches 96, 101*f*
 derivatives of 98
 formation of 97*f*
Branchial cleft cyst 108
Branchial groove 97, 97*f*
 fate of 97, 98*f*
Bright-field binocular microscope
  82, 83*f*
Brush 140
Buccal developmental groove 21
Buccal mucosa 219
Buccal surface 5
Buccinator muscle 66*f*
 positions of 67*f*
Bud stage 112, 113*f*
Bundle bone 201, 202*f*

## C

Cancellous bone 200
Canine 2, 139, 169
 eruption of 29*t* 78*f*
 measurement of 29*t*

Cap stage 112, 114*f*
Capsule 228
Carbohydrate 236
Cardiac plate 95*f*
Carving maxillary first
 molar, steps of 54*f*
 premolar, steps of 54*f*
Carving permanent maxillary
 canine, steps for 53*f*
 central incisor, steps for 53*f*
Cavity preparation 166
Cell 85, 170
 bodies 157
 absence of 178
Cellular cementum 132, 179, 180*f*,
  181*t*
 arrangement of 180*f*
 formation of 132*f*
Cellular change 174
Cemental matrix 183
Cementicles 194, 195*f*
Cementing interrod substance 144
Cementoblast 121*f*, 132, 182, 183, 192
Cementoclasts 192
Cementocyte 181*f*
Cementodentinal junction 182*f*, 183
Cementoenamel junction 5, 153,
  153*f* 177, 178, 183, 203*f*
 variations of 154*f*
Cementogenesis 131
Cementoid tissue 184
Cementum 1, 123*t*, 177, 177*f*, 183,
  185, 186
 chemical composition 177
 classification of 182
 clinical considerations 184
 development of 131
 function 177
 hyperplasia 184
 hypertrophy 184
 physical characteristics 177
 scanning electron microscopy 181
 secondary 132
 structure 178
 types of 178, 183
Central fossa 7, 7*f*
Central incisor 138, 139, 169
Centric occlusion 73
Cephalometric landmarks 80*f*
Cephalometry 80
Cervical
 enamel 153
 line 5
 loop 118*f*
  enamel epithelia of 119
 region 146

Cervix 5
Cheek, blood supply of 57
Chemical composition 143
Chondroitin 173
Cingulum 5
Circumpulpal dentin 161
Circumvallate papillae 220, 223*f*
Cleft
  lip 108
  mandible 108
  palate 108
Clotting time 237
Collagen fibers 160, 187
Condylar guidance 75
Confocal scanning microscope 83
Connective tissue
  cells 186
  elements 234
Coronal pulp 168, 169
Cortical plates 202, 202*f*
Cranial base, growth of 106
Cranial fossa, anterior 70*f*
Cranial vault, growth of 106
Craniocaudal folding begins 95*f*
Crown 4, 6
Crypt 6
  floor, bone deposition on 135*f*
Crystals, arrangement of 146*f*
Cusp 6
  ridges 9

## D

Dark ground illumination 82
Dead tract 165, 166*f*
Deciduous canine 14
  eruption of 15*t*
  measurement table of 15*t*
  tooth bud of 111*f*
Deciduous central incisor, tooth bud of 111*f*
Deciduous dentition 1, 10, 76
Deciduous incisors 11
  eruption of 11*t*
  measurement table of 12*t*
Deciduous lateral incisor, tooth bud of 111*f*
Deciduous mandibular
  canine 16
  central incisor 13
  first molar 20
  lateral incisor 14
  second molar 21
Deciduous maxillary
  canine 14
  central incisor 11
  first molar 16
  lateral incisor 12
  second molar 18
Deciduous molars 16
  eruption of 16*t*
  measurement table of 17*t*
  premolars beneath divergent roots of 134*f*

Deciduous occlusion, changes in 76
Deciduous predecessor 134*f*
Deciduous teeth 3, 4, 10, 111*f*, 139, 141, 147*f*, 183
  bud 111*f*
  importance of 10
  morphology of 2*f*
  remnants of 141
  retained 141
  shedding of 139
  submerged 141
Defense cells 172, 172*f*, 193, 193*f*
Dehydration 86
Delayed eruption 141
Dental
  caries 164
  epithelium 113, 114
  follicle 118, 118*f*
  formula 3
  hard tissue, resorption of 140*f*
  lamina 110*f*, 111, 137
  fate of 111
  papilla 118, 119, 169
Denticles 174
Dentin 1, 123*t*, 157, 167, 183
  chemical composition 157
  clinical considerations 166
  color 157
  development of 128, 130*f*
  different forms of 160
  formation of 119, 171
  forming cells 164
  ground section of 166
  hardness 157
  innervation of 163
  physical characteristics 157
  physiologic secondary 161
  radio density 157
  reactionary 131
  reparative 164, 165*f*
  sclerotic 166, 166*f*
  sialoprotein 129
  specific gravity 157
  structure of 157
  tubular configuration of 167
  vitality of 164
Dentinal tubules 158, 161*f*, 162, 163
  lateral branches of 159*f*
  S-shaped curvature of 158*f*
Dentinocemental junction 160, 162, 164*f*
Dentinoenamel junction 153, 153*f*
Dentinogenesis 129, 129
Dentition 6, 76*f*
Dentogingival junction 222, 224
  development of 136*f*
Depression 63
Desmolytic stage 125
Desmosome 211*f*
Developing tooth, part of 121*f*
Diastema 6
Digestion 236
Digestive function 207

Direct neural stimulation 163
Distal step terminal plane 77*f*
Distal terminal bars 126
Ductal system 233
Ducts
  branching of 227
  presence of 227

## E

Early bell stage 115*f*, 116, 117*f*
  enamel organ in 116
Eccentric occlusion 73
Ectoderm 94*f*
Ectodermal grooves, obliteration of 96*f*
Electron microscope 145
Embedded denticle 175, 175*f*
Embrasure 6, 6*f*
Embryo, folding of 94
Embryonic disk 93*f*
Enamel 1, 140, 143, 155, 156
  age changes of 155
  color 143
  cord 116
  cuticle 155
  density 143
  development of 123
  epithelium 155
    reduced 136
  formation 119
  forming cells 119
  hardness 143
  hypocalcification 128
  hypoplasia 128
  knot 115
  lamellae 152, 153, 153*f*
  matrix
    formation of 125
    maturation of 127, 128*f*
    mineralization of 127
  navel 116
  niche 115, 115*f*
  organ
    formation 168
    part of 114, 115*f*
  pearl 184
  permeability 143
  physical characteristics 143
  prism formation 125*f*
  proteins 144
  rod 127*f*, 144, 145*f*-147*f*
    alternate deviation of 147*f*
    curvature of 147*f*
    direction of 146
  septum 116
  small protuberance of 184
  solubility 143
  specific gravity 143
  spindle 152, 152*f*
  structure of 144
  tufts 151, 151*f*
Enamelins 126, 144
Endoderm 94*f*

# Index

Endoplasmic reticulum 113, 171
Endosteum 199
Enumeration 66, 69
Enzyme 236
   collagenase 192
Eosinophils 173
Epithelial attachment 225
Epithelial cell 110, 136
Epithelial diaphragm
   formation of 121$f$
   proliferate, tongue-like
      extensions of 122$f$
   surface view of 122$f$
Epithelial pearls 218
Epithelium 219
   junction of 214, 214$f$, 215$f$
Eruption 133
   aberrations in 141
Eruptive tooth movement 133, 134
Ethmoidal air cell 70$f$
Ethmoidal sinuses 69
Excretion 237
Extracellular filaments 136
Extrinsic fiber cementum 182

## F

Face
   blood supply of 56
   development of 90
   growth of 106
   sensory nerve supply of 60, 60$f$
   veins of 56$f$
Facial cleft 108
   lateral 108
Facial processes 95$f$
   fusion of 96$f$
False denticles 174, 175$f$
Fédération Dentaire Internationale
   Approved System 4
Fibers 173, 187
   alveolar group of 190$f$
   dense group of 189
Fibroblast 136, 172, 191, 192
   cell membrane 136
Fibronectin 136
Fibronexus 136, 138
Fibrosis 174
Fifth pharyngeal pouch 99
Filiform papillae 220, 221$f$
First molar 139, 169
First pharyngeal pouch 97
First premolar 139, 169
Fissural cyst 108
Fissure 7
Fistulas 108
Fluorescence microscope 83
Fluorides 143
Flush terminal plane 77$f$
Foliate papillae 220
Foregut endoderm, derivatives of 94
Fossa 7
Fourth pharyngeal pouch 99

Free denticle 175, 175$f$
Free gingiva 218
Frontal bone 70$f$
Frontal sinuses 69
Frontomaxillary suture 106
Fungiform papillae 220, 222$f$

## G

Gingiva 218
   surface characteristics of 218$f$
Gingival fibers 189, 189$f$
Gingival group 188
Gingival sulcus 222, 224$f$
   development of 224, 224$f$
Glands 227
   classification of 227
Globular process 96
Glycoprotein 173, 191
Glycosaminoglycans 116, 191
Gnarled enamel 147, 148$f$
Gnathion 80
Golgi apparatus 171
Golgi material 113, 129
Gonion 80
Granular cell layer 212
Groove 7, 7$f$
Growing tooth germ 135
Gubernacular cord 137, 137$f$
Gum pads 75$f$, 76$f$

## H

Hard palate 217, 217$f$
Hard tissue
   formation 122
   progresses, formation of 121$f$
Haversian system 200$f$
Hemidesmosome 211$f$
Hertwig's epithelial root sheath 119,
   122, 131, 132, 183, 184, 193,
   194
   elongation of 121$f$
   fate of 122
Hindgut endoderm, derivatives of
   95
Howship's lacunae 192, 192$f$
Hunter-Schreger bands 150, 151,
   151$f$
   significance of 151
Hyaluronic acid 173
Hydrodynamic theory 163
Hypercementosis 184, 184$f$
   localized 184
Hypermineralized dentin 159

## I

Incisal guide angle 75
Incisal ridge 9
Incisive papilla 217
Incisors 2
   crowns, distal flairing of 78$f$
   eruption of 24$t$
   lateral 138, 139, 169

Inflammatory cell infiltration 176
Infraorbital nerve 59$f$
Initial osteogenesis, site of 103$f$
Inner enamel epithelium 114, 116,
   155
Inner epithelial cells 120
Intercalated ducts 233, 233$f$
Intercellular substance 173
Interglobular dentin 162, 163$f$
Intermediate cell layer 212
Intermediate cementum 183
Intermediate mesoderm 94
Intermediate plexus 190, 191$f$
Internal enamel epithelium
   determines crown pattern,
   cell division of 117$f$
Interradicular fiber 190$f$
Interstitial cementicles 194
Intertubular dentin 159, 159$f$
Intra-articular disk 62
Intratubular dentin 159
Intrinsic fiber 182
   cementum 183

## J

Jaw
   blood supply of 56
   bones, parts of 201
   development of 101
Joint capsule 62
Junctional epithelium 224, 224$f$
   development of 224, 224$f$

## K

Keratinized oral epithelium 209

## L

Labial mucosa 219
Labial pits 108
Lamellae 153
Lamina
   densa 215
   lucida 215
   propria 215
      junction of 214, 214$f$, 215$f$
Langerhans cell 213
Late bell stage 119, 120$f$, 121$f$
Lateral plate mesoderm 94
Leeway space 79$f$
Left maxillary second premolar 35$f$
Light microscopy 82
Line angle 4
Linea alba 209
Lingual fossa 7, 7$f$
Lingual thyroid 108
Lingula 104$f$
Lining mucosa 208, 213, 213$f$, 219
Lips
   blood supply of 57
   vermilion zone of 219
Lower arch 6
Lower deciduous molars 17$t$

Lower face 107
Lower jaw, blood supply of 56
Lubrication 207
Lymph
   drainage 71
   vessels 174
Lymphocyte 173, 213

## M

Macrophage 193
   colony-stimulating factor 118
Macrostomia 108
Malassez epithelial rests 193, 193*f*
Mamelons 7, 8*f*
Mandible
   development of 102
   different developmental blocks for 104*f*
   formation 103*f*
   nerve supply of 59
Mandibular
   canine 31, 31*t*
   central incisors 28
   condyle 61
      histology of 64*f*
   deciduous
      canines 16*t*
      molar 22
   first premolar 36
   fossa 61
   incisor 24, 25*t*
   lateral incisors 28
   left second premolar 38*f*
   molars 40, 134
   ossification, spread of 104*f*
   premolars 33*t*, 38*t*
   right first premolar 36*f*
   second premolar 37
   teeth, nerve supply of 59
Mantle dentin 160
Marginal ridge 8, 9*f*
Masseter muscle, positions of 67*f*
Mast cells 173, 193
Mastication, muscles of 61, 66
Masticatory mucosa 208, 213, 213*t*, 216
Matrix formation 131
Maxilla
   alveolar process of 70*f*
   development of 105
   nerve supply of 58
Maxillary artery 57*f*
Maxillary canine 31
Maxillary central incisor 13
Maxillary deciduous molar 19
Maxillary first
   molar, carving of 55
   premolar 32
Maxillary incisor 24
Maxillary lateral incisor 13
Maxillary left first premolar 32*f*
Maxillary molars 40

Maxillary premolar 33*t*
   carving of 54
Maxillary second premolar 34
Maxillary sinus 69, 70*f*, 71*f*
   CT scan of 71*f*
   lining of 72*f*
Maxillary teeth 169
   nerve supply of 58
Maxillary tuberosity 134*f*
Meckel's cartilage 104, 104*f*
Medial pterygoids muscle 66, 66*f*
Median line 8
Median palatine cyst 108
Melanocyte 213
Menton 80
Merkel cells 213
Mesenchymal cells 173
Mesial 8
   drift 79
   step terminal plane 77*f*
   surface 8
Mesoderm 92, 92*f*, 94*f*
   differentiation of 94*f*
   subdivisions of 93
Microscopy 82
Microstomia 108
Middle superior alveolar nerve 59*f*
Midgut endoderm, derivatives of 94
Milk dentition 1
Mineralization 131
   pattern of 128*f*
Mitochondria 113
Mixed acini 232*f*
Mixed dentition 77
Mixed fiber cementum 182
Molars 2
   eruption of 39*t*
   measurement table of 39*t*
   pulps 168
Monocytes 140
Monson curve 74
Morphology 4, 227
Morula 90, 90*f*
Mouth
   floor of 219
   opening 67
Mucoperiosteum 216
Mucosa
   structure of 216
   types of 208*f*
Mucous acini 229, 229*f*
Mucous cell 229, 231, 231*t*
Muscles 63
Myoepithelial cells 231, 232*f*

## N

Nasal cavity 70*f*
Nasmyth membrane 225
Neck 5
Neighboring cell 179
Nerve fibers, types of 174
Neural crest cells 93, 93*f*
Neural groove, formation of 93*f*

Neural plate 95*f*
   formation of 93*f*
Neural tube 93*f*
   somites on either side of 94*f*
Nonamelogenins 144
Nonfunctional occlusion 73
Nonfunctional teeth 184
Nonkeratinized oral epithelium 212
   histology of 213*f*
Nonkeratinocytes 213
   characteristics of 214*t*
Normal dentin 164, 165*f*
Notochord 92, 92*f*

## O

Oblique ridge 9*f*
Occlusal surface 8
Occlusion 8, 73
   development of 75
   plane of 74
Odontoblast 129*f*, 140, 161*f*, 166, 170, 171*f*
   cell 158*f*, 166
   differentiation of 129, 129*f*
   layer 163
   life cycle of 130*f*
   process 160, 160*f*
Odontoclast activity 140*f*
Oncocytes 233
Oral cavity 138, 208*f*
   development of 90
   different regions of 216
Oral epithelium 136, 209, 213, 214*t*
Oral mucosa 207, 207*t*
   classification of 208
   component tissues of 209
   functions of 207
   lamina propria of 216*t*
   organization of 208
Oral mucous membrane 207
Oral tissues 1
   study of 82
Orbit 70*f*
Orbitale 80
Organic matrix 141
   deposition of 129
   mineralization of 130
Orodental tissues
   innervation of 58
   venous drainage of 58
Orofacial development, early 95
Orthodontic tooth movement 189
Orthokeratinized oral epithelium, histology of 210*f*
Osteoblasts 191, 198, 198*f*
Osteoclast 192, 198, 199*f*
Osteocytes 198, 198*f*
Osteoprogenitor cells 199
Outer enamel epithelium 113, 118
Overbite 79*f*
Overjet 79*f*
Owen contour lines 162
Oxytalan fibers 191

## Index

### P

Pain transmission, theories of 163
Palate
  blood supply of 57
  development of 101
  sensory nerve supply of 59*f*
Palatine
  processes, fusion of 102*f*
  rugae 218
  shelves, fusion of 102*f*
Palmer notation 3
Paraffin-embedding procedure 85
Parakeratinized oral epithelium,
    histology of 210*f*
Paranasal sinuses 69
Paraoral tissues 1
Paraxial mesoderm 93
Parazones 151
Parlodion-embedded specimens,
    preparation of sections of 87
Passive eruption 133
Pellicle 155
Perikymata 150*f*
Periodic acid Schiff 194
Periodontal collagen 187
Periodontal ligament 119, 141, 182,
    186, 191, 192 194, 195
  cells of 191, 192*f*
  fibers of 187
  functions 186
  ground substance of 191
  myelinated 194
  nerves of 194
  nonmyelinated 194
  principal fibers of 188*f*
  structure 186
  traction 138
Periodontium 1, 56, 186, 195
  blood supply of 57
Periosteum 199
Peritubular dentin 159, 159*f*
  formation 131
Permanent canines 29, 77
Permanent dentition 1, 79, 139
Permanent incisors 24, 77, 134*f*
Permanent mandibular
  canine 30
  central incisor 27
  first molar 44
  lateral incisor 28
  second molar 48
  third molar 49
Permanent maxillary
  canine 29, 31*t*
    carving of 52
  central incisor 24
    carving of 52
  first molar 40
  lateral incisor 26
  second molar 42
  third molar 43
Permanent molars 39, 78, 133
Permanent occlusion, changes in 79

Permanent teeth 3, 4, 10*t*, 24, 147*f*
  bud 111*f*
  contact area of 5*f*
  tooth morphology of 2*f*
Phagocytosis 193
Pharyngeal pouches 97, 97*f*, 98*f*
  fate of 97
Phase-contrast microscope 82, 83*f*
Physiologic tooth movement, phase
    of 135
Pit 8
  and groove 8*f*
Placenta 91
Plaque 155
Plasma cells 173
Pogonion 80
Polarizing microscope 84
Posterior wall 70
Posteruptive phase 137
Posteruptive tooth movement 133,
    135, 138
Precision rotary microtome 86*f*
Predentin 160, 160*f*
Predentinal tubule 171
Preeruptive tooth movement 133
Premature eruption 141
Premolars 2, 32
  eruption of 32*t*
  measurement of 32*t*
Prickle cell layer 212
Primary apical foramen 121*f*
Primary cementum 131
Primary dentin 160, 161
  interface 161
Primary dentition 1, 10, 138
Primary epithelial band 110, 110*f*
Primary palate 102*f*
Primary taste sensations, distribution
    of 222*f*
Primary teeth 10, 10*t*, 168
Primate spaces 76*f*
Primitive streak 91, 92*f*
Prochordal plate 91, 91*f*
Progenitor cells 193
Progenitor population 209
Prosthetic concept 73
Proteins 236
Proteoglycans 184, 191
Protraction 63
Protrusion 63
Proximal root concavity 8
Proximal surface 8
Pterygoid, lateral 66
Pterygopalatine
  fossa 59*f*
  suture 107
Pulp 1, 168
  anatomy 168
  anlage 168
  cavity 8, 169*t*
  chamber 168
  defense cells of 172*f*
  function of 168
  histology of 170*f*, 171*f*

  organ 173
  sensory nerves in 168
  stone 174, 175
  structural features 170
Pulpal nerve 174

### R

Radicular dentin, sclerosis of 166
Radicular pulp 168
Refractive index 143
Resorption tunnel 205
Resorptive cells 192
Resting lines 205, 205*f*
Reticulin fibers 191
Retraction 63
Retzius lines 148, 149, 149*f*
Retzius striae 149, 149*f*
Rods
  direction of 147*f*
  groups of 146
  keyhole appearance of 145*f*
  sheath 144, 147
Roof 70
Root 4
  canal 168
  completion of 160
  elongation of 122*f*
  formation of 119
  growth 122, 137, 138*f*

### S

Saliva 235
  functions of 236
  quantity of 235
Salivary glands 227, 235*t*
  classification of 227, 227*t*
  development of 107
  general organization of 228*f*
  secretory elements of 228*f*
  structural pattern of 228
Salter incremental lines 181, 182*f*
Scanning electron microscope 85
Second molar 139, 169
Second pharyngeal pouch 99
Second premolar 139, 169
Secondary attachment epithelium
    225
Secondary dentin 161, 161*f*
  formation 131
  interface 161
Secretion
  control of 237
  types of 227
Secretory cells 228
  damage of 227
Sella point 80
Sensation 207
Serous acini 230, 230*f*
Serous cells 230, 231, 231*t*
Serous crescent 231, 232*f*
Sharpey's fibers 179, 181, 188
  insertion of 182
Silver nitrate 143

Simple diaphragm 122f
Sinistroflexion 146
Skin 207, 207t
Skull
   anterior part of 70f
   development of 105
   subdivisions of 105f
Soft palate 219
Somites, subdivisions of 94f
Specialized mucosa 208, 220
Spee curve 74, 74f
Sphenoidal sinuses 69
Spongy bone 200, 203, 203f
Stellate reticulum 114, 116
Stomatodeum, boundaries of 95f
Stratum
   basale 209
   corneum 212
   germinativum 211
   granulosum 212
   intermedium 116, 155
   spinosum 212
Striated ducts 233, 234f
Subodontoblastic layer 171
Succedaneous dentition 1
Sulcular fluid 224
Sulcus 9
   deepening of 225
Sulfated enamel proteins 127
Superficial cell layer 212
Supermentale 80
Supernumerary tooth 122
Supplemental groove 7
Supporting cells 220
Sustentacular cells 220
Swelling 111f
Sympathetic nerves 174
Synovial membrane 62
Synthetic cells 191

## T

Taste 236
   bud 220, 223f
   cells 220
Temporalis muscle, positions of 67f
Temporomandibular joint 61, 61f, 63f, 105
   development of 105
Temporomandibular ligament 62
Tensile strength and compressibility 143, 157
Terminal excretory ducts 234, 235f
Tertiary dentin 131, 162
   formation 131
Thermal regulation 207

Third arch, overgrowth of 100f
Third molar 139, 169
Third pharyngeal pouch 99
Three germ layers, derivatives of 92
Thyroglossal duct cyst 108
Tissue
   culture 85
   preparation 110
   processing 171
   repair 237
Tomes' granular layer 162, 163, 164f
Tomes' processes 125f
Tongue 221f
   blood supply of 57
   development of 99f
   dorsal surface of 220
   final disposition of 101f
   formation of 99
   origin of different parts of 100f
   ventral surface of 219
Tooth
   arterial supply of 56
   blood supply of 56
   carving
      equipment for 52f
      method of 52
   concentric growth of 133
   development 110
      bud stage of 113f
      cap stage of 114f
      different stages of 112
      early bell stage of 117f
      initiation of 111
   eruption of 136f, 137
   formation, chronology of 11t, 15t, 16t, 24t, 29t, 32t, 39t
   functions of 3
   germ, histodifferentiation of 119
   innervations of 56
   integrity, maintenance of 237
   long axis of 135
   longitudinal ground section of 88f
   mechanism of eruption of 137, 138f
   morphology of 4
   movement, histology of 135
   parts of 1f
   position 189
   preparation of ground sections of 87
   pulp 169
   region of 153
   sequence of eruption of 139f
   shedding of 133

   surfaces of 4
   wearing down of 166
Trabeculae 228
Transduction theory 164
Transmission electron microscope 84
Transparent dentin 166
Transseptal fibers 189f
Transseptal group 188, 189
Transverse ridge 9, 9f
Triangular fossa 7, 7f
Triangular ridge 9, 9f
Trigeminal nerve
   branches of mandibular division of 60f
   distribution of 58f
   mandibular division of 60f
   maxillary division of 59f, 60f
   ophthalmic division of 60f
True denticles 174, 175f
Trunk 9
Tubercle 9
Tuftelin 126, 127

## U

Ultraviolet microscope 83
Universal system 3
Upper arch 5
Upper deciduous molars 17t
Upper face 106
Upper jaw, blood supply of 57

## V

Vascular pressure 138
Vasoactive intestinal polypeptide 237
Vestibular fornix 219
Vitamins 236
Volkmann's canals 200f
von Ebner incremental lines 162, 162f
von Korff fibers 130f

## W

Weil's zone 170
Wilson curve 74

## Y

Yolk sac 91

## Z

Zsigmondy's method 3
Zygomaticomaxillary suture 107
Zygomaticotemporal suture 107
Zygote 90, 90f

EU GSPR Authorised Reprsentative
Logos Europe, 9 rue Nicolas Poussin
1700, La Rochelle, France
Phone: +33 (0) 6 67 93 73 78
E-mail: contact@logoseurope.eu

www.ingramcontent.com/pod-product-compliance
Ingram Content Group UK Ltd.
Pitfield, Milton Keynes, MK11 3LW, UK
UKHW050429150426
5217IPUK00019B/1301